ROONEY'S
GUIDE TO THE
DISSECTION OF THE HORSE

Seventh Edition

Paul G. Orsini, D.V.M.
Diplomate, American College of Veterinary Surgeons
Diplomate, American Veterinary Dental College
Director of Veterinary Anatomy
School of Veterinary Medicine
University of Pennsylvania
Philadelphia, Pennsylvania

W. O. Sack, D.V.M., Ph.D., Dr.med.vet.
Professor em. of Veterinary Anatomy
College of Veterinary Medicine
Cornell University
Ithaca, New York

With 110 drawings by Michael A. Simmons, MFA

Veterinary Textbooks, Ithaca, New York

Revised Reprinting 2003

Published and distributed by: Veterinary Textbooks
36 Woodcrest Avenue
Ithaca, NY 14850

Library of Congress Catalogue Card Number 00-131199

ISBN 0-9601152-4-2

GENERAL HORSE DATA

Scientific name: *Equus caballus*

(Genus) ↗   ↖ (Species)

Belongs to: Class *Mammalia*, Order *Perissodactyla*, Family *Equidae*
Living relatives: (same Order) *Tapir, Rhinoceros;* (same Genus) *Zebra, Donkey*

Vertebral Formula: C7, T 18, L6, S5, Cd 15-21 *(Arabs and donkeys often only L5)*

Separate bones in skeleton: *about 175; when the bones forming the skull, and the auditory ossicles are counted the total is about 205.*

Dental Formula: Permanent $2(I\frac{3}{3}\ C\frac{1}{1}\ P\frac{3\ or\ 4}{3}\ M\frac{3}{3}) = 40\ or\ 42$

Deciduous $2(Di\frac{3}{3}\ Dc\frac{0}{0}\ Dp\frac{3}{3}) = 24$

Amount of circulating blood: *7-8% of bodyweight; 35-40 Liters in a 1,000 lb (451kg) horse*

Rate of hoof growth: *about 1 cm per month*
Body temperature: *38° C (100° F)*
Pulse rate: *about 24-40 per minute*
Respiration rate: *about 14 per minute*

Estrous cycle: *The mare is seasonably polyestrous. She comes in heat every three weeks during Spring and early Summer.*
First heat: *If born in the Spring, the following Spring. If born in the Fall, the second Spring.*
Length of gestation: *315-365 days; average 341 days*

Preface

A renewed change of authorship made necessary a revised reprinting of this guide. Dr. Sue Hackett, who only four years ago took on the continuance of Rooney's Guide, left her academic position and entered veterinary practice. Dr. Paul Orsini of the Pennsylvania Veterinary School has agreed to take her place. He is a veterinarian and an experienced veterinary anatomist whose position at Penn allows him to do also clinical work. With this reprinting following the previous printing by only two years, we left text and figures unchanged, except for correcting recently uncovered minor errors and typos. ***Page and Figure numbers therefore remain the same.***

In line with the present practice at many schools to introduce students to clinical material early in the curriculum, our guide treats the animal body topographically. By examining body parts, such as neck, thorax, limbs, head, etc., it is thought that the study of the horse's structure may be more readily related to clinical work. This view is augmented by the shaded paragraphs with clinical content that will enliven the anatomical work on the cadaver and, we hope, encourage discussion among students and with instructors. For the same reason, the guide provides detailed instruction for the palpation of the live animal, a skill that is important in the physical examination of patients unable to verbalize their ills. We set certain less important material in small type without disturbing the dissection sequence. Instructors may skip over these sections to finish their course in the time they have been allotted. To shorten time for review, paragraphs that do not contain anatomical information have been set in italics. The limbs may be dissected on fresh post mortem room specimens. The point where this can be started most suitably is mentioned on page 85R for the hindlimb and page 113L for the forelimb.

The suggestions made by M. Susan Hackett, DVM, PhD for the previous printing and those received from Alastair G. Watson, DVM, PhD, are greatly appreciated.

Figures 1-3, 1-10, 3-5, 3-6, 3-7, 4-17, 5-1, 5-21, 6-28, and 7-2, kindly supplied by Professor A. Horowitz, were modified from Ellenberger and Baum by him, and drawn by David Stewart Geary.

Philadelphia , PA and Ithaca, NY   Paul Orsini
August, 2003   W. O. Sack

Contents

Glossary of some Anatomical and Lameness Jargon in the Horse

(Compiled by M. Susan Hackett, DVM, PhD.)

For better or worse, people who own or work around horses are notorious for the jargon they use to describe various parts of the horse or disease conditions. Veterinarians working with horses should be familiar with them. (See also the back of the back cover.)

Ankle---Fetlock; metacarpo/metatarsophalangeal joint.

Blood spavin---Distention of the cranial branch of the medial saphenous vein, forming a soft enlargement where it crosses over the dorsomedial aspect of the tibiotarsal joint.

Bog spavin---Descriptive term for chronic distention of the tibiotarsal joint with synovial fluid, causing a swelling that is most obvious on the dorsomedial aspect of the hock joint.

Bone spavin, also True or Jack spavin---Osteoarthritis involving the distal intertarsal and/or tarsometatarsal joints, often resulting in new bone growth that is located on the dorsomedial surface of the hock over the involved joints.

Bowed tendon---Inflammation of the deep and/or superficial flexor tendons, usually due to excessive strain; characterized acutely by diffuse swelling that is warm and painful to the touch and chronically by a thickened tendon that is commonly adhered to surrounding structures and prone to reinjury.

Bucked shins or Shin splints---Dorsal metacarpal disease; a painful condition most commonly seen in young racehorses in association with strenuous exercise; subperiosteal hemorrhage and stress microfractures located on the dorsal aspect of the large metacarpal bone related to cyclical compression loading and bone remodeling.

Buttress foot---Pyramidal disease; new bone growth in the region of the extensor process of the distal phalanx; an advanced form of low ringbone.

Cannon bone---Large metacarpal or metatarsal bone.

Capped hock---Subcutaneous calcaneal bursitis resulting from direct trauma.

Club foot---A foot with an axis of 60° or more to the ground; in foals, abnormal upright foot conformation is observed secondary to excessive flexion of the coffin joint due to the pull of a "contracted" deep digital flexor tendon.

Coffin joint---Distal interphalangeal joint; completely enclosed within the hoof capsule.

Contracted tendons---A descriptive term that refers to various flexural deformities of the limbs that may be either congenital or acquired; in acquired disease, the flexural deformity is most commonly observed at the coffin joint (club foot) or as abnormal angulation of the pastern and fetlock joints; normal limb alignment is prevented by an apparent relative shortening of some combination of the deep digital flexor tendon, superficial digital flexor tendon, and interosseus, however the nature of the primary defect is not well understood.

Corn---Bruising of the sole at the angle formed by the wall and bar, usually due to stepping on a stone or improper shoeing.

Coronary band---The dermis (corium) of the coronary and perioplic regions in association with the stratum germinativum of the coronary and perioplic epidermis; the coronary cushion lies deep to the coronary band, forming a distinct ridge that fits into a corresponding depression on the inside of the proximal part of the hoof wall; often used interchangeably with the coronet, although the coronary band is not a structure that is visible on the outside surface of the foot.

Coronet---The junction of the haired skin with the hoof.

Cribbing---A vice in which a horse arches its neck and swallows air; a horse that cribs will usually have to bite a solid object, such as a manger, to achieve the abnormal posture; causes excessive and uneven wear of the incisor teeth and has been associated with chronic colic and weight loss.

Croup---The highest part of the rump of a horse.

Curb---Enlargement at the plantar surface of the calcaneus due to inflammation and thickening of the plantar ligament that covers the bone.

Fistulous withers---Infection involving the supraspinous bursa thought to be traumatic in origin; of public health importance because *Brucella abortus* is sometimes cultured from the lesion.

Foot---The foot of the horse is regarded as the hoof and its contents.

Founder---Laminitis.

Gonitis---Inflammation of the stifle joint; it is not really a diagnosis, just a description of a general region of involvement.

Gravel---Drainage at the coronet subsequent to a puncture wound or other damage at the white line; at one time it was thought to be due to proximal migration of a piece of gravel, however it is actually due to pus following the path of least resistance when sensitive tissue deep to the white line becomes infected.

Heaves, also Chronic obstructive pulmonary disease and Broken wind---A chronic respiratory disease seen in adult horses and characterized by bronchitis and bronchiolitis; common clinical signs are a cough, poor exercise tolerance, and loud abnormal breath sounds; a "heave line" is sometimes seen that follows the costal arch and develops as the external abdominal oblique muscle hypertrophies secondary to chronic forced expiration.

High ringbone---New bone growth occurring on the distal end of the proximal phalanx and/or the proximal end of the middle phalanx (involves the pastern joint).

Hock---Tarsus.

Hook bone, or Hooks---Coxal tuber; the term is used more often with reference to cattle.

Hunter's bump---Subluxation of the sacroiliac joint, seen externally as a displacement (asymmetry) of one or both sacral tubers.

Jack tendon, also Cunean tendon---Medial tendon of insertion of the cranial tibial muscle; occasionally it is resected to relieve pain associated with cunean bursitis or bone spavin.

Knee---Carpus.

Low ringbone---New bone growth occurring on the distal end of the middle phalanx and/or the proximal end of the distal phalanx, involving the coffin joint.

Occult, or Blind spavin---Clinical features of bone spavin, but without radiographic evidence to confirm the diagnosis.

Pastern joint---Proximal interphalangeal joint.

Pin bone---Ischial tuber, the term is used more often with reference to cattle.

Poll evil---Infection with necrosis of tissue in and around the cranial nuchal bursa; mostly of historic importance, it is rarely diagnosed today.

Prescapular lymph node---Superficial cervical lymph node.

Prefemoral lymph node---Subiliac lymph node.

Quittor---Necrosis of one or both cartilages of the hoof due to trauma.

Roarer, also Idiopathic laryngeal hemiplegia---Hemiparesis or paralysis of the left vocal fold that commonly results in exercise intolerance and/or abnormal inspiratory noise during exercise; clinical signs are caused by failure to abduct the vocal fold because of denervation atrophy of the cricoarytenoideus dorsalis secondary to degeneration of the recurrent laryngeal nerve; affected horses are usually 16 hands or taller (a hand equals 4 inches).

Seedy toe---Abnormal horn present at the white line; observed in association with chronic laminitis as a result of separation of the sensitive and insensitive laminae.

Shin---Dorsal surface of the large metacarpal or metatarsal bone.

Shoe boil, or Capped elbow---Olecranon bursitis at the point of the elbow secondary to the trauma of being hit by the shoe of the affected limb.

Sidebones---Ossification of the collateral cartilages, usually in the forelimbs.

Splint bones---Rudimentary metacarpal or metatarsal bones II and IV.

Splints---A swelling most commonly observed on the medial surface of the forelimb between the second and third metacarpal bones; *true splint* refers to a tear of the interosseous ligament associated with obvious pain and swelling on the abaxial (outer) surface of the splint bone (an interosseous ligament binds each splint bone to the large metacarpal bone); *blind splint* refers to an inflammatory process of the interosseous ligament that is harder to detect because the swelling occurs on the axial (inner) surface of the splint bone.

Spur vein---The lateral thoracic vein extending caudally from the point of the elbow on the lateral and ventral aspect of the thorax.

Stifle---Femorotibial and femoropatellar joints; same joint as the human knee.

Stringhalt---Involuntary flexion of the hock that affects one or both hindlimbs at the walk or trot; generally seen as isolated cases with unknown etiology in the United States, but outbreaks have been reported in New Zealand and Australia that are thought to be due to a plant or mycotoxin consumed during pasture grazing; in isolated cases it may be confused with intermittent upward fixation of the patella.

Suspensory ligament---Interosseus muscle.

Sweeney---Loss of muscle mass in the infra- and supraspinatus muscles secondary to suprascapular denervation.

Thoroughpin---Idiopathic synovitis of the tarsal sheath resulting in synovial effusion and distention of the sheath without inflammation, pain, or lameness.

Throatlatch area---Ventral retropharyngeal region; the name comes from a part of the tack, i.e. the strap that passes under the throat and helps to hold a bridle or halter in place.

Thrush---Degenerative condition of the frog affecting the central and lateral grooves characterized by the presence of black necrotic material and a foul odor; predisposing causes include standing on dirty bedding and neglecting to frequently pick out the foot.

Thumps---Sudden bilateral (occasionally unilateral) movement of the horse's flanks each time the heart beats; due to phrenic nerve stimulation causing the diaphragm to contract (synchronous diaphragmatic flutter); results from electrolyte imbalances that occur with extreme physical exertion or from hypocalcemic tetany.

Tying-up syndrome---Also referred to as exercise-related myopathy, exertional rhabdomyolysis, azoturia, paralytic myoglobinuria, and Monday-morning disease; a complex disease affecting the skeletal muscles most often following prolonged, or intense physical activity; muscle cramping and fasciculations occur and an af-fected horse will have a stiff, stilted gait and be reluctant to move.

Viborg's triangle---A region in the lateral retropha-ryngeal area used for surgical access to the guttural pouch; boundaries are the mandible cranially, the linguofacial vein ventrally, and the tendon of the sterno-cephalicus dorsocaudally.

Whorlbone disease---Trochanteric bursitis; poorly-defined entity thought to arise secondarily to hock lameness; most commonly diagnosed in Standardbreds and thought to be due to a change in gait that causes abnormal stress in region of the trochanteric bursa, which lies between the tendon of the accessory head of the middle gluteal muscle and the low cranial part of the greater trochanter.

Withers---The highest part of the back; formed by the long spinous processes of T2-8 between the scapular cartilages.

Windpuffs, or Wind galls--Chronic distention with synovial fluid of the palmar (or plantar) recess of the fetlock joint; also refers to chronic distention of various tendon sheaths when the distention is not associated with lameness (such as swelling of the digital flexor tendon sheath at the level of the fetlock).

Wind-sucking---Usually used in reference to pneumo vagina, although it may also refer to cribbing; involuntary aspiration of air into the vagina of the mare so that it is chronically distended; associated with poor conformation of the perineum and is the cause of infertility because of fecal contamination of the repro-ductive tract.

Introduction

Both horses and ponies can be studied with this guide; measurements are given for horses and should be halved for ponies. The dissection requires about 65 laboratory hours, and about 75 hours if the sections printed in small type are also done.

Students require a scalpel, rat-tooth thumb forceps, a stiff and a flexible probe, and a pair of straight scissors about 6 inches (15 cm) long with a pointed and a blunt tip. Large tools such as saws, large knives, wood chisels, mallets, and hoof nippers should be available in the laboratory. At Cornell, the large tools are in the course lockers which in addition contain skeletal material (distal portion of fore and hindlimbs and a right or left half of a skull) a dried hoof, wet sections of the horse's foot, a few teeth, and a pliable larynx in a jar. All students are required to wear gloves and some form of eye protection during dissection. This is particularly important while opening the thoracic and abdominal cavities when splashing can occur.

Structures of importance are printed in bold type; these should be studied with the aid of a textbook. Numbers *in the margins* key the dissection to the text and figures of TEXTBOOK OF VETERINARY ANATOMY, 2nd. ed. by Dyce, Sack, and Wensing (W.B. Saunders, Co., 1996.)

THE SPECIMEN—It may be useful to describe briefly how an animal as large as a horse is preserved for dissection. It is hoped that an appreciation of the large amount of work and material that goes into the preparation of each specimen will lead students to dissect it with care and to prolong its usefulness by keeping it well wrapped between laboratory periods.

The horse is brought to the ground and is fully anesthetized with a suitable anesthetic given to effect. The horse lies in lateral recumbency while a mid-cervical incision is made parallel and dorsal to the external jugular vein. The common carotid artery is identified, exteriorized, and cannulated. The horse—while remaining fully anesthetized—is bled through the cannula until death occurs. After the horse has died, a large hook is driven through the spinous processes of the sacrum, and a second one is placed in the caudal part of the neck to support the front by the laminar part of the nuchal ligament. Then the horse is raised to the standing position by two hoists attached to the hooks. The head is supported by a cradle and pulled forward and upward by a hook placed behind the skull. A mixture of 6% formalin, 2% phenol, and 30% ethanol is injected under 6 lbs. pressure through the cannula into the vascular system; and while this is being done the animal is thoroughly washed. The appearance of white foam at the nostrils, presumably due to the rupture of small vessels in the lungs, signals that the injection is coming to an end.

On average, a medium-sized horse requires about 80 liters of embalming fluid (1 L/10 lbs. of body weight). A large hypodermic needle or a small trocar is inserted through the right flank into the base of the cecum to allow some of the intestinal gas that rapidly accumulates after death to escape. (The needle is usually left in place until the horse is brought into the dissection laboratory.) A few days later, either Latex or a mixture of boiled carpenter's glue and red household dye (about 8 - 10 L) is injected under 6 lbs. pressure through the cannula to render the arteries visible and easier to dissect. The body openings, including the eyes, are covered with petroleum jelly and the specimen is then stored in a humidity-controlled cooler until dissection begins.

Embalming, like anesthesia, is not an exact science; and for no obvious reason an occasional horse is not as well preserved as the others. The problem areas are the intestines, the muscles of the back, and the distal parts of the limbs; sometimes a vessel in the thorax ruptures and much of the arterial marker escapes into the pulmonary cavity.

WRAPPING THE SPECIMEN—Horses are too large to be totally covered with plastic. Therefore, only the part that has been exposed is wrapped— the undisturbed skin, except that covering the distal parts of the limbs, prevents drying for a time.

How the dissected portion of the body is to be wrapped is shown in Fig. 1-11. A moist cloth goes on the exposed surface, the moisture is prevented from escaping by a sheet of plastic, and the plastic is held in place by the skin which is on the outside and allowed to dry. It is important during the dissection to keep the wrappings moist with mold-inhibiting solution and to store them *off the floor* to avoid bacterial and fungal contamination that is then transferred to the horse.

SEQUENCE OF DISSECTION—The abdominal and thoracic viscera of specimens as large as the horse cannot be preserved as well as those of smaller animals, and it is best to study them as soon as possible and leave the head and the limbs, which generally keep better, to the last. The neck is dissected first and while this is done the head is removed and stored in a cooler where it is more easily protected from drying. Then the forelimbs are removed and stored, and the thoracic cavity and its contents are studied. Then follows the abdominal cavity and its contents of which only the stomach, liver, and spleen are kept for review; the intestines usually have to be discarded. After that the dissection proceeds to the pelvis, reproductive organs, and udder, and then to the hindlimb. At the end the forelimb and the head are dissected.

The viscera of ponies, most of the time, are well preserved. The order of dissection may therefore be changed to one that gives more weight to anatomical relationships: neck, head (detached and split), forelimb, thorax, abdomen, pelvis, hindlimb.

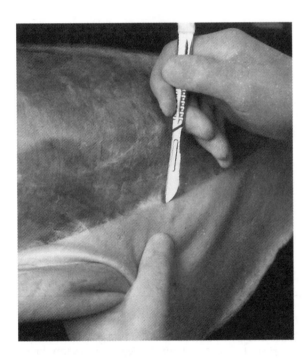

When dissecting horses or cows, large pieces of skin have to be reflected. As shown in the photograph to the left, keep the bevel of the scalpel against the deep surface of the skin and make long even strokes. The white superficial fascia stays on the animal. The deep surface of the skin is bluish and contains many fine arteries and veins.

It is well to remind veterinary students that the dissection of the horse (or of a ruminant) not only helps to understand the structure of these animals, but significantly reinforces what was learned about the anatomy of the dog or cat. Domestic mammals, on the whole, are not as dissimilar as they appear at first glance.

1

NECK

Purpose and Plan of the Dissection

1---To see the clinically very important (external) jugular vein and the muscles that form the jugular groove.

2---To see esophagus, trachea, and accompanying vessels and nerves in the visceral space ventral to the vertebrae.

3---To demonstrate the thyroid gland at the cranial, and the superficial cervical lymph nodes at the caudal end of the neck.

4---To see the extrinsic forelimb muscles present in the neck, the muscles dorsal to the vertebrae that support the heavy head, and the ventral strap muscles and the clinically important fascial layers separating some of these.

5---To demonstrate the well developed nuchal ligament.

6---To show the position of the cervical vertebrae in the laterally flattened neck, especially at the junction with the thorax where the vertebrae are more ventrally placed than is usually assumed.

Plan. *After removal of the skin and study of the superficial muscles, nerves (optional), and jugular vein, various neck muscles are transected and reflected to expose the organs in the visceral space ventral to the vertebrae, and the large nuchal ligament dorsal to the vertebrae. The head is detached at the level of C3 and stored for later study.*

(Paragraphs set in italics give dissection instruction; they contain no anatomical information.)

Cut off the mane with scissors. Palpate the nuchal crest on the back of the skull and incise the skin, just lateral to the mane, from this crest to the transverse plane of the shoulder joint (Fig. 1-1). Do not remove the median strip of skin from which

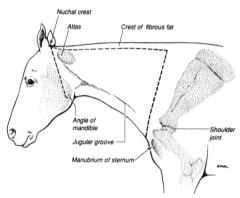

FIGURE 1-1. Skin incisions on the neck.

the large, coarse hairs of the mane arise. Make a transverse skin incision from the cranial end of the first incision to the midventral line, passing just caudal to the base of the ear and over the angle of the mandible. Make another transverse incision from the caudal end of the first incision cranial to the shoulder joint to the palpable manubrium of the sternum. Reflect the skin to the ventral midline leaving the underlying superficial fascia on the neck.

Note the lymphatics that converge toward the **superficial cervical lymph nodes** to be seen later cranial to the shoulder joint (Fig. 1-2).

The **cutaneus colli muscle** of the horse, unlike the extensive platysma of the dog, is a relatively small V-shaped muscle arising from the manubrium of the sternum. Its fibers diverge dorsocranially to the sides of the neck, thinning

6
9
R

---

*Numbers in the margins: plain numbers refer to the text, and numbers with a line below refer to page numbers of Figures in TEXTBOOK OF VETERINARY ANATOMY, 2nd. ed. by Dyce, Sack, and Wensing (1996).

3

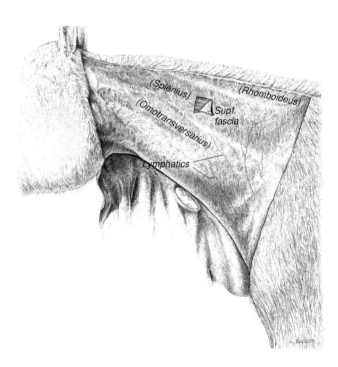

FIGURE 1-2. Skin removed from lateral surface of the neck. Some of the muscles are visible through the superficial fascia. The (common) carotid artery was exteriorized and cannulated for embalming through the hole in the reflected skin.

out and blending into the superficial fascia (Fig. 1-3). Beginning on the lateral border of the muscle close to the manubrium, and working medially and cranially (to about the middle of the neck), reflect the muscle to its origin on the manubrium and leave it hanging (Fig. 1-4). This reflection exposes the **external jugular vein** in the jugular groove.

Work under the middorsal strip of skin from caudal to cranial, removing the mane, skin, and the thick **crest** of fat down to the funiculus nuchae (Fig. 1-5). The latter is the most dorsal, cord-like part of the **nuchal ligament** which will be seen in its entirety later (Fig. 1-21). Reflect the crest to the poll and remove it. This fibrous yellow crest of fat is thickest over the wider caudal portion of the funiculus, both structures becoming thinner as they approach the poll.

The following pattern for a typical spinal nerve will be used in the dissection of the cervical, thoracic, and lumbar nerves.

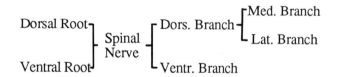

Study the break-up of a **typical cervical spinal nerve** in Fig. 1-6 to understand which of the above branches supply the skin and where they become subcutaneous, and which supply muscles; and on your specimen find the stumps of some of the ventral cutaneous nerves that are shown and numbered in Fig. 1-7.

Ask an instructor which of the un-shaded sections set in small type throughout this guide are to be done.

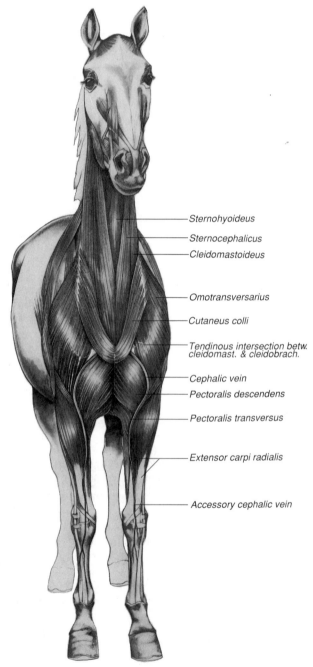

FIGURE 1-3. Superficial muscles and veins. (From Ellenberger-Dittrich-Baum by Horowitz/Geary.)

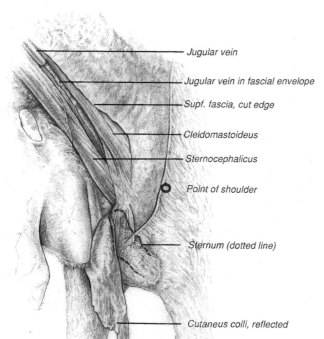

FIGURE 1-4. Caudal half of jugular groove exposed by the reflection of the cutaneus colli; left craniolateral view.

The following section is concerned with the **CUTANEOUS NERVES OF THE NECK.**

The removal of the crest will have exposed some of the *dorsal cutaneous branches of the cervical nerves* (Fig. 1-6/a) which emerge, together with small arteries along the lateral edge of the funiculus nuchae (Fig. 1-5). Usually only one or two short stumps are found; no matter, as long as it is understood that these nerves supply the skin over the dorsolateral region of the neck. The dorsal branch of C1 emerges from the alar foramen of the atlas. The *lateral branches of the dorsal branches of the cervical nerves* (Fig. 1-6/7) are motor to the dorsolateral muscles of the neck and are not visible at this stage.

Dissection in the superficial fascia will expose the *ventral cutaneous branches of cervical nerves 2-6* as they emerge through the cleidomastoideus (Fig. 1-7). The large C6 appears just cranial to the shoulder joint and sends several branches to the skin over the shoulder and pectoral muscles. C4 is near the middle of the neck, and C2 appears just caudoventral to the palpable *wing of the atlas.* C2 also gives rise to the *great auricular nerve* which passes to the parotid region and convex surface of the ear just cranial to the wing of the atlas (Fig. 1-7). This series of nerves supplies the skin over the ventrolateral region of the neck as shown in Figure 2-14. C1 does not have a ventral cutaneous branch; its ventral branch supplies the ventral strap muscles attaching to the larynx and hyoid apparatus.

The *ventral branches of the cervical nerves,* before reaching the skin, innervate the ventral cervical muscles (except the sternocephalicus and cleidomastoideus which are supplied by the accessory nerve). C6, C7, and C8 join T1 and T2 to form the *brachial plexus.*

The purpose of the following dissection is to

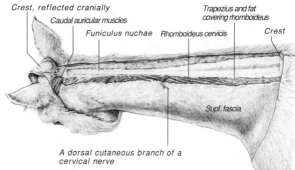

FIGURE 1-5. Funiculus nuchae exposed by the removal of the fatty crest in the dorsal border of the neck.

demonstrate the disposition of the deep **CERVICAL FASCIA** and the "envelopes" it forms around various muscles and other structures in the ventral part of the neck (Fig. 1-8/heavy black lines).

The fascial envelopes depicted in the transverse section of the neck (Fig. 1-8) are important in the diagnosis and treatment of abscesses (or tumors) in that they contain, or influence the direction of spreading, fluids resulting from inflammatory processes in the neck. For example, an inflammatory process resulting from a choke may break through the esophageal wall and be channeled by the surrounding deep fascia directly into the thoracic cavity.

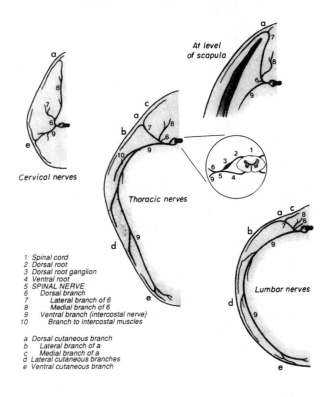

1 Spinal cord
2 Dorsal root
3 Dorsal root ganglion
4 Ventral root
5 SPINAL NERVE
6   Dorsal branch
7   Lateral branch of 6
8   Medial branch of 6
9   Ventral branch (intercostal nerve)
10   Branch to intercostal muscles

a Dorsal cutaneous branch
b   Lateral branch of a
c   Medial branch of a
d Lateral cutaneous branches
e Ventral cutaneous branch

FIGURE 1-6. Distribution of the spinal nerves in neck, thorax, and flank; schematic.

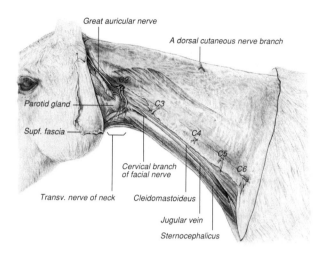

FIGURE 1-7. Jugular groove and ventral cutaneous branches of cervical nerves exposed by the reflection of the superficial fascia.

(If your horse is suspended by a large hook at the caudal part of neck, the hook unfortunately distorts the muscles in this area.) Deep to the origin of the **trapezius** (cervical part) on the funiculus nuchae the cervical part of the **rhomboideus** may be palpated. Make a longitudinal incision down to the rhomboideus near its caudal end and with scissors cut the trapezius and the fascial envelope of the rhomboideus, extending the cut to the cranial end of the rhomboideus. The caudal end of this envelope will be exposed when the withers are dissected (Fig. 2-2).

Locate the **JUGULAR GROOVE** and palpate the muscle forming its dorsal border. This is the **cleidomastoideus** which extends to the mastoid process of the skull. Continuous with the cleidomastoideus dorsally and usually visible through the superficial fascia is the **omotransversarius** which attaches on the transverse processes of the more cranial cervical vertebrae. Palpate the oblique line formed by the **wing of the atlas**, the "transverse process" of C1; this is a prominent, palpable landmark in the live horse. The cleidomastoideus is continued at the shoulder joint by the cleidobrachialis which attaches on the deltoid tuberosity and crest of the humerus. Do not dissect these attachments but visualize them on your specimen. The cleidomastoideus and cleidobrachialis represent the **brachiocephalicus** in the horse; together with the omotransversarius they form a large unit that advances the forelimb or, when the limb is fixed, move the neck laterally (Fig. 1-10).

Free the dorsal border of the omotransversarius with a shallow cut and reflect the border ventrally. This exposes the large **accessory nerve** (XI) as it

traverses the space between omotransversarius and trapezius in the caudal part of the neck to innervate the trapezius.

The muscular body of the **splenius** and the **serratus ventralis cervicis** are now exposed. The fibers of the two muscles are nearly parallel and it is difficult now to determine where one begins and the other ends. They will be considered in more detail later.

Return to the jugular groove. The muscle forming its ventral border is the **sternocephalicus** which extends from the manubrium to the mandible (Fig. 1-10). Having established the width of the groove, carefully incise the superficial fascia longitudinally in the middle of the groove and expose—but do not open—the **external jugular vein** from the linguofacial vein to as close

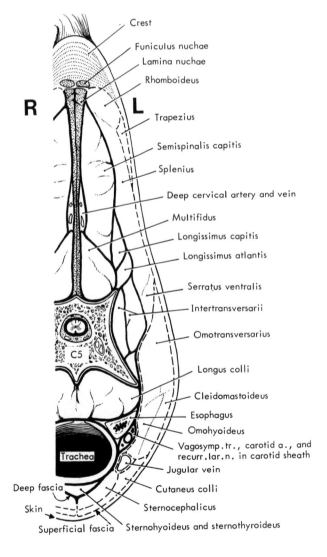

FIGURE 1-8. Transverse section of the neck at C5. (After Habel, 1981).

longitudinal cut 4 cm* dorsal and parallel to the jugular groove from about the level of C3 to the caudal skin incision. In the middle of the neck pass your fingers from below between the omohyoideus and the cleidomastoideus until the longitudinal cut is encountered. Transect the cleidomastoideus at this point and, separating it from the underlying omohyoideus, reflect the caudal stump until the superficial cervical lymph nodes are exposed. If carefully done, the cleidomastoideus and omohyoideus separate well; the omohyoideus has wide flat bundles.

Again in the middle of the neck find the ventral border of the omohyoideus and work your fingers under it, between the muscle and the carotid sheath. Transect the omohyoideus, up to the longitudinal cut made previously to separate cleidomastoideus and omotransversarius. Reflect the caudal stump of the omohyoideus, severing some of its dorsal bundles along the longitudinal cut, and noting that the omohyoideus passes *deep* to the superficial cervical lymph nodes (Fig. 1-12/4,15).

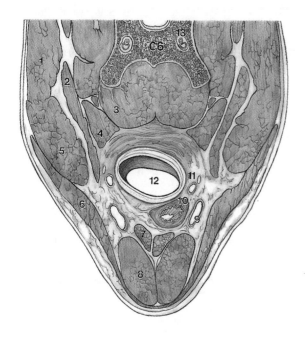

1. Omotransversarius
2. Omohyoideus
3. Longus colli
4. Scalenus
5. Cleidomastoideus
6. Cutaneus colli
7. Sternothyroideus and sternohyoideus, fused
8. Sternocephalicus
9. Jugular vein
10. Esophagus
11. Vagosympathetic trunk and carotid artery
12. Trachea
13. Vertebral vessels

FIGURE 1-9. Transverse section at C6 of the ventral part of the neck. Note that, just cranial to the thoracic inlet, the esophagus can position itself ventral to the trachea. The jugular vein and carotid artery lie in fat deep to the thin cutaneus colli.

to the thoracic inlet as possible. The jugular vein lies in a distinct fascial envelope which may contain dried blood that escaped during a recent venipuncture. Pull the vein laterally and incise the medial wall of the envelope exposing the **omohyoideus** (not present in the dog) which lies deep to the vein in the cranial half of the neck. The superficial fascia has to be reflected cranially to expose the linguofacial vein and the ventral end of the parotid gland which will be used as a landmark later (Fig. 1-13/9).

In order to expose the carotid sheath and deeper structures in the **VISCERAL SPACE** the cleidomastoideus and the deeper lying omohyoideus will have to be transected and reflected. To begin with we have to locate the dorsal border of the cleidomastoideus; this is difficult because it is fused with the omotransversarius that lies dorsal to it. To save time the division between the latter two muscles is best made artificially by a

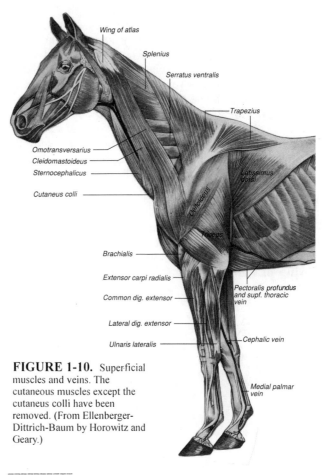

FIGURE 1-10. Superficial muscles and veins. The cutaneous muscles except the cutaneus colli have been removed. (From Ellenberger-Dittrich-Baum by Horowitz and Geary.)

Wing of atlas
Splenius
Serratus ventralis
Trapezius
Latissimus dorsi
Omotransversarius
Cleidomastoideus
Sternocephalicus
Cutaneus colli
Deltoideus
Triceps
Brachialis
Extensor carpi radialis
Common dig. extensor
Lateral dig. extensor
Ulnaris lateralis
Pectoralis profundus and supf. thoracic vein
Cephalic vein
Medial palmar vein

---

* Students working on ponies should halve the measurements given in this guide for full-grown horses.

The deep fascia forming the **carotid sheath** (another fascial envelope; Fig. 1-8) is deep to the omohyoideus in the groove between the trachea and the longus colli and scalenus muscles. The common carotid artery is usually visible before the sheath is opened. In the cranial half of the neck the omohyoideus is interposed between the jugular vein and the structures in the sheath.

Venipuncture in the horse is preferred in the cranial half of the neck because the jugular vein is not obscured by the cutaneus colli and because of the dubious assumption that the omohyoideus protects the common carotid artery from a misdirected needle. The mishap of inadvertently puncturing the carotid artery has disastrous consequences with some injectables. It should be remembered that the jugular vein in the cranial half of the neck lies directly under the skin.

Open the carotid sheath exposing the **common carotid artery** and the **vagosympathetic trunk** dorsal to it. The **recurrent laryngeal nerve** is ventral to the artery (Fig 1-12/11,12,13). Tag both nerves close to the thoracic inlet. Replace all structures, reconstructing the carotid sheath and the jugular groove.

The **sternocephalicus** arises from the manubrium of the sternum fused with its fellow of the opposite side (Fig. 1-3). They separate halfway up the neck and finally pass under the parotid gland and linguofacial vein to be inserted on the caudel border of the ramus of the mandible (Fig. 1-13/11). Clean the muscle from the manubrium to the parotid gland. Determine the course of the tendon of insertion by tensing the muscle and palpating through the parotid gland. The triangle formed by the linguofacial vein, the ramus of the mandible, and the tendon of the sternocephalicus is known as **Viborg's triangle** (/8).

A greatly enlarged guttural pouch and the related retropharyngeal lymph nodes are accessible surgically through Viborg's triangle. A *normal* guttural pouch is a considerable distance dorsomedial to the triangle.

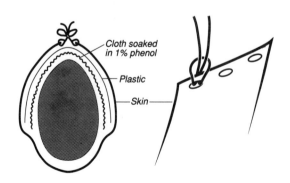

FIGURE 1-11. How to wrap neck and trunk.

Find the thin **sternohyoideus** and **sternothyroideus muscles**; this is not easy, because they have been mutilated when the carotid artery was cannulated for exsanguination and embalming. The muscles lie in an envelope of deep fascia on the ventral surface of the trachea between the two sternocephalicus muscles (Fig. 1-8). Isolate them to where the sternohyoideus fuses with the omohyoideus. These muscles extend into the inter-mandibular space to be inserted on the thyroid cartilage and on the basihyoid bone; the insertions will be seen with the dissection of the larynx. The schematic ventral view of the muscles in Fig. 1-14 will make their complex connections plain.

Tracheotomy, cutting an opening into the ventral surface of the trachea, most often is an emergency operation in cases of proximal airway obstruction, usually in the larynx. The tube that is inserted into such an opening is about an inch (2.5 cm) in diameter. Palpate tracheal cartilages 4-6 and perform a tracheotomy at that level. Which muscles have to be spread in the midline?
Discuss with your group or with an instructor why clinicians prefer this location for a tracheotomy over one in the middle or caudal end of the neck.

The **esophagus** should still be enclosed in its envelope of deep fascia. Open the envelope and note that it forms also the deep wall of the carotid sheath and thus is a barrier between an inflammatory process in the esophagus and the important structures in the carotid sheath (Fig. 1-8). Trace the esophagus through the visceral space. Since it passes from the dorsal to the left aspect of the trachea, students on the right side will not find it in the caudal part of the neck. Incise the lateral wall of the esophagus and note the two layers of striated muscle and the tough longitudinally folded mucosa. The striated muscle ends at the base of the heart. (See Fig. 1-9 that shows an unexpected position of the esophagus (/10) at the thoracic inlet.)

Examine the **trachea.** It also lies in a envelope of deep fascia. This is continuous at the thoracic inlet with the endothoracic fascia and could conduct an inflammatory process affecting the trachea into the thoracic cavity. The trachea is flattened dorso- ventrally and lies against the ventral surface of the longus colli (Fig. 1-8). Transect the trachea at about C4 and note its caliber and cross-sectional appearance.

Preserving the accessory nerve, transect the omotransversarius in the middle of the neck and reflect the caudal stump to the caudal skin incision, severing the muscle from the transverse process of C4. The more proximal segments of the ventral branches of the cervical nerves 4-6 may now be seen, and the superficial cervical lymph

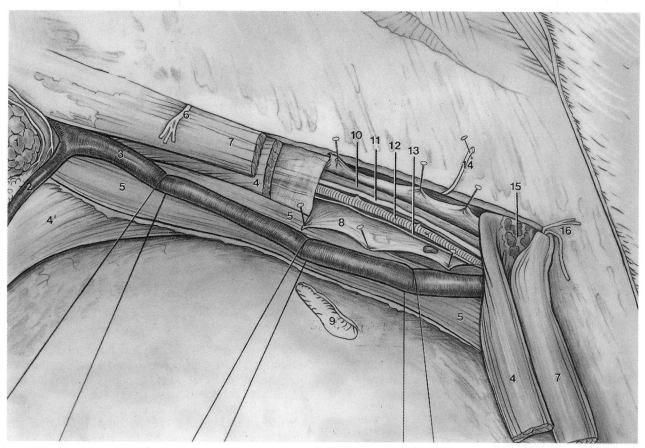

1.	Parotid gland	6.	C3
2.	Linguofacial vein	7.	Cleidomastoideus
3.	Jugular vein	8.	Carotid sheath, reflected
4.	Omohyoideus		by pins
4'	Combined omo- and sterno-	9.	Midventral skin incision
	hyoideus		for exsanguination
5.	Sternocephalicus	10.	Esophagus

11.	Vagosympathetic trunk	14.	C5
12.	Common carotid artery	15.	Supf. cervical lymph nodes
13.	Recurrrent laryngeal nerve	16.	C6

FIGURE 1-12. Deep dissection of the visceral space in the caudal part of the neck, lateral view.

nodes though imbedded in fat are now fully exposed.

The **superficial cervical lymph nodes** lie between the cleidomastoideus and omotransversarius laterally and the omohyoideus medially on the cranial border of the subclavius (Fig. 1-15/ 8). They receive lymphatics from the neck, thorax, shoulder, and arm and send efferents to the caudal deep cervical lymph nodes to be seen later at the thoracic inlet.

The prescapular branch of the **superficial cervical artery** passes dorsally through the superficial cervical lymph nodes (Fig. 1-16); don't look for it. The short superficial cervical artery (to be seen later) passes cranially from the subclavian as the latter winds around the first rib. It also releases a deltoid branch which accompanies the **cephalic vein** (a branch of the

jugular) in the groove between descending pectoral and brachiocephalic muscles (Fig. 1-3). Expose the cephalic vein and deltoid branch dorsal or deep to it, about 8 cm ventral to the disappearance of the jugular vein.

The cephalic vein and accompanying deltoid branch, both sizable vessels, bleed profusely when a horse lacerates itself in this area by a projecting object on a fence or wall.

In the following dissection the cranial stumps of the cleidomastoideus and omotransversarius are removed to allow exposure of the accessory nerve to where it divides into dorsal and ventral branches. This also exposes the thyroid gland and the cranial deep cervical lymph nodes.

Reflect the cranial stumps of the omotransversarius and cleidomastoideus cranially, separating the latter from the omohyoideus which

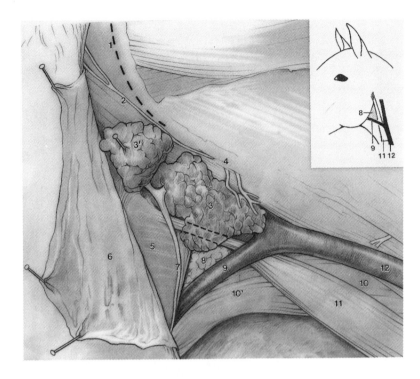

1. Palpable wing of atlas
2. Great auricular nerve
3. Parotid gland, reflected with parotidoauricularis at 3'
4. C2
5. Masseter on caudal border of mandible
6. Superficial fascia, reflected
7. Parotid duct
8. Viborg's triangle
9. Linguofacial vein
10. Omohyoideus
10' Combined omo- and sternohyoideus
11. Sternocephalicus
12. Jugular vein

FIGURE 1-13. Superficial dissection of the retromandibular space to show Viborg's triangle. The inset outlines the borders of the triangle.

should stay in place for the time being. Find the dorsal branch of the accessory nerve on the deep surface of the omotransversarius, free it from the muscle, and pin the nerve to the splenius. You

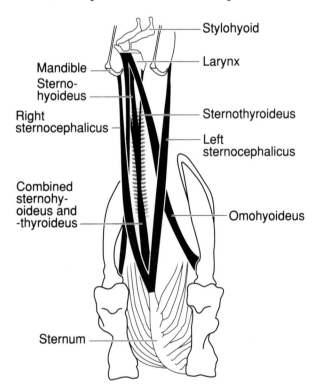

FIGURE 1-14. The relationship of the strap muscles ventral and lateral to the trachea; left craniolateral view. The right and left sternocephalicus muscles have been separated to expose muscles and trachea lying deep to them. (Modified from B. and B. Premiani: *El Caballo,* Buenos Aires, Ediciones Centauro, 1957.)

may have encountered several large nerves while reflecting the muscles. They are cutaneous branches of C2 that pass through the muscles and to the ear (great auricular nerve) and to the ventral part of the neck (transverse nerve of neck); they are shown in Figs. 1-7 before, and 1-17 after the muscle reflection; it is not necessary to preserve them. Reflect the muscles sufficiently to cut the omotransversarius off the wing of the atlas and the cleidomastoideus tendon a little farther forward just dorsal to the parotid gland and remove the two muscles.

The fleshy longus capitis is now exposed running longitudinally on the lateroventral aspect of the vertebrae (Fig. 1-17). It extends from the transverse processes of vertebrae 3, 4, and 5 to the muscular tubercles on the base of the skull (see skeleton). Just examine these attachments by palpation.

The junction of head and neck is of considerable clinical importance in the horse because of the presence of the larynx, the guttural pouches, the atlanto-occipital space and joint, and a concentration of major nerves, vessels, and lymph nodes. All of these structures will be encountered gradually but it will be helpful, even at this stage, to study transverse sections of this area from time to time to become familiar with the crowded relationships that exist here. Figure 1-18 depicting the level of the atlas shows the topography of many of the structures that have already been seen.

Trace the **accessory nerve** cranially under the wing of the atlas to where it is joined by the ventral branch, and then expose the ventral branch for a short distance. Find the musculotendinous junction of the sternocephalicus deep to the

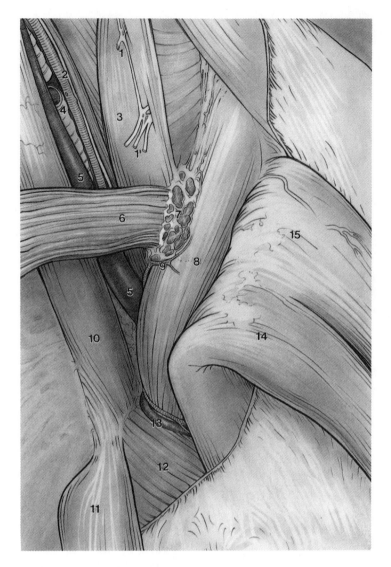

1. C5, C6 at 1'
2. Common carotid a. and vagosympathetic trunk
3. Ventral scalenus
4. Trachea
5. Jugular vein
6. Omohyoideus
7. Superficial cervical lymph nodes
8. Subclavius
9. Prescapular branch of superficial cervical artery
10. Sternocephalicus
11. Cutaneus colli, reflected
12. Pectoralis descendens
13. Cephalic v. and deltoid branch of supf. cervical a.
14. Cleidomastoideus
15. Omotransversarius

FIGURE 1-15. Deep dissection at the junction of neck and trunk to demonstrate the superficial cervical lymph nodes; craniolateral view.

ventral end of the parotid gland and expose the ventral branch of the accessory nerve again as it enters the dorsomedial surface of this junction to innervate the muscle (Fig. 1-17/10).

Bilateral neurectomy of the ventral branch of the accessory nerve and resection of the sternohyoideus, sternothyroideus, and omohyoideus muscles (the modified Forssell's operation) is one surgical method in the treatment of crib-biting. The ventral branch of the accessory nerve is accessible surgically and has been used in the diagnosis of equine motor neuron disease.

Reflect the cranial stump of the omohyoideus ventrally off the carotid sheath and trachea. Make a longitudinal cut over the carotid artery and reflect the sheath, exposing the vagosympathetic trunk dorsal to the artery and the recurrent laryngeal nerve ventral to the artery (Fig. 1-17). The recurrent nerve should be traced to the caudal pole of the thyroid gland and tagged there. (The

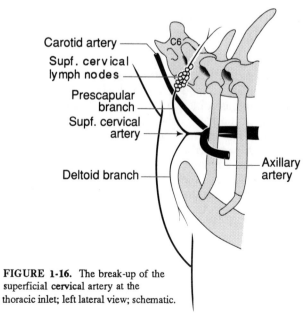

Carotid artery
Supf. cervical lymph nodes
Prescapular branch
Supf. cervical artery
Deltoid branch
C6
Axillary artery

FIGURE 1-16. The break-up of the superficial cervical artery at the thoracic inlet; left lateral view; schematic.

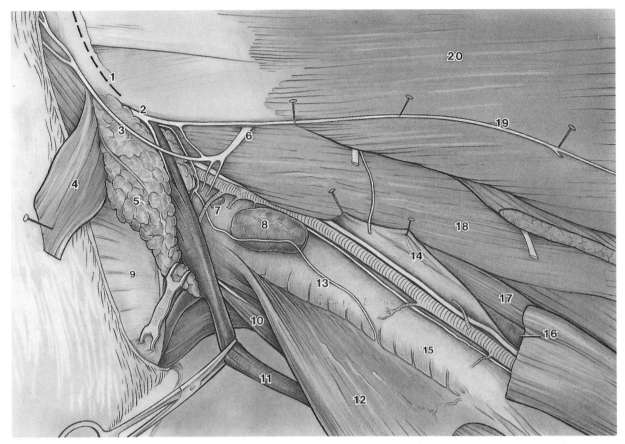

1. Wing of atlas
2. Accessory nerve
3. Great auricular nerve
4. Parotidoauricularis, reflected
5. Parotid gland
6. C2
7. Cranial deep cervical lymph nodes
8. Thyroid gland
9. Masseter
10. Sternocephalicus and ventral branch of accessory nerve entering it
11. Jugular vein
12. Omohyoideus, reflected
13. Ventral branch of C1
14. Carotid sheath, opened to expose (from dorsal to ventral) vagosympathetic trunk, common carotid
artery, recurrent laryngeal nerve
15. Trachea
16. Esophagus
17. Longus colli
18. Longus capitis
19. Dorsal branch of accessory nerve
20. Splenius

FIGURE 1-17. Deep dissection of the visceral space in the cranial half of **the neck,** lateral view.

tag—or at least its string—will be very helpful in re-identifying this nerve when the larynx is studied later.)

The lobe of the **thyroid gland** lies on the lateral surface of the first few tracheal cartilages. It is ovoid, convex (and thus palpable in the live animal) and is joined to the lobe of the opposite side by a narrow isthmus (don't look for the isthmus). The **cranial deep cervical lymph nodes** are variably distributed in the area, most often between the thyroid gland and the carotid artery (Fig. 1-18/22). They receive afferents from the mandibular and retropharyngeal lymph nodes, the deeper areas of the head, pharynx, guttural pouches, and larynx. They send efferents to the middle and caudal deep cervical lymph nodes.

Both internal (IV) and external (III) **parathyroid glands** are present, but don't look for them. The internal glands usually lie in the vicinity of the cranial pole of the thyroid gland;

the external glands lie on the ventral surface of the trachea farther down the neck.

While the following dissection of the large **NUCHAL LIGAMENT** is done, one student can begin removing the skin of the thorax (next chapter) as outlined in the paragraph "The high ridge formed . . . ." on page **17,** and is finished on p. **18** at the start of the small type.

Reflect the exposed portion of the trapezius to the caudal skin incision, cutting it around the hook in the neck. Free the cervical part of the rhomboideus from the funiculus nuchae and from the dorsal border of the splenius and reflect it also to the caudal skin incision. Free the triangular cervical portion of the serratus ventralis by severing its origins on the transverse processes of the last four or five cervical vertebrae—you may need an instructor to help you to distinguish this muscle from the splenius. Cut the serratus around the hook and reflect it to the caudal skin incision.

Sever the dorsal attachments of the splenius to the funiculus nuchae from withers to poll. Transect the **splenius** as far caudally as possible and reflect it ventrally off the underlying **semispinalis capitis** (Fig. 1-19/6). The semispinalis capitis is easily recognized by the numerous oblique tendinous intersections in its dorsal part. Transect and reflect the semispinalis capitis in the same manner as the splenius.

The **nuchal ligament** is now fully exposed (Figs. 1-20 and 1-21). The funicular part is a smooth, bright-yellow double cord of connective tissue that arises from the back of the skull and is continued over the thorax by the supraspinous ligament. The paired, fenestrated sheets of the laminar part arise from the spinous processes of T2 and T3 and from the funiculus and attach on the spinous processes of C2-5. Do not work out the attachments. The ligament helps support the heavy head while its elasticity allows the head to be lowered so the mouth can reach the ground.

The **deep cervical artery** may have been reflected off the laminar part of the nuchal ligament with the semispinalis capitis. It is distributed over the surface of the lamina, supplying the adjacent muscles and the dorsal portion of the neck (Fig. 1-20/ 4).

Both branches of the dorsal branches of the cervical nerves are now also visible—perhaps also on the deep surface of the semispinalis. The medial branches pass dorsally on the ligament to the skin on the dorsum of the neck; the lateral branches are distributed to the lateral cervical muscles (Fig. 1-6).

A **caudal nuchal bursa** may be present between the funiculus and the strong insertion of the laminar part of the ligament on the spinous process of the axis (Fig. 1-21).

Some veterinarians use the neck muscles dorsal to the vertebrae for intramuscular injections. Put the reflected muscles back against the nuchal ligament to obtain a measure of their combined thickness, and note that the deep cervical artery and vein and accessory nerve could (possibly) be injured

After consulting an instructor, remove the head by sawing between the axis and C3. Wrap and store the head after identifying it by carving the number of your horse into the lower part of the masseter on both sides. (The heads will be split and returned to you later.)

Ask an instructor whether the front of your horse needs to be rehung

before the forelimbs are removed during the dissection of the thorax.

If rehanging is needed, palpate the rounded knobs of the <u>articular</u> processes between C3 and C4, and between C4 and C5 (see demo specimen of cervical vertebrae). Ventral to the C4/C5 articular processes is the intervertebral foramen between these two vertebrae. To locate it on your specimen, plunge the post mortem knife (course locker) horizontally into the foramen from left to right. Unhook the front hoist so the horse rests on

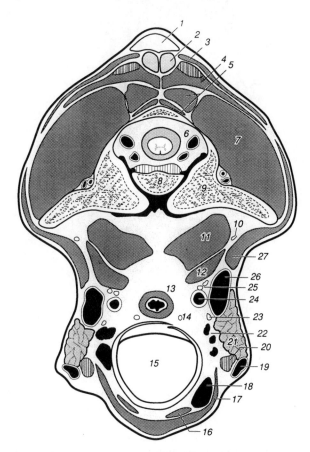

1. Crest	15. Trachea
2. Funicular part of nuchal lig.	16. Sternothyroideus
3. Splenius	17. Combined omo- and sterno-
4. Semispinalis capitis	hyoideus
5. Rectus capitis dorsalis, major	18. Thyroid gland
and minor, on dorsal arch of	19. Linguofacial vein
atlas	20. Tendon of sternocephalicus
6. Epidural fat	21. Parotid gland
7. Obliquus capitis caudalis	22. Cranial deep cervical lymph
8. Dens of axis	nodes
9. Atlas	23. Ventral branch of spinal
10. Dorsal branch of spinal	accessory nerve
accessory nerve	24. Common carotid artery
11. Longus colli	25. Vagus and sympathetic
12. Longus capitis	trunk
13. Esophagus	26. Maxillary vein
14. Recurrent laryngeal nerve	27. Cleidomastoideus and omo-
	transversarius

FIGURE 1-18. Transverse section of the neck at the level of the wing of the atlas. (Modified after Sisson and Grossman, 1953.)

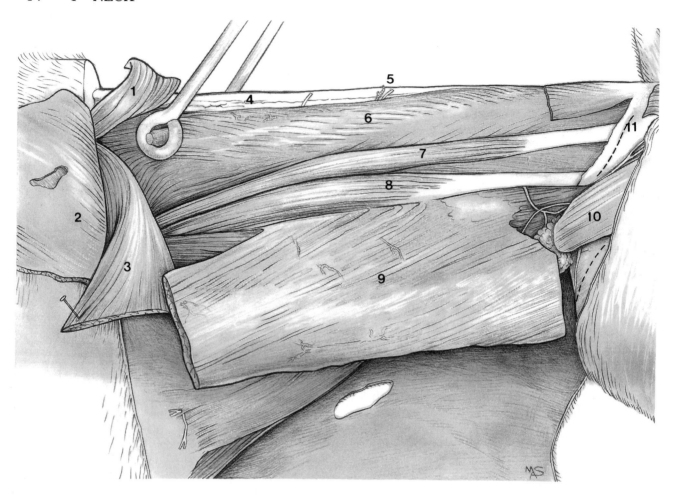

1.	Cervical rhomboideus	5.	Dorsal cutaneous nerve and
2.	Cervical trapezius		arterial branches
3.	Cervical serratus ventralis	6.	Semispinalis capitis
4.	Funiculus nuchae	7.	Longissimus capitis

8.	Longissimus atlantis	10.	Parotidoauricularis
9.	Splenius	11.	Wing of atlas

FIGURE 1-19. Deep dissection of dorsal part of neck; lateral view.

its forelimbs; remove the hook from the nuchal ligament, withdraw the post mortem knife and insert the tip of the hook horizontally into the intervertebral foramen, holding the eye of the hook ventral to the longus colli. Hammer the hook horizontally through left and right foramina so the eye of the hook ends up in the midline ventral to the longus colli. Attach the hoist and elevate the horse with the forelimbs about 5 cm off the ground. Leave the horse like that for the remainder of the lab to settle the hook into place.

Examine also the *cervical vertebrae* on a skeleton or on a demo specimen. Malformations of the articular processes may result in pressure on the spinal cord and clinical signs of ataxia ("wobbles"). Certain forms of ataxia (dynamic stenosis of the cord, for instance) are treated surgically by fusing neighboring vertebrae. This is done via a ventral approach—through the visceral space of the neck.

Exercises on the Live Animal

Students at Cornell should view the videotape on the NECK in the series <u>Equine Anatomy Reviewed on the Live Animal</u> before attempting these palpations.

1---Find the jugular groove and raise the jugular vein. Occlude the vein long enough (at least 10 seconds) to see it actually swell and fill the groove. Try to feel the esophagus in the caudal 10-15 cm of the left jugular groove.

2---Visualize the course of the accessory nerve and of the deep cervical vessels in relation to IM injections that some veterinarians perform in the upper part of the neck.

3---Palpate the ventral surface of the trachea and note that this is easier in the cranial half of the neck, because the trachea is covered here only by

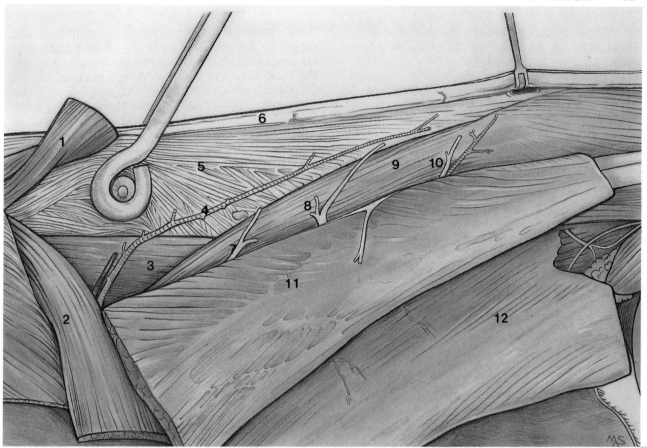

1. Cervical rhomboideus
2. Cervical serratus ventralis
3. Longissimus cervicis
4. Deep cervical artery
5. Lamina nuchae
6. Funiculus nuchae, and caudal nuchal bursa where the funiculus is elevated
7. C5
8. C4
9. Intertransversarius muscles
10. C3
11. Semispinalis capitis
12. Splenius

FIGURE 1-20. Deep dissection of dorsal part of neck exposing the nuchal ligament; lateral view.

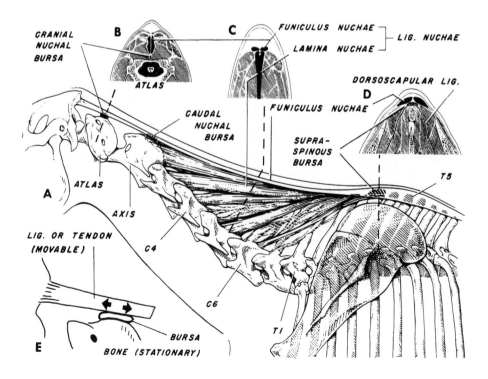

FIGURE 1-21. Nuchal ligament and associated bursae. (Drawn by L. Sadler.)

the thin sternohyoideus and -thyroideus muscles. These must be separated in the midline when a tracheotomy is performed.

4---Carefully grasp the trachea and palpate cranially until the wider cricoid cartilage of the larynx can be felt. At this level find the convex, fluctuating thryoid gland; it feels like half a walnut.

5---On the flat cranial surface of the trunk find the manubrium sterni and lateral to it the groove between brachiocephalicus and descending pectoral muscle. Remember that the cephalic vein and the deltoid branch of the superficial cervical artery lie in the depth of the groove.

6---Palpate the sternocephalicus throughout its length. Extend the head to demonstrate the tendon of insertion. Distend the jugular vein at the same time and outline Viborg's triangle.

7---Palpate the wing of the atlas, and below it the soft ventral end of the parotid gland. The caudal edge of the mandible is also easily found.

8---At the caudal end of the neck roll the chain of superficial cervical lymph nodes under the tips of your fingers. You are palpating through the wide band of muscle formed by brachiocephalicus and omotransversarius.

THORAX

Purpose and Plan of the Dissection

1---To learn what forms the withers and to see the supraspinous bursa and adjacent muscles, and the dorsoscapular ligament within the withers.
2---To demonstrate the line of pleural reflection and the basal border of the lung.
3---To see the heart and great vessels in situ and to learn how much of the heart is covered by the forelimb.
4---To note the position of the lungs and the size of the lung fields that are available for auscultation on the sides of the animal.
5---To see the autonomic ganglia in the cranial part of the thorax, the vagus and sympathetic trunk and their branches, and the phrenic nerves at the level of the heart (partly optional).
6---To see the interior of the heart and the topography of its valves.

Plan. After removal of the skin and study of the superficial muscles and nerves (optional), the withers are dissected in greater detail. Intercostal muscles caudal to the forelimb are removed to expose the lungs after which the forelimb is detached and stored. The large serratus ventralis and the remaining intercostal muscles are removed and the concentration of structures (some optional) at the thoracic inlet are studied. Certain ribs and the lungs are removed and the topography of the heart and other mediastinal structures is studied in situ. *Finally, the heart is removed, and heart and lungs are examined on the table.*

The high ridge formed by the long spinous processes of T2-8 between the scapular cartilages marks the **withers** (Fig 1-21).

Incise the skin on the dorsal midline (Fig. 2-1) over the withers to the last thoracic vertebra (palpate the last rib or estimate from a skeleton). Make an incision along the curve of the last rib to about 20 cm ventral to its costochondral junction. Reflect the skin ventrally off the thorax to the level of the shoulder joint. Make a horizontal skin incision from the point of the shoulder (greater tubercle of humerus) over the caudal border of the triceps to the axillary skin fold. In the end, the skin should be reflected to an oblique line running from the axilla to the ventral end of the caudal transverse incision.

Reflecting skin and cutaneous muscles together saves time. The cutaneous muscles begin to appear as faint bands on the undersurface of the skin as you reflect it. There is usually a layer of fat deep to the cutaneous muscle that obscures the latissimus dorsi and other muscles of the thorax. Therefore, remove also the layer of fat with the

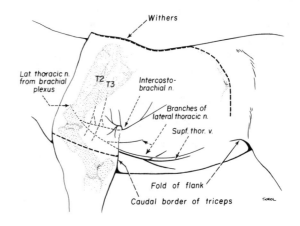

FIGURE 2-1. Skin incisions on the thorax and the distribution of the lateral thoracic nerve.

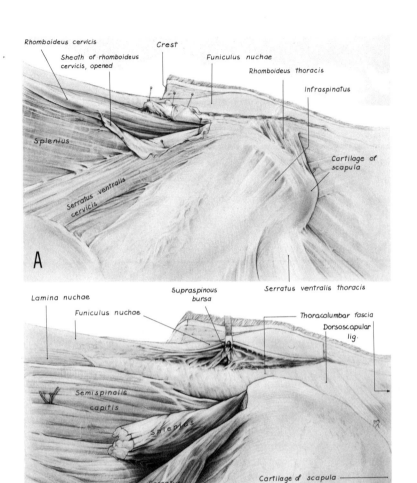

Rhomboideus cervicis

Sheath of rhomboideus cervicis, opened

Crest

Funiculus nuchae

Rhomboideus thoracis

Infraspinatus

Splenius

Serratus ventralis cervicis

Cartilage of scapula

A

Lamina nuchae

Supraspinous bursa

Serratus ventralis thoracis

Funiculus nuchae

Thoracolumbar fascia

Dorsoscapular lig.

Semispinalis capitis

Splenius

Serratus ventralis cervicis

Cartilage of scapula

L. SADLER

B

FIGURE 2-2. Withers, left lateral view. *A:* Sheath of rhomboideus opened and pinned back. *B:* Rhomboideus cervicis and thoracis removed to expose the dorsoscapular ligament; the wide funiculus nuchae raised and the supraspinous bursa opened.

cutaneous muscle caudal to the caudal border of the triceps. The **cutaneous muscles** (cutaneus omobrachialis over the triceps and cutaneus trunci extending from the triceps to the thigh) twitch the skin to remove irritants (insects, for example). The latter muscle is innervated by the lateral thoracic nerve (from the brachial plexus; Fig. 2-1) that courses with the superficial thoracic vein, to be seen shortly.

As the reflection proceeds you will notice a bundle of vessels with a medium-sized vein appearing from under the caudal border of the triceps, opposite the ventral border of the latissimus dorsi. These vessels must be cut, because the vein is not the very much larger **superficial thoracic (spur) vein** (Fig. 1-10) which is subcutaneous near the point of the elbow (tuber olecrani) and accompanies the lateral border of the pectoralis profundus. When this large vein has been reached, the skin reflection is complete (Fig. 2-1).

Ask an instructor which of the un-

shaded sections set in small type throughout this guide are to be done.

CUTANEOUS AND OTHER SUPERFICIAL NERVES OF THE THORAX. The *dorsal cutaneous branches* of the thoracic nerves (Fig. 1-6/a) emerge over the dorsal edge of the scapular cartilage and along the dorsal border of the latissimus dorsi. They innervate the fascia and skin of the dorsal portion of the thorax. The medial branches of the dorsal branches are motor and deep. The *lateral cutaneous branches* (/d), seen in two rows on the lateral surface of the thorax ventral to the latissimus, are branches of the intercostal nerves (ventral branches of the thoracic nerves; /9).

Find the **lateral thoracic nerve** that accompanies the spur vein; it arises from the brachial plexus and provides by direct branches and indirectly by communication with branches of the intercostobrachial nerve the motor innervation of the cutaneus trunci. In the axilla it gives off a branch that joins the lateral cutaneous branches of intercostal nerves 2 and 3 to form the **intercostobrachial nerve,** which emerges along the ventral border of the latissimus dorsi to supply the motor innervation of the

3
1
3
L

cutaneus omobrachialis and the dorsal part of the cutaneus trunci, and to innervate the skin of the shoulder and arm. The radiating branches of this nerve were cut in the previous skin reflection (Figs. 2-1 and 2-14). Other branches of the lateral thoracic nerve enter the cutaneus trunci between the latissimus dorsi and the pectoralis profundus. Also in the axilla, the caudal pectoral nerves diverge ventrally from the lateral thoracic nerve and enter the pectoralis profundus. The lateral thoracic nerve continues in the cutaneus trunci to the flank. The lateral cutaneous branches of the intercostal nerves cross the branches of the lateral thoracic and run with them for short distances; but then they pass through the cutaneus trunci to innervate the skin.

Transect the latissimus dorsi along the caudal border of triceps and trapezius and reflect it dorsally. Then sever its dorsal attachment to the thoracolumbar fascia and discard the muscle. A part of the serratus ventralis thoracis is now exposed (Fig. 1-10).

Withers

Identify and isolate the ventral borders of both the cervical and thoracic trapezius. Detach (cut) the entire muscle from its origin on the funiculus nuchae and from its insertion on the scapular spine and remove it. Remove also any of the fatty crest that remains on the funiculus.

The following description of the supraspinous and dorsoscapular ligaments should be read before proceeding with the dissection: The **supraspinous ligament** runs cranially in the middorsal line from the sacrum to the withers, giving origin laterally to the thoracolumbar fascia. It consists of a cord of white fibrous tissue and is closely attached to the summits of the vertebral spinous processes.

Before reaching the withers the ligament widens and at T4 is continued on each side of the midline by the paired **funiculus nuchae**, the yellow elastic cord previously seen to extend to the skull. At the withers the funiculus is wide and flat and covers the dorsal border of the rhomboideus thoracis. The **thoracolumbar fascia** is much thicker here and from its lateral surface releases the **dorsoscapular ligament**. This extends ventrolaterally to be inserted on the deep surface of the scapula where it interdigitates by numerous elastic lamellae with the scapular insertion of the serratus ventralis (Fig. 2-3/5'). The thoracolumbar fascia continues cranially to the level of T1 and is continued by the splenius; the semispinalis capitis arises from a deep lamina of the thoracolumbar fascia.

The **rhomboideus thoracis** has been exposed by the removal of the trapezius. It arises from the lateral surface of the dorsoscapular ligament and inserts with the rhomboideus cervicis on the deep surface of the scapular cartilage. Ventral to the

rhomboideus cervicis the serratus ventralis cervicis is exposed as it passes to its insertion on the deep surface of the scapula. The fascial sheath surrounding the rhomboideus cervicis has already been opened when we examined the neck muscles. Open also the caudal part of the sheath; it extends to the level of the supraspinous bursa to be seen presently (Fig. 2-2/A).

Fistulous withers is a chronic inflammatory disease affecting the supraspinous bursa and adjacent tissues. It may be caused by trauma to the region or by infection of the bursa itself. One of the known infectious organisms, *Brucella abortus*, is a zoonotic agent capable of causing "undulant fever" in humans, especially veterinarians treating fistulous withers.

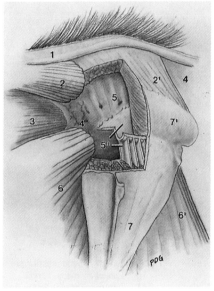

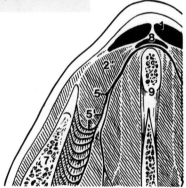

1. Funiculus nuchae
2. Rhomboideus cervicis (thoracis at 2')
3. Splenius
4. Thoracolumbar fascia
5. Fibrous part of dorsoscapular lig. (5' elastic part)
6. Serratus cervicis (thoracis at 6')
7. Scapula (7' scapular cartilage)
8. Supraspinous bursa
9. Spinous processes

FIGURE 2-3. *Top:* Dissection of the dorsoscapular ligament, a lateral offshoot of the thoracolumbar fascia; craniolateral view. Portions of the rhomboideus and serratus ventralis muscles have been removed. (From P. D. Garrett (1990), with permission.) *Bottom:* Transverse section of the withers at the level of the supraspinous bursa (8).

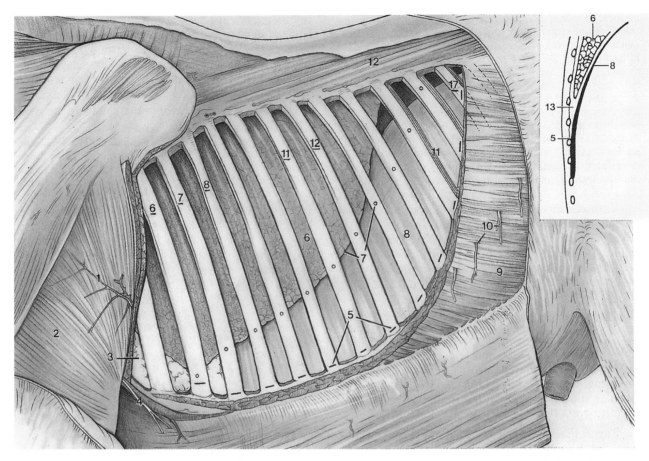

1.	Intercostobrachial nerve	6.	Caudal lobe of lung	12.	Longissimus dorsi
2.	Triceps	7.	Basal border of lung		
3.	Pericardium	8.	Diaphragm	13.	Costodiaphragmatic recess
4.	Lateral thoracic nerve and	9.	External abdominal oblique		
	supf. thoracic vein	10.	Lateral cutaneous nerves		
5.	Line of pleural reflection	11.	Intercostal vessels and nerve		

FIGURE 2-4. The caudal lobe of the lung exposed through the intercostal spaces. The underlined numbers mark the ribs. The inset shows the costodiaphragmatic recess (13) in dorsal (horizontal) section.

By careful cutting and scraping, completely **remove the rhomboideus muscle from the surface of the dorsoscapular ligament.** Clean also more cranially to see the origin of the splenius. By blunt dissection, work carefully between the funiculus nuchae and the spinous processes of T2 and 3 to find the **supraspinous bursa** in a mass of fat and connective tissue (Figs. 2-3/8 and 2-2/B). The bursa is normally dorsal to the dorsoscapular ligament, but may vary in position and size, extending sometimes laterally between the trapezius and rhomboideus muscles.

Incise the thoracolumbar fascia from the caudal end of the scapular cartilage to the caudal skin incision parallel to the dorsal midline and reflect it ventrally. This will reflect also the thin serratus dorsalis which should be removed with the fascia. The narrow iliocostalis, characterized by its long flat tendons, is now exposed and should be removed, exposing the ribs to the lateral edge of the longissimus.

Thoracic Wall

The purpose of the following dissection is to demonstrate the line of pleural reflection and the basal border of the lung. At the **line of pleural reflection** (Fig. 3-5) the costal pleura on the lateral wall of the thorax becomes continuous with the pleura on the diaphragm (diaphragmatic pleura). The line extends along the eighth and ninth costal cartilages, crosses the costochondral junction of the ninth rib, and passes dorsocaudally in a gentle curve and at progressively increasing distances from the costochondral junctions of the succeeding ribs. It reaches the middle of the cranial border of the last rib and turns craniomedially ending at the vertebral end of the last (17th) intercostal space.

The line of pleural reflection is clinically important because it is the limit of the pleural cavity. A needle inserted craniodorsal to it will enter the pleural cavity, whereas a needle inserted caudoventral to it will pass through the costal part of the diaphragm into the peritoneal cavity. Anatomically, the thoracic and pleural cavities are not exactly coextensive, nor are the abdominal and peritoneal cavities exactly coextensive. The diaphragm separates the thoracic and abdominal cavities, while the diaphragm together with the pleura, peritoneum, and intervening connective tissues separates the pleural and peritoneal cavities.

The following dissection exposes lung and diaphragm through the intercostal spaces by removing the intercostal muscles. The intercostal vessels and nerves which follow the caudal border of the ribs will also be removed, *but should be preserved in intercostal spaces 15-17* (Fig. 2-4/11).

Caution: The diaphragm is closely applied to the costal pleura in the last few intercostal spaces and should not be mutilated. Begin in the dorsal end of the 15th intercostal space and remove the intercostal muscles, endothoracic fascia, and costal pleura. Probe with one finger in the pleural cavity for the caudal and ventral limits of the **costodiaphragmatic recess** where the removal of the intercostal tissues should stop. The costodiaphragmatic recess is the potentional space between the costal and diaphragmatic pleura (Fig. 2-4/inset). Remove the remaining tissues of the 15th intercostal space: dorsally to the edge of the longissimus and ventrally to the line of pleural reflection, completely opening the intercostal space. Repeat the process for each of the intercostal spaces not covered by the forelimb (also the 16th and 17th). Remove the external abdominal oblique and serratus ventralis where they overlie the intercostal spaces to be opened. Probe the pleural reflection in each space before

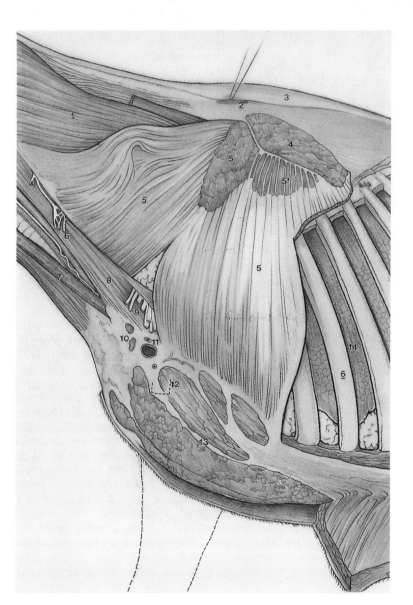

1. Splenius
2. Supraspinous bursa
3. Funiculus nuchae
4. Rhomboideus thoracis
5. Serratus ventralis
5' Elastic lamellae of dorsoscapular lig. interdigitating with serratus ventralis
6. C6
7. Jugular vein dorsal to sternocephalicus
8. Scalenus ventralis
9. Brachial plexus
10. Caudal deep cervical lymph nodes
11. Subclavian artery and vein
12. Position of ventral end of first rib
13. Stumps of pectoral muscles on sternum
14. Caudal lobe of lung

FIGURE 2-5. Deep dissection after the removal of the left forelimb. The underlined number marks a rib.

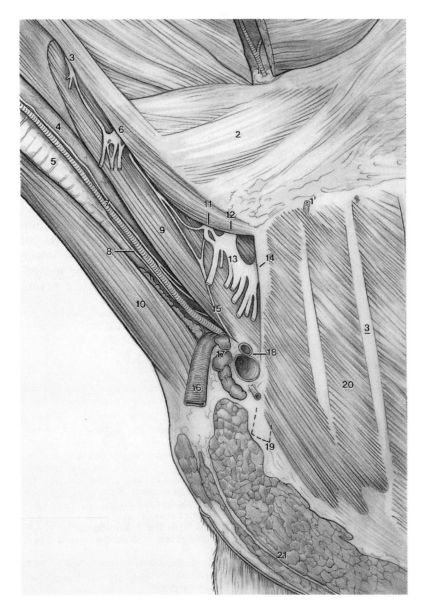

1. Deep cervical artery
1' Stump of dorsal scapular artery
2. Longissimus cervicis
3. C5
4. Esophagus
5. Trachea
6. C6
7. Carotid artery and vagosympathetic trunk
8. Recurrent laryngeal nerve
9. Scalenus ventralis
10. Sternocephalicus
11. C7
12. C8
13. Brachial plexus
14. T1 and T2
15. Root of phrenic nerve
16. Jugular vein, reflected ventrally
17. Caudal deep cervical lymph nodes
18. Subclavian artery and vein
19. Position of ventral end of first rib
20. External intercostal muscle
21. Stumps of pectoral muscles on sternum

FIGURE 2-6. Structures at the thoracic inlet, the left forelimb has been removed; left lateral view. The underlined number marks a rib.

cutting the intercostal tissues. The edge of the muscles left in place over the ventral ends of the intercostal spaces marks the line of pleural reflection (Fig. 2-4/5).

The **basal border of the lung** is now visible (Fig. 2-4/7). In the live horse it curves from the costochondral junction of the 6th rib, through the middle of the exposed part (from back muscles to costal arch) of the 11th rib, to the margin of the back muscles in the 16th intercostal space. (The thumb rule "6,11,16" is often used to remember these landmarks.) In the embalmed specimen the lung is usually shrunken and the basal border is slightly off caudally. Mark the basal border of the lung as given for the live horse on the ribs for later reference.

Mark also the position of the caudal border of the triceps on the ribs. In the normal standing

position the **olecranon** is usually in the transverse plane of the fifth costochondral junction and the triceps line coincides roughly with the fifth intercostal space.

To remove the forelimb: Elevate the cranial end of the specimen and push the foot medially. Using a large knife (larger than your post mortem knife) cut the serratus ventralis from the scapula and scapular cartilage, keeping the knife as close to the scapula as you can. Free the subclavius from the neck and leave it on the limb. Work down between the scapula and thorax until the roots of the brachial plexus and the axillary vessels are encountered. Expose these structures by forcefully displacing the loose areolar tissue (in which they are embedded) with your fingers and show the structures to the other members of your group. *It is especially important for the later dissection of the forelimb to make the remaining cuts as close to the ribs and sternum as possible. Therefore, sever the nerves and axillary vessels* close to the first rib. *Now cut the pectoral muscles and skin from the manubrium sterni to the olecranon,* keeping the knife close to the sternum and thorax *to leave as much muscle on the limb as possible.*

Before storing the limb, look at the deep surface of the scapula and observe the yellow elastic lamellae of the **dorsoscapular ligament** interdigitating with strips of the serratus ventralis. See the lamellae also on the trunk (Fig. 2-5/5'). The description of how the dorsoscapular ligament inserts on the scapula may make more sense to you now (Fig. 2-3).

Remove the **serratus ventralis** from its origins on the cervical vertebrae and ribs. Visualize this muscle on the skeleton. It forms, with the contralateral muscle, an elastic sling suspending the thorax between the forelimbs. Its insertion on a small area of the scapula acts as a fulcrum around which the forelimb swings during locomotion. Remove also what is left of the rhomboideus and the portion of the iliocostalis that was deep to the serratus.

Find the **ventral scalenus** and clean its lateral surface, preserving the roots of the phrenic nerve which obliquely cross this surface on their way to the thoracic cavity. The ventral scalenus extends from the first rib to the transverse processes of the last few cervical vertebrae (Fig. 2-6/9). The dorsal scalenus, which originates from the lateral surfaces of the ribs (dog, ox), is absent in the horse.

The roots of the **phrenic nerve** pass around the ventral border of the scalenus and unite as they approach the thoracic inlet. The phrenic nerve thus formed enters the thoracic cavity within the mediastinum where it will be traced later (Fig. 2-12).

THE ROOTS OF THE BRACHIAL PLEXUS AND OF THE PHRENIC NERVE. Find the large nerve trunks of the *brachial plexus* passing between the ventral scalenus and the much smaller middle scalenus dorsal to it. Remove the middle scalenus dorsal to the nerve trunks, cutting it from the first rib and reflecting it in dorsocranial direction. Most of the roots of the brachial plexus are now exposed (Fig. 2-6/11-14). The thickest root is the ventral branch of T1; it passes around the cranial border of the first rib. About 3 cm cranial to it is the ventral branch of C8, which is a little thinner. The ventral branch of C7 is about half as thick as C8.

Trace the *phrenic nerve* root, crossing the scalenus about 6 cm cranial to the first rib, to the ventral branch of C7. The phrenic nerve root from C6 crosses the muscle farther cranially, running almost parallel to its fibers. The root from C5 is not always present.

Locate the **caudal deep cervical lymph nodes**. They are variably distributed around the thoracic inlet on the ventral surface of the trachea among the muscles and vessels. They drain the head, neck, thorax, and forelimb largely through the cranial and middle deep cervical, superficial cervical, cranial mediastinal, and axillary nodes. Efferents join the thoracic and right lymphatic ducts which carry the lymph to the veins at the thoracic inlet.

Pick up the **recurrent nerve** where it was tagged previously in the neck. Trace it to the thoracic inlet deep to the common carotid artery, and note its close relationship to the caudal deep cervical lymph nodes.

If they have not been cut off with the forelimb, the prescapular and deltoid branches of the **supf. cervical artery** may now be traced to their origin from the parent artery (Fig. 2-12).

Trace the **deep cervical and dorsal scapular arteries** proximally to their emergence from the thoracic cavity through the first and second (sometimes third) intercostal spaces, respectively (Fig. 2-12). The deep cervical artery was last seen on the side of the nuchal ligament near the median plane; it emerges from the dorsal end of the first intercostal space and passes *deep* to the shiny longissimus cervicis which is just dorsal to the first few ribs. This muscle has to be resected to expose the artery. The dorsal scapular artery is *superficial* to the longissimus, but may have been removed with the serratus ventralis. It sometimes leaves an impression on the longissimus but its stump should certainly be present (Fig. 2-7/11).

Remove the intercostal muscles that were covered by the limb. The entire lung should now be visible.

With your finger probe the cranial extent of the **pleural cavity**. On the left the pleura is reflected directly from the mediastinum to the first rib. On the right the pleura forms two cul-de-sacs (cupulae pleurae); one extends about 3 cm cranial to the first rib on the deep surface of the scalenus, the other is a little shorter and is ventral to the level of the cranial vena cava.

The **cardiac notches of the lungs** can also be seen now. They allow the pericardial pleura to contact the costal pleura in intercostal spaces 3 - 6 on the left and spaces 3 and 4 on the right. Slight variations exist, especially in ponies.

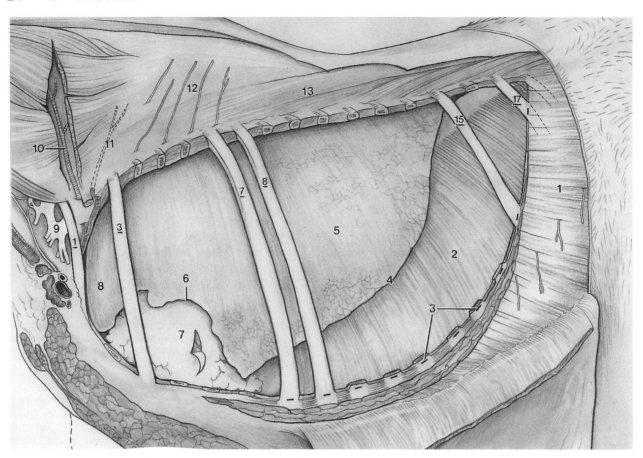

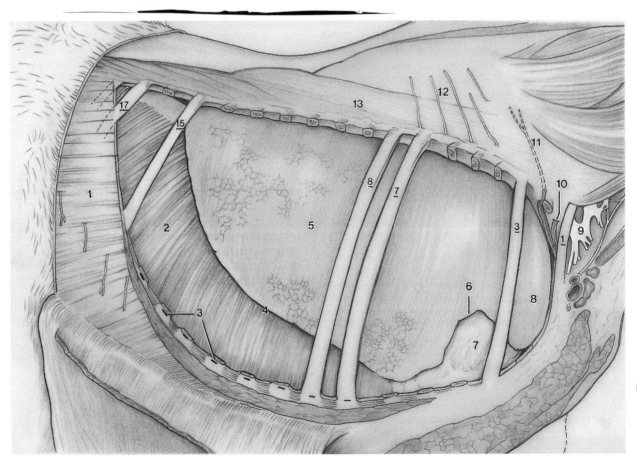

Thoracic Viscera

The **HEART**, more vertical than in the dog, lies between intercostal spaces 2 and 6. The **apex** is opposite the last segment of the sternum and slightly cranial to the sternal attachment of the diaphragm. The distance from apex to **base** is usually two thirds of the dorsoventral diameter of the thorax. More than half of the heart lies to the left of the median plane. Except for a small area on the left, the heart is covered by the forelimb in the normal standing position (Fig. 3-5). Verify the location of the heart by palpation through the intercostal spaces.

Auscultation of the heart is important in cardiac evaluation of a patient. Certain points (puncta maxima) near the caudal border of the triceps have been determined for listening most advantageously to the sounds of the four heart valves. These points of maximum audibility are roughly as follows:

1. Left AV valve (bicuspid or mitral): *Left side,* low in the 5th intercostal space caudodorsal to the olecranon.

2. Aortic valve: *Left side,* high in the 4th intercostal space just below a horizontal line through the shoulder joint (roughly through the middle of the first rib).

3. Pulmonary valve: *Left side,* low in the 3rd intercostal space.

4. Right AV valve (tricuspid): *Right side,* low in the 3rd or 4th intercostal space.

Find these points on your specimen. You will notice that most of them lie cranial to the triceps line you marked. Therefore, when the heart of a live horse is auscultated the stethoscope has to be pushed under the triceps, or the forelimb has to be pulled cranially.

Pass a scalpel through the intercostal space at each of these points and make several stab incisions (close together) through the pericardium and into the heart wall. We will see the actual relationship between these surface points and the valves when the heart is opened.

Remove all the ribs except 1, 3, 7, 8, 15, 17 and 18. Cut them with heavy clippers or with the tip of your saw at the lateral border of the longissimus and at the line of pleural reflection. It is important to keep especially ribs 7 and 8 in place. Large horses have been seen to have their back break and to collapse in the middle when these ribs were inadvertently removed.

The **LUNGS** of the horse have a simpler lobation than the lungs of the other domestic mammals. The cardiac notch divides the lung into cranial and caudal lobes (Figs. 2-7 and 2-8). The right lung has an accessory lobe and is considerably larger than the left.

The surface projection of the lung has to be known when the lung is to be examined by percussion and auscultation. Being roughly triangular, the projection's cranial limit is the triceps muscle, dorsally it is bounded by the lateral edge of the back muscles, and the basal border of course forms the third border (Fig. 3-5). Since the lung is thin at the basal border, lung sounds stop a few cm proximal to this border so that the "audible" lung field is a little smaller than the projection. In normal breathing, the basal border moves about 5 cm. When a horse is excited or has the "heaves", the lungs are inflated considerably beyond the normal.

Before the **REMOVAL OF THE LUNGS,** students of both sides should see the caudal vena cava when the caudal lobe of the RIGHT lung is raised, and should notice that the accessory lobe of that lung is located medial to the vein and medial to the caval fold that connects the vein with the floor of the thoracic cavity.

Now remove both lungs by cutting the pulmonary arteries and veins and the principal bronchus at the hilus without injury to the phrenic nerve and the base of the heart.

The **mediastinum** containing heart, great vessels, trachea, and esophagus (also thymus in the foal) is now in full view, and the mediastinal pleura covering these structures is still intact.

Locate the following structures cranial to the heart, i.e., in the cranial mediastinum, *on the right side* : (For the left side see further on.)

1. Cranial vena cava

2. Costocervical trunk (arterial): follow Fig. 2-10, cut away the veins (/8, 9, 10) and see the costocervical trunk (/15)

3. Deep cervical artery (/16)

1.	External abdominal oblique	7.	Heart, in Fig. 2-7 mediastinal
2.	Diaphragm		pleura and pericardium are
3.	Line of pleural reflection		fenestrated
4.	Basal border of lung	8.	Cranial lobe of lung
5.	Caudal lobe of lung	9.	Brachial plexus
6.	Cardiac notch	10.	Deep cervical artery

11.	Dorsal scapular artery	
12.	Lat. branches of dors.	medial to scapula
	branches of spinal nerves	13. Longissimus dorsi

FIGURES 2-7 and 2-8. Lung and heart *in situ*; lateral views. The underlined numbers mark the ribs.

4. Vertebral artery (/17)

5. Azygous vein: on the right as in the dog (/stump near 20)

6. Phrenic nerve: passes caudoventrally over the cranial vena cava, the heart, and then *ventral* to the lung root with the caudal vena cava to the diaphragm.

7. Trachea: palpate its rings dorsal to the heart.

8. Vagus: passes caudodorsally over the lateral surface of the trachea and then *dorsal* to the lung root.

9. Loose part of cranial mediastinum : ventral to great vessels, slightly to the left of the median plane; contains thymus tissue in young subjects.

10. Cranial mediastinal lymph nodes: scattered in the *dorsal* part of the cranial mediastinum and continuous cranially with the caudal deep cervical nodes. Imbedded in fat, difficult to see. They drain the pleura, pericardium, heart, trachea, esophagus, and tracheobronchial lymph nodes. Efferents pass to the caudal deep cervical lymph nodes and to the thoracic duct. Palpate the lymph nodes deep to rib 1.

Locate the following structures cranial to the heart, i.e., in the cranial mediastinum, *on the left side* :

1. Costocervical trunk (arterial): follow Fig. 2-9, cut away the veins, and find costocervical trunk (/11)

2. Deep cervical artery (/12)

3. Vertebral artery (/13): its origin may be concealed by the first rib.

4. Phrenic nerve (/28): passes caudoventrally over the base of the heart and then *ventral* to lung root. to the diaphragm .

5. Vagus (/26): best seen as it crosses the palpable left subclavian artery, then passes *dorsal* to the lung root.

6. Loose part of cranial mediastinum: ventral to great vessels; contains thymus tissue in young subjects.

7. Cranial mediastinal lymph nodes: scattered in the *dorsal* part of the cranial mediastinum and continuous cranially with the caudal deep cervical nodes. Imbedded in fat, difficult to see. Same drainage as on right side (see previous item 10).

8. Aortic arch (/19): large hard tube just cranial to lung root.

9. Trachea (/4): palpate its rings between aortic arch and costocervical trunk.

10. Esophagus(/3):palpate dorsolateral to trachea, disappears with trachea medial to aortic arch.

On the right side look again at the dorsally open space between caval fold and caudal mediastinum that housed the accessory lobe of the right lung. In the intact animal the caudal mediastinum ventral to the esophagus is pushed well over to the left by the accessory lobe. Pick up this mediastinum and note its fenestrations.

Cut the ventral and middle scalenus muscles (Fig. 2-6) from their origin on the first rib and remove the rib with bone cutters or saw. *Do not destroy structures deep to the rib.*

The purpose of the following dissection is to expose the **AUTONOMIC GANGLIA AND VAGAL AND SYMPATHETIC TRUNKS** in the cranial part of the thoracic cavity. The caudal cervical and first two thoracic ganglia are fused to a variable degree and are referred to as the cervicothoracic ganglion (G' in Figs. 2-9 and 2-10).

Locate the thoracic origin of the longus colli. The thoracic **sympathetic trunk** may be seen between the lateral edge of the muscle and the necks of the ribs. Incise the pleura dorsal to the trunk from the first to the sixth ribs. Carefully reflect the pleura ventrally off the trunk and continue the reflection to the level of the phrenic nerve. Trace the sympathetic trunk cranially and, as it disappears deep to the costocervical, deep cervical, and vertebral vessels, cut these vessels successively, pinning their dorsal stumps up so as to obtain an unobstructed field. Remove also the cranial mediastinal lymph nodes as necessary.

Medial to the first rib the sympathetic trunk is joined by large communicating branches from C8, T1, and T2 forming the prominent **cervicothoracic ganglion·** At the craniodorsal angle of the ganglion the vertebral nerve arises and accompanies the vertebral artery and vein into the neck (Figs. 2-9/22 and 2-10/23). It carries postganglionic sympathetic fibers to the cervical nerves.

Pick up the vagosympathetic trunk in the neck and note its division into vagus and sympathetic trunk as it approaches the thorax. Trace the **sympathetic trunk**, the dorsal of the two, caudally (removing the scalenus as necessary) to expose the **middle cervical ganglion** at the cranial border of the first rib (removed). From the middle cervical ganglion the sympathetic trunk continues dorsally and joins the cervicothoracic ganglion at the origin of the vertebral nerve. The sympathetic trunk thus zig-zags at the first rib; this is accentuated however by the suspension of the front of this heavy specimen solely by the neck.

Clean the lymph nodes and fascia in the area. Identify some of the **cardiac nerves** (there are about seven on each side) arising from the middle cervical and cervicothoracic ganglia and from the thoracic sympathetic trunk and vagus. Several of the cardiac nerves communicate with similar nerves

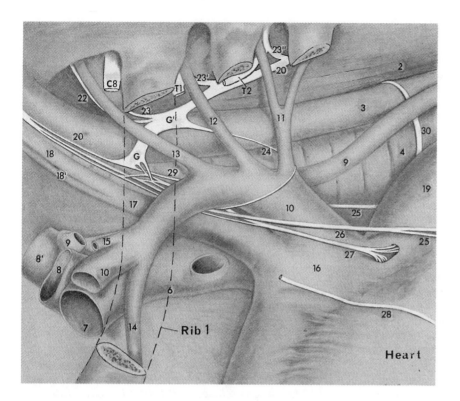

2. Longus colli
3. Esophagus
4. Trachea
6. Cranial vena cava
7. Left subclavian vein
8, 8' Left and right external jugular veins
9. Thoracic duct
10. Left subclavian artery
11. Costocervical trunk
12. Deep cervical artery
13. Vertebral artery
14. Internal thoracic artery
15. Superficial cervical artery
16. Brachiocephalic trunk
17. Bicarotid trunk
18, 18' Left and right carotid arteries
19. Aorta
20. Sympathetic trunk
22. Vertebral nerve
23, 23' 23" Communicating branches
24. Ansa subclavia
25. Recurrent laryngeal nerve
26. Vagus
28. Phrenic nerve
27, 29, 30 Cardiac nerves
G. Middle cervical ganglion
G' Cervicothoracic ganglion

◄ Cran.

FIGURE 2-9. Vessels and nerves of the cranial mediastinum; left lateral view. C8, T1, T2 are brachial plexus roots. (Modified from Hopkins '37.)

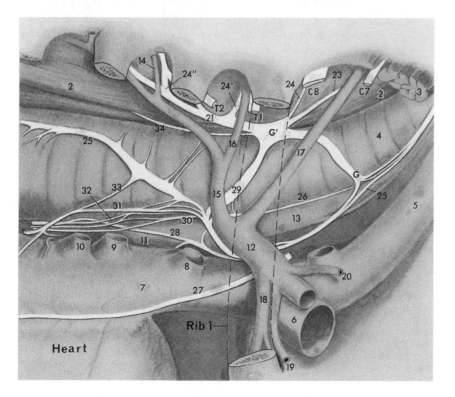

2. Longus colli
3. Scalenus ventralis
4. Trachea
5. Right external jugular vein
6. Right subclavian vein
7. Cranial vena cava
8. Stump of vertebral vein
9. Stump of deep cervical vein
10. Stump of costocervical vein
11. Brachiocephalic trunk
12. Right subclavian artery
13. Bicarotid trunk
14. Dorsal scapular artery
15. Costocervical trunk
16. Deep cervical artery
17. Vertebral artery
18, 19 Internal and external thoracic arteries
20. Superficial cervical artery
21. Sympathetic trunk
23. Vertebral nerve
24, 24', 24" Communicating branches
25. Right vagus
26. Recurrent laryngeal nerve
27. Phrenic nerve
28, 30-34 Cardiac nerves
29. Caudal limb of ansa subclavia
G. Middle cervical ganglion
G' Cervicothoracic ganglion

FIGURE 2-10. Vessels and nerves of the cranial mediastinum; right lateral view. C7, C8, T1, T2 are brachial plexus roots. (Modified from Hopkins '37.)

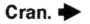 **Cran. ►**

of the other side before passing to the heart (Figs. 2-9/27, 29, 30 and 2-10/28, 30-34).

Trace the **VAGUS** to its bifurcation into dorsal and ventral branches at the level of T6. Right and left ventral branches unite at this level to form the **ventral vagal trunk** which passes caudally ventral to the esophagus. The dorsal branches unite farther caudally dorsal to the esophagus and form the **dorsal vagal trunk**. The vagal trunks accompany the esophagus through the diaphragm and carry parasympathetic nerve supply to the abdominal viscera. The ventral branches of the vagus give rise to a plexus on the bifurcation of the trachea from which the lungs and esophagus are supplied (Fig. 2-11/10, 8,12).

The recurrent laryngeal nerves are branches of the vagus nerves. The **right recurrent laryngeal nerve** (don't look for it) leaves the right vagus at the level of the first rib and loops around a branch of the subclavian artery to run up the neck where it was tagged. The **left recurrent laryngeal nerve** (find it) arises farther caudally than the right one,

namely at the base of the aortic arch. It is small but is easily traced as it passes from lateral to medial around the arch of the aorta, also to pass up the neck (Fig. 2-11/4). *Tag the nerve at the aortic arch.* Palpate the bifurcation of the trachea caudal to the base of the aortic arch—at the level of T6. The tracheobronchial lymph nodes you may feel here will be exposed on these organs after they have been removed from the cadaver.

The **thoracic duct** is visible dorsal to the aorta (Figs. 2-9/9 and 2-11/7). It is related medially to the intercostal vessels and lymph nodes. The duct may be unilateral on the right or left, or bilateral. The **bronchoesophageal artery** may be seen arising from the aorta at the sixth thoracic vertebra (Fig. 2-11/17). Passing ventrally, it crosses the right surface of the aorta where it can be palpated from the right side of the horse. Insert one finger medial to the right azygous vein and run it along the right side of the aorta. The artery is about 4 mm in diameter before it branches to supply the esophagus and the lungs.

To remove the HEART and other structures of the mediastinum: Ligate the caudal vena cava twice and transect between the ligatures. Transect the esophagus close to the esophageal hiatus of the diaphragm. In the thoracic inlet loosen the large veins and arteries, the esophagus, and the trachea from the ribs, sternum, and longus colli. Here also you must cut (close to the ribs) the vertebral, deep cervical, costocervical, and internal thoracic vessels and then pull everything into the thoracic cavity and out on the left side. Cut the aorta free from the thoracic vertebrae and transect it at the diaphragm. Free the mediastinum from the thoracic floor. The strong **sternopericardiac ligament** is represented by the adhesion of the fibrous pericardium to the caudal part of the sternum; it needs to be broken down with your fingers. Now remove the mediastinal viscera *en masse.*

Arrange the **heart** on the table so that its right side is up. Incise the **pericardium** from apex to base and remove it by cutting its attachment all around the base of the heart.

The **coronary groove** marks the division between the atria and the ventricles. Passing from the coronary groove to the apex of the heart are the **subsinuosal** (on the *right* side) and **paraconal** (on the *left* side) **interventricular grooves**. They mark the position of the interventricular septum. Remove some of the fat from the coronary and subsinuosal interventricular grooves and locate the right coronary artery, the large middle cardiac vein, and the thin cardiac nerves accompanying these vessels. Don't spend too much time looking for the nerves; they are often elusive. (The middle cardiac vein lies next to the right coronary artery

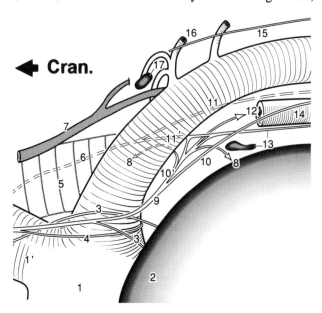

← **Cran.**

1, 1' Aortic arch and brachio-cephalic trunk	branches of left vagus
2. Cranial lobe of left lung reflected caudally	11, 11' Dorsal and ventral branches of right vagus
3. Cardiac nerves	12. Branch to esophagus
4. Left recurrent laryngeal nerve	13. Ventral vagal trunk and a tracheobronchial lymph node
5. Trachea	
6. Right vagus	14. Esophagus
7. Thoracic duct	15. Sympathetic trunk
8. Branches to right and left lung	16. A dorsal intercostal artery
9. Left vagus	17. Bronchoesophageal artery and a cranial mediastinal lymph node
10, 10' Dorsal and ventral	

FIGURE 2-11. The distribution of the vagus nerves at the level of the aortic arch; left lateral view. The cranial lobe of the left lung has been reflected caudally.

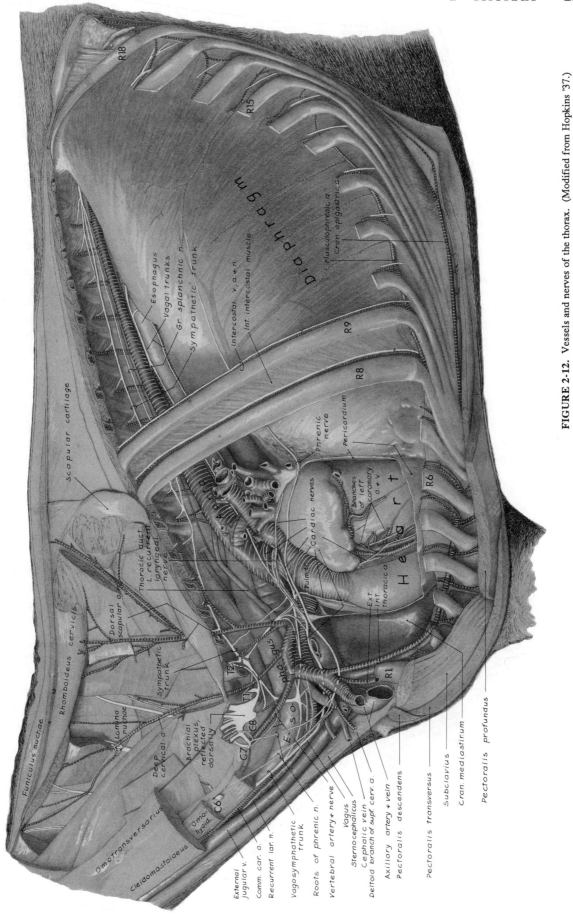

FIGURE 2-12. Vessels and nerves of the thorax. (Modified from Hopkins '37.)

in the subsinuosal interventricular groove.)

Turn the heart over so that its left side is up. Remove some fat from the coronary and paraconal interventricular grooves and locate the left coronary artery and its branches and the great cardiac vein.

Find the **left recurrent laryngeal nerve** which was tagged at the base of the aortic arch. Clean the nerve as it curves around the aorta in close relationship to the **left tracheobronchial lymph nodes**. Do not trace the nerve any farther. Verify its continuity with the previously tagged cervical recurrent nerve by tensing the latter.

Inflammation of the tracheobronchial lymph nodes causing degeneration of the left recurrent laryngeal nerve is one of several unsubstantiated theories concerning the etiology of laryngeal hemiplegia ("*roaring* "). In a "roarer" partial paralysis of certain laryngeal muscles allows the vocal fold(s) to become slack and to swing into the air current that passes through the larynx on inspiration. The characteristic roaring sound is due to the vibration of the lax vocal fold(s).

Turn the heart again so its right side is up. With scissors incise the right wall of the cranial vena cava, through the right atrium, and out the caudal vena cava. Open the atrium widely, clean out the clotted blood or color mass and examine the **right AV (tricuspid) valve**. Locate the **fossa ovalis** in the **interatrial septum** just dorsal to the opening of the **coronary sinus**, which is the short collecting trunk of the large cardiac veins you have just seen in the coronary and interventricular grooves.

Incise the wall of the right ventricle from the atrium to the apex between the two interventricular grooves and clean out the ventricle. Examine the **right AV valve, chordae tendineae, papillary muscles**, and the **septomarginal band** which carries Purkinje fibers of the conducting system from the **interventricular septum** to the outside wall of the ventricle.

Turn the heart once more so its left side is up. Beginning at one of the left pulmonary veins, cut through the lateral wall of the left atrium and then turn the knife toward the apex of the heart, opening the left ventricle between the two interventricular grooves. Examine the cusps of the opened **left AV (bicuspid or mitral) valve** and explore the approach to the **aortic valve** craniomedial to the left AV valve. The aortic valve will be seen later. The left AV and aortic valves are the common sites of valvular lesions (endocarditis) in the horse.

Clean the surface of the pulmonary trunk and aorta and find the **ligamentum arteriosum**, the remnant of the large fetal **ductus arteriosus**, connecting the two. Isolate the **pulmonary trunk**

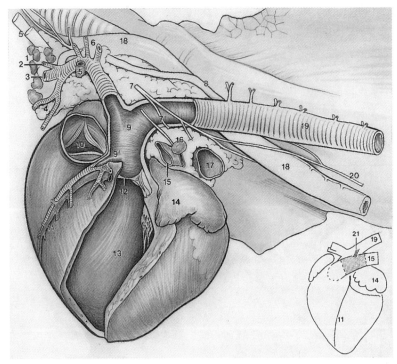

1. Caudal deep cervical lymph nodes
2. Superficial cervical artery
3. Left subclavian artery
4. External and internal thoracic arteries
5. Veins
6. From proximal to distal: costocervical trunk, deep cervical, and vertebral arteries
7. Left vagus (7' recurrent laryngeal nerve)
8. Thoracic duct
9. Latex in aortic arch at junction with brachiocephalic trunk
9' Origin of left coronary artery
10. Pulmonary valve
11. Descending branches of left coronary vessels in paraconal interventricular groove
12. Latex-filled aortic valve
13. Interventricular septum facing opened left ventricle
14. Left auricle
15. Pulmonary trunk
16. Tracheobronchial lymph node
17. Left principal bronchus
18. Esophagus
19. Descending aorta
20. Dorsal vagal trunk
21. Ligamentum arteriosum

FIGURE 2-13. Pluck with aortic arch and left ventricle opened, and a segment of pulmonary trunk removed as shown in inset.

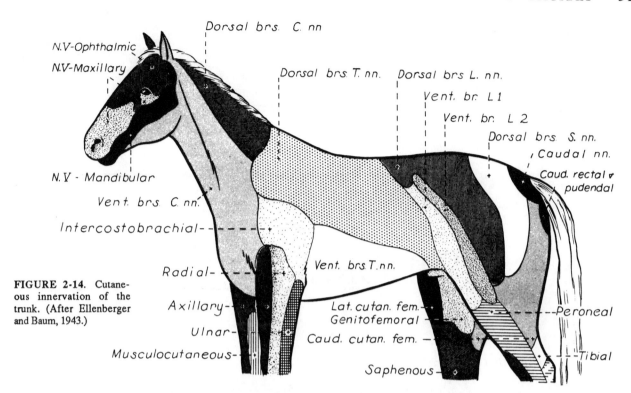

Dorsal brs. C. nn

N.V-Ophthalmic
N.V-Maxillary

Dorsal brs. T. nn.   Dorsal brs L. nn.

Vent. br. L1

Vent. br. L 2

Dorsal brs. S. nn.

, Caudal nn.

Caud. rectal &
pudendal

N. V - Mandibular

Vent. brs. C. nn.

Intercostobrachial-

Radial-

Vent. brs T. nn.

Axillary-

Lat. cutan. fem.-
Genitofemoral-
Caud. cutan. fem. -

Peroneal

Ulnar-

Musculocutaneous-

Saphenous-

Tibial

FIGURE 2-14. Cutaneous innervation of the trunk. (After Ellenberger and Baum, 1943.)

distal (caudal) to the lig. arteriosum and transect it. Transect it again 8 cm proximal to the first transection, close to the base of the heart (Fig. 2-13/inset). Cut the lig. arteriosum and remove the segment of pulmonary trunk. Clean both stumps of clotted blood and examine the **pulmonary valve.** Removing a segment of pulmonary trunk has exposed the origin of the aorta, which should be cleaned.

Beginning at the apex of the heart, incise the wall of the left ventricle again, but this time close to the paraconal interventricular groove and toward the origin of the aorta, opening also the **aortic valve.** For better exposure of the valve remove also the left wall of the aortic arch and brachiocephalic trunk which leaves its cranial surface (Fig. 2-13/9). Examine the aortic valve and look for the **origins of the coronary arteries.**

With the left side of the heart facing you, find the three stab incisions you made at the points of maximum audibility; also find the one on the right side for the right AV valve. How close to the actual valves were they? The true lateral projections of the valves upon the chest wall are not necessarily the points of maximum audibility probably because the sounds are deflected when they encounter tissues of different densities.

Exercises on the Live Animal

Students at Cornell should view the videotape on the THORAX in the series <u>Equine Anatomy</u>

<u>Reviewed on the Live Animal</u> before attempting these palpations.

1---In the neck, palpate the groove between the rhomboideus and splenius and follow it to the scapula. Palpate the prominent caudal angle of the scapula and then the dorsal border of the scapular cartilage. Opposite the high point of the withers palpate the (horizontal) groove between the cartilage and the (expanded) funiculus nuchae. Visualize the supraspinous bursa deep to the funiculus.

2---Palpate the caudal border of the triceps and the olecranon.

3---With the aid of Fig. 1-10 attempt to raise the superficial thoracic vein which may be used for venipuncture in thin horses.

4---Palpate the greater tubercle of the humerus (point of shoulder); this is more easily done if a skeleton is nearby.

5---Palpate the last rib and then, palpating cranially, determine which rib is the 9th. This sounds easy, but it isn't.

6---Referring to (Fig. 3-5), trace the line of pleural reflection. What is its significance?

7---Referring to page 22 outline the basal border of the lung, and by palpating the edge of the back muscles visualize the area of lung available for auscultation.

8---Referring to Fig. 3-5, determine how much of the heart is not covered by the forelimb. Attempt to put a fingertip on the points of maximum audibility of the heart valves to realize how far under the triceps a stethoscope has to be pushed.

3

ABDOMEN

Purpose and Plan of the Dissection

1---To see the extent of the abdominal muscles and their aponeuroses and the distribution of the lumbar nerves (optional), and to note the position of the subiliac lymph nodes.

2---To learn the normal position of the abdominal organs, taking into account that the intestines especially can move.

3---To appreciate which abdominal organs lie within the thoracic cage (and are inaccessible) and which portions of these are, in addition, covered by the lungs.

4---To learn which abdominal organs are attached to the abdominal wall and are thus restricted in their movements, and which portions of others lie relatively free and can change their position.

5---To study the disposition of the greater omentum (optional) and to see the epiploic foramen.

6---To understand the complex arrangement of the large intestine and to appreciate its bulk and how much of the available space it occupies.

7---To see the arteries that supply the intestines and the disfigured (parasitized) cranial mesenteric artery from which they arise.

8---To learn that only a small portion of the abdominal cavity and its contents are within reach in rectal palpation

Plan. After the reflection of the abdominal muscles in the flank the abdominal cavity is opened and most of the diaphragm is removed to permit study of the abdominal organs in situ. The liver, small intestine, small colon, cecum and large colon, and kidneys are removed in succession to be studied on the table. The thorax is removed by

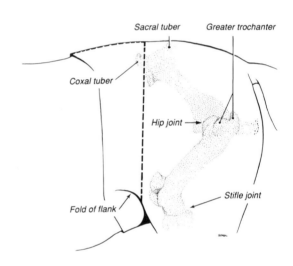

FIGURE 3-1. Skin incisions on the flank.

transecting the back at the level of the last rib; the specimen then consists of pelvis and hindlimbs, suspended by only one hoist. Then follows study of ovaries, uterine tubes, uterine horns, and tissues that suspend them, and the peritoneal pouches that separate rectum, reproductive tract, and bladder in the pelvic cavity.

Flank, Abdominal Muscles, and Lumbar Nerves

Palpate the coxal tuber and the large stifle joint ventral to it. Just cranial to the stifle is the **fold of the flank** (Fig. 3-1) which contains the folded-over cutaneus trunci to be seen shortly.

Continue the dorsal midline incision to the transverse plane of the coxal tuber. Make a

32

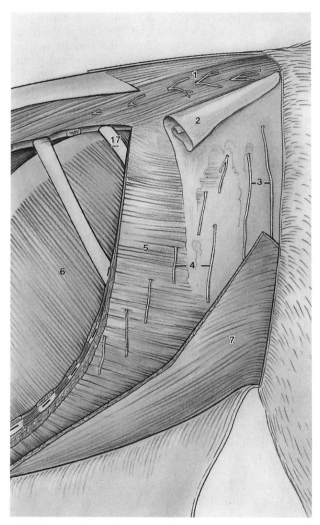

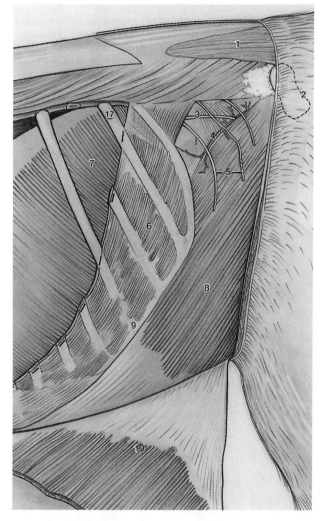

1. Dorsal cutaneous branches
2. Thoracolumbar fascia, reflected off the longissimus muscle
3. Lateral cutaneous branches L1 and L2
4. Lateral cutaneous branches

    T17 and T18
5. External abdominal oblique muscle
6. Diaphragm
7. Cutaneus trunci

FIGURE 3-2. Flank with skin and most of the cutaneus trunci reflected; left lateral view. The underlined number marks a rib.

1. Most cranial extent of gluteus medius
2. Position of coxal tuber
3. Ventral branch of T18
4. One of the cranial branches of the deep circumflex iliac artery supplying the flank
5. Lateral cutaneous branches

    T18 and L1
6. Internal intercostal muscle
7. Diaphragm
8. Internal abdominal oblique
9. Costal arch
10. External abdominal oblique, reflected

FIGURE 3-3 Flank. The external abdominal oblique has been reflected to expose the internal oblique; left lateral view. The underlined number marks a rib.

transverse skin incision over the tuber to the caudal end of the flank fold and then to within 20 cm of the ventral midline. Reflect this and the large, previous skin flap ventrally off the abdominal wall. Preserve the superficial nerves. Note that the **cutaneus trunci** is present only for a short distance dorsal to the flank fold. *Reflect it with the skin.*

Incise the thoracolumbar fascia a few cm lateral to the dorsal midline and reflect it ventrally to the lateral edge of the longissimus muscle where the fascia should be cut off and discarded. The **CUTANEOUS NERVES OF THE LUMBAR REGION AND FLANK** are now exposed. Their stumps are easily found; tracing them any distance is difficult.

The *dorsal cutaneous branches* of the last thoracic and the lumbar nerves emerge through the longissimus and ramify over the back and over the dorsal portion of the flank (Fig. 3-2/1).

The *lateral cutaneous branches* emerge through the external abdominal oblique muscle which the recent skin reflection partially exposed. That from L2 emerges about 6 cm cranioventral to the coxal tuber and passes ventrally. Find its stump in the superficial fascia. That from L1 appears about 6 cm cranioventral to the previous nerve and follows a similar course. The lateral cutaneous branch of T18 emerges through the external oblique just caudal to the costochondral junction of the 18th rib (palpate). These branches thus appear on an oblique line from the coxal tuber to the costal arch. The remaining lateral cutaneous branches (T17, T16, and so forth) emerge close to their respective costochondral junctions (Fig. 3-2/3,4). Note that there are often two lateral cutaneous nerves per spinal nerve.

The ventral cutaneous branches shown in Fig. 1-6/e emerge near the ventral midline and need not be exposed.

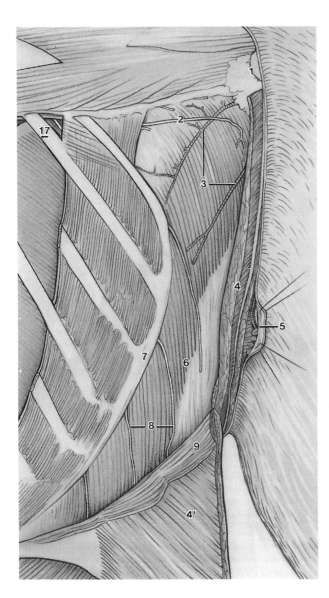

1. Coxal tuber
2. Ventral branch of T18
3. Cranial branches of the deep circumflex iliac artery
4. Internal abdominal oblique, reflected at 4'
5. Skin reflected to expose caudal branch of the deep circumflex iliac artery, lateral cutaneous femoral

nerve, and the subiliac lymph nodes
6. Transversus abdominis
7. Costal arch
8. Ventral branches of T15 and T16
9. Lateral edge of rectus abdominis reflected with internal oblique

FIGURE 3-4. Flank. The internal abdominal oblique has been reflected to expose the transversus abdominis; left lateral view. The underlined number marks a rib.

Much of the **external abdominal oblique** muscle is exposed (Fig. 3-2/5). It arises from the lateral surface of the ribs and the thoracolumbar fascia along a curved line from the triceps to the 18th rib. It is inserted directly on the coxal tuber and, by means of an extensive aponeurosis, on the linea alba (abdominal tendon), and on the prepubic tendon and the iliac fascia (pelvic tendon). Do not attempt to work out these insertions now. The musculoaponeurotic junction forms a curve, parallel to the curved line of origin, from the coxal tuber to the ventral end of the 5th rib.

The external oblique is covered by the thick, yellow elastic **abdominal tunic** (tunica flava abdominis). This strong, modified deep fascia assists the abdominal muscles in supporting the heavy viscera.

Detach the external oblique at its lumbar origin and from the last two or three ribs and bluntly dissect ventrally between external and internal oblique muscles. Remove fat and identify the dorsal border of the internal oblique. The nerves crossing this border are lateral cutaneous branches of T18 - L2 that pierce the external oblique to reach the skin (Fig. 1-6/d).

Palpate the **subiliac lymph nodes** on the cranial edge of the tensor fasciae latae dorsal to the stifle. They drain the superficial parts of hip, thigh, and flank, and send efferents to the lateral iliac lymph nodes within the abdomen. The **lateral cutaneous femoral nerve**, formed by the ventral branches of L3 and L4, lies deep to the nodes. It is accompanied by the **caudal branch of the deep circumflex iliac artery** (Fig. 3-4/5).

Make a transverse incision 2 cm cranial to the corresponding skin incision through the aponeurosis of the external oblique from the tuber coxae to the stifle. Reflect the external oblique ventrally, cutting it from the lateral surfaces of the ribs and pulling through it the lateral cutaneous branches of T18-L2.

Examine the **internal abdominal oblique**. It lies deep to the external oblique with its fibers coursing cranioventrally from the tuber coxae and dorsal part of the pelvic tendon of the external oblique aponeurosis (inguinal ligament). The muscle inserts on the last rib and preceding costal cartilages (Fig. 3-3/8). The aponeurosis of the internal oblique fuses with that of the external oblique to form the external lamina of the **rectus sheath** which ends at the linea alba and caudally on the prepubic tendon. Reflect the internal oblique in the same manner as the external, severing its origin at the coxal tuber.

The **transversus abdominis** is now exposed. On its surface course the ventral branches of the last few thoracic nerves and of L1 and L2. Only the thoracic nerves are visible; the lumbar nerves are hidden by the muscles of the thigh (Fig. 3-4/6). The large vessels encountered in the reflection of the internal oblique and on the surface of the transversus belong to the **cranial branch of the deep circumflex iliac.**

Replace all the muscles and determine the lines of transition between the muscular and aponeurotic parts. It is *important to know* what structures are encountered by a surgical incision at any given point.

> The musculoaponeurotic junction of the external abdominal oblique muscle is known also as the "heave line". It is greatly exaggerated in subjects showing marked expiratory abdominal breathing (heaves).
>
> The abdominal tunic that adheres to the superficial surface of the external abdominal oblique muscle needs to be carefully sutured in the closure of abdominal surgical incisions.

Abdominal Topography

Free the transversus abdominis from the ends of the lumbar transverse processes; incise it along the last rib and the caudal transverse incision and reflect it ventrally to the reflected internal and external oblique muscles. The peritoneum may have been reflected with the transversus. If not, incise and reflect it as you did the muscles. Fat horses have a layer of fat between peritoneum and transversus; remove it. Remove also the remaining intercostal tissues and the diaphragm from the intercostal spaces, and remove the ventral ends of ribs 9-14 and 16, cutting them at their costochondral junctions so that only the costal arch remains.

Remove the rest of the diaphragm, preserving a 10 cm wide median strip containing the esophagus and the caudal vena cava (Fig. 3-10). Palpate the right and left **triangular ligaments of the liver** and preserve them. The right ligament closely attaches the right lobe of the liver to the costal part of the diaphragm. The left attaches the left lobe to the tendinous center of the diaphragm. Also, palpate and preserve the gastrophrenic ligament attaching the dorsal part of the greater curvature of the stomach to the crura of the diaphragm.

The abdominal viscera will be studied primarily from a *topographic* viewpoint. It is important, therefore, that all students in the group participate in studying the abdominal organs on both sides *before* their step-by-step removal to examine them on the table. The topographic relationships that are of importance in surgery and diagnosis will be emphasized. Remember that there are several diagnostic approaches to the abdomen:

1. Palpation, percussion, and auscultation of the lateral and ventral abdominal walls
2. Palpation per rectum
3. Exploratory celiotomy
4. Abdominocentesis
5. Radiography
6. Ultrasonography
7. Endoscopy.

The **spleen** is located in close relation to the greater curvature of the stomach. It curves obliquely cranioventrally from its base under the last three or four ribs to the blunt apex at the ventral third of the ninth to twelfth intercostal spaces. The spleen in your specimen may not conform to this position; it may lie more ventrally due to the general sagging of the viscera or it may be greatly enlarged (splenomegaly) that occurs with anesthesia when barbiturates are part of it.

Pull the base of the spleen cranially. The **left kidney**, imbedded in a mass of retroperitoneal fat (adipose capsule), lies ventral to the last rib and the first two or three lumbar transverse processes. It is more caudally placed than the right kidney and is palpable per rectum (Fig. 3-20/10).

Palpate the dorsal attachment of the spleen. It fixes the base of the spleen to the left kidney (renosplenic lig.) and to the left crus of the diaphragm (phrenicosplenic lig.). The **gastrosplenic ligament** passes from the hilus of the spleen to the greater curvature of the stomach. It blends with the other splenic ligaments dorsally and is continuous with the greater omentum ventrally.

On the right the **liver** extends from the level of the seventh or eighth rib to contact the **right kidney** which is ventral to the last two or three ribs and the first lumbar transverse process. (Do not disturb organ relationships by searching too vigorously for the kidney. It may have sagged slightly cranioventrally with the rest of the viscera). Most of the liver lies to the right of the median plane; only the left lobe lies cranial to the stomach and spleen on the left side. (Figs. 3-6 and 3-7). Relate the marks you made on the ribs for the basal border of the lung to the liver to establish how much of it is covered by the lungs.

Palpate the **coronary ligament** of the liver by passing your fingers medially between the remnant of the diaphragm and the liver. Where your fingers are stopped, the visceral peritoneum of the liver is continuous with the parietal peritoneum of the diaphragm. This reflection is the coronary ligament; it is present on each side of the caudal vena cava, and ventral to the vein it releases the falciform ligament (Fig. 3-10/6). On each side the coronary ligament can be traced dorsally to the **right and left triangular ligaments**

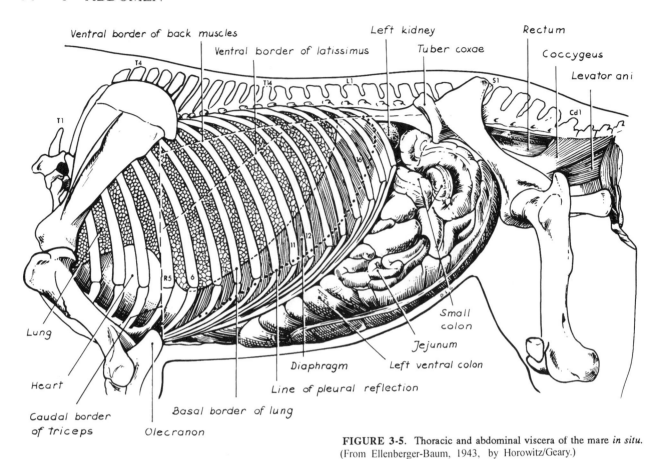

FIGURE 3-5. Thoracic and abdominal viscera of the mare *in situ.* (From Ellenberger-Baum, 1943, by Horowitz/Geary.)

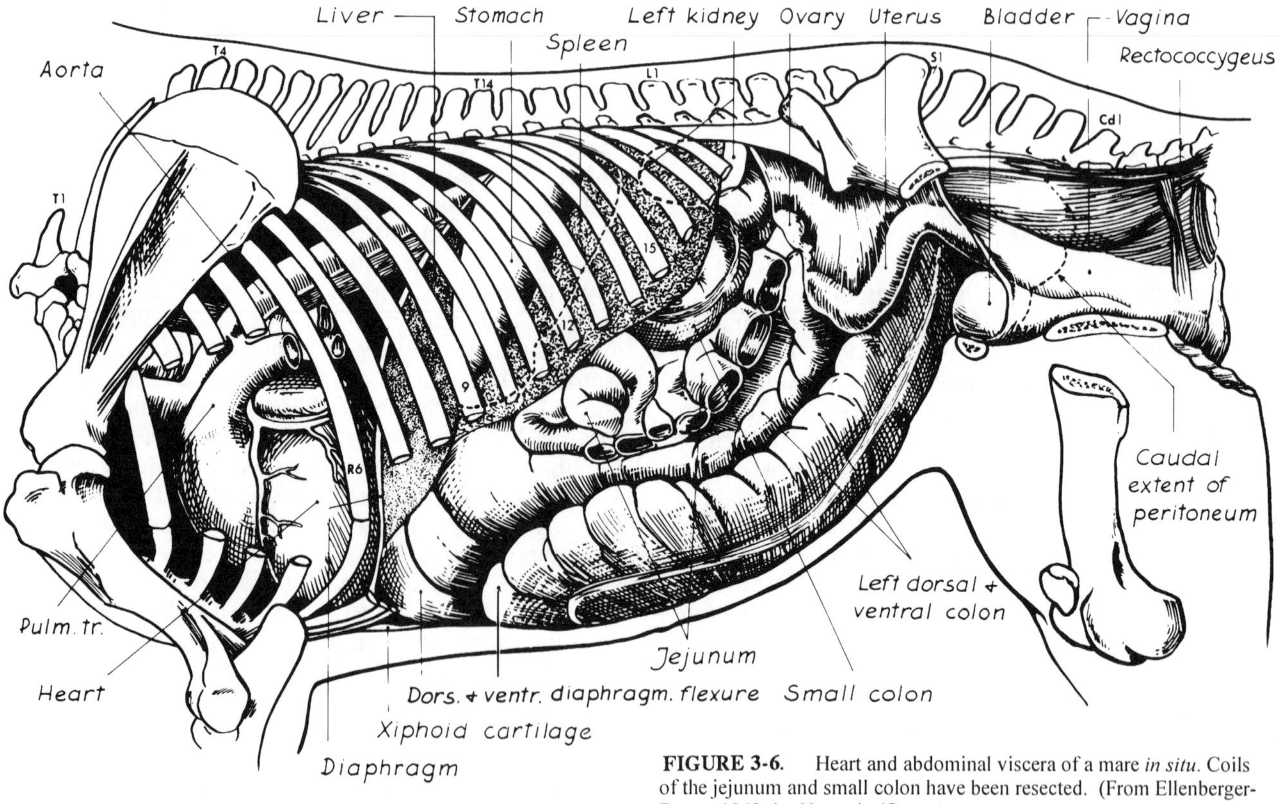

FIGURE 3-6. Heart and abdominal viscera of a mare *in situ.* Coils of the jejunum and small colon have been resected. (From Ellenberger-Baum, 1943, by Horowitz/Geary.)

that are more easily demonstrated and attach the liver to the diaphragm at more lateral levels. The **falciform ligament**, a remnant of the fetal ventral mesentery, runs from the umbilical fissure (of the liver) to the umbilicus. In its free margin is the **round ligament** of the liver, the vestige of the fetal umbilical vein.

Knowing the **normal position of the liver** is important for determining whether it is enlarged or to perform a biopsy. The following facts have to be kept in mind:

1. The liver does not reach the ventral abdominal wall at any point.
2. In the normal adult the liver is entirely within the thoracic cage (Fig. 3-7)
3. In the foal the liver is larger relative to body size than in the adult. Therefore, the liver may extend beyond the costal arch.
4. The lung overlies the liver on both sides of the body.
5. Ultrasonography of the liver is a practical technique that can yield information on the overall size of the organ, the parenchymal texture, and the appearance of blood vessels. The bulk of the normal adult liver is on the right side from the 7th to the 15th intercostal spaces.

The **descending duodenum** can be seen emerging from under the right lobe of the liver and passing caudodorsally suspended by a short **mesoduodenum**. Raise the liver and follow the duodenum and mesoduodenum cranially (Fig. 3-8/5,5'). The **epiploic foramen**, a dorsoventrally compressed slit, is located on the visceral surface of the liver above the porta. Insert only one finger, as the cranial and caudal boundaries are easily torn and unnecessarily enlarge the foramen. The dorsal border of the foramen is formed by the caudate process of the liver and, closer to the median plane, by the caudal vena cava. The ventral border is formed by the right lobe of the pancreas and, again more medially, by the portal vein (Fig. 3-11/arrow). Now raise the more cranial part of the liver and palpate the lesser omentum running from the visceral surface of the liver to the lesser curvature of the stomach and to the cranial part of the duodenum. The caudal part of the lesser omentum is the hepatoduodenal ligament; it forms the cranial border of the epiploic foramen.

It happens sometimes that a loop of jejunum herniates through the epiploic foramen—in either direction. If from

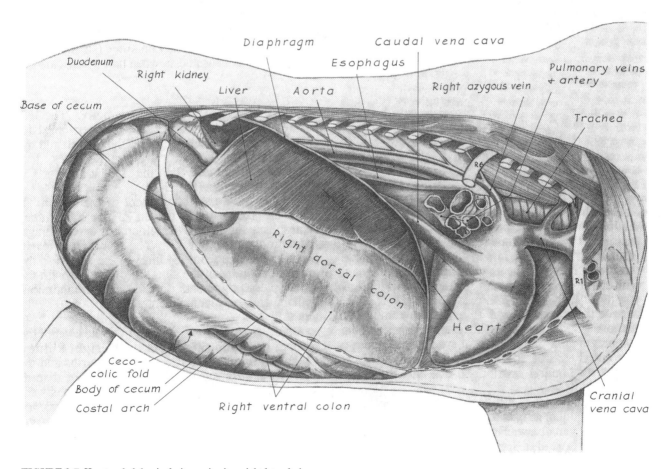

FIGURE 3-7. Heart and abdominal viscera *in situ;* right lateral view. (From Ellenberger-Baum, 1943, by Horowitz/Geary.)

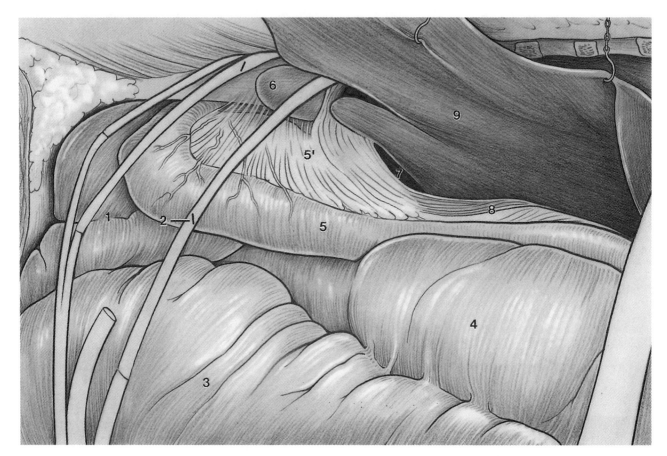

1. Base of cecum
2. Previous mark on the 15th rib to indicate line of pleural reflection
3. Right ventral colon
4. Right dorsal colon
5. Descending duodenum (mesoduodenum at 5')
6. Right kidney
7. Epiploic foramen
8. Hepatoduodenal ligament
9. Right lobe of liver, reflected dorsally

FIGURE 3-8. Epiploic foramen exposed by the dorsal reflection of the liver.

medial to lateral, the loop must tear the greater omentum or push it ahead of itself. If from lateral to medial, the loop has farther to travel; it passes cranially ventral to the stomach, then dorsally and to the right between stomach and liver along the lesser omentum, and enters the foramen to end up within the omental bursa.

At this point a brief **DESCRIPTION OF THE INTESTINAL ARRANGEMENT** of the horse may prove helpful in the dissection to follow: The **duodenum** arises from the stomach and passes caudally on the right of the root of the mesentery. Then, after climbing over the top of the base of the cecum (which occupies the right flank), it curves from the right to left caudal to the mesentery and passes cranially on the left side of the mesentery to become the jejunum ventral to the left kidney. The **jejunum** lies in numerous coils on the left side of the abdomen, finally ending as the **ileum**, which passes from left to right caudal to the root of the mesentery and ventral to the duodenum to enter the base of the **cecum** at its lesser curvature. The right ventral colon, the first part of the **ascending colon**, arises from the lesser

cecal curvature lateral to the ileocecal junction and, after a complex turn to be seen later, passes cranioventrally. At the diaphragm, it turns to the left to become the left ventral colon which passes caudodorsally to the pelvic inlet. Here the left ventral colon flexes upon itself, forming the left dorsal colon. The latter returns to the diaphragm and turns to the right to form the very large right dorsal colon. This is continued by the **transverse colon** that passes from the right to left cranial to the root of the mesentery. (The relationship of the duodenum, ileum, and transverse colon to the root of the mesentery and the cranial mesenteric artery is a constant one in the domestic mammals and is the result of an embryological twist of the developing intestinal loop; Fig. 3-9.) The long **descending colon** arises form the transverse colon and becomes the **rectum** at the pelvic inlet. Unfortunately, the intestines cannot be studied and removed in the same sequence.

The **CECUM** has the shape of a printed comma when "seen" from the left side of the animal; it consists of base, body, and apex (Fig. 3-16). The base of the cecum lies at the pelvic inlet to the right of the median plane and against the paralumbar fossa. In preserved subjects it unfortunately is collapsed. The gas that lies dorsal to the ingesta in the intact animal expands after death and has to be released, deflating the organ.

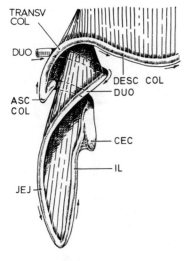

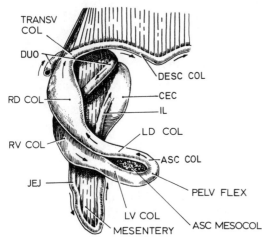

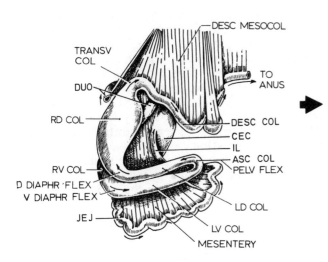

Dorsally, the base of the cecum is attached to the ventral surface of the right kidney, pancreas, and liver (Fig. 3-7). The **body** of the cecum extends obliquely cranioventrally toward the diaphragm. The blind **apex** usually lies a short distance caudal to the xiphoid cartilage. Verify the position of the apex by passing the hand under the large mass of the right dorsal and ventral colon.

To locate the **cranial mesenteric artery**: Incise the peritoneum between the descending duodenum and the right kidney. Dissect bluntly with the fingers through the areolar tissue attaching the base of the cecum to the ventral surface of the right kidney. This exposes: ventrally—the **portal vein** passing over the dorsal surface of the pancreas; dorsally—the **caudal vena cava**; medially—the **root of the mesentery** (Fig. 3-11). Palpate the root of the mesentery which lies ventral to the first lumbar vertebra. The hard, rough cord in the mesentery is the cranial mesenteric artery intimately covered by the combined celiac and cranial mesenteric ganglia and nerve plexus. (Fig. 3-15/6). Palpate the origin of the artery from the aorta and expose its most proximal 2-3 cm for a later transection. Palpate now also the celiac artery which arises from the aorta a short distance cranial to the cranial mesenteric and immediately trifurcates (Fig. 3-16/inset/14).

Ascending and transverse **COLON** of the horse are usually referred to as the **large colon**, the descending as the **small colon**.

The **right ventral colon** arises from the lesser curvature of the base of the cecum opposite the last rib. It makes a tight turn with a dorsocaudal convexity (to be seen later) and then passes cranially on the ventral body wall to the diaphragm. It is closely attached to and usually covered by the larger right dorsal colon. At the diaphragm the right ventral colon bends upon

FIGURE 3-9. Three stages in the development of the equine intestinal tract; left lateral view. Cranial is to the left. The arrows indicate the direction from stomach to anus. (After Horowitz, 1965; drawn by D.S. Geary.)

Top: The clockwise rotation (in dorsal view) of the original loop has already occurred. The cecum begins to enlarge, and the ascending colon forms a loop of its own that grows ventrally and to the left, cranial to the root of the mesentery.

Middle: The cecum is relatively large and its apex grows cranially on the right side of the mesentery. The loop of ascending colon has elongated and been deflected to the left side and caudally by the diaphragm.

Bottom: The loop of the ascending colon bends on itself forming dorsal and ventral diaphragmatic flexures. The left parts of the loop lie on the left side, the right parts on the right side of the mesentery. The descending (small) colon increases in length.

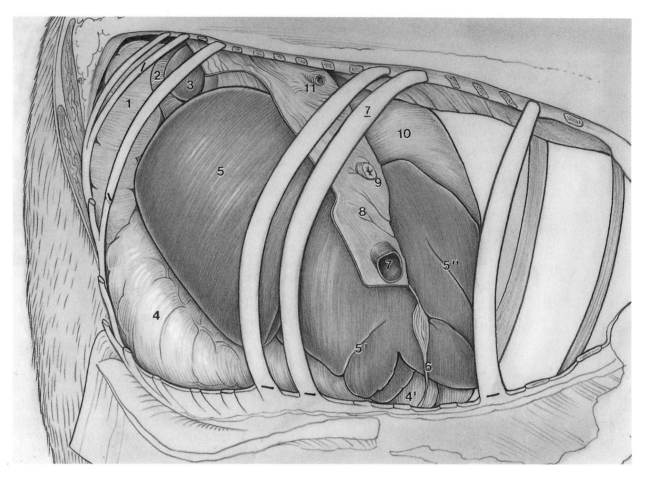

1. Base of cecum
2. Descending duodenum
3. Right kidney
4. Right ventral colon (dorsal diaphragmatic flexure at 4')
5. Right lobe of liver (quadrate lobe at 5' left lobe at 5")
6. Falciform ligament
7. Caudal vena cava
8. Strip of diaphragm
9. Esophagus
10. Stomach
11. Aorta

FIGURE 3-10. Abdominal viscera after the removal of the diaphragm; right craniolateral view. The underlined number marks a rib.

itself, forming the **ventral diaphragmatic** (sternal) **flexure,** to become the **left ventral colon.** Follow the left ventral colon caudally into the pelvic inlet. Raise the coils of small intestine and small colon in the left flank and locate the left ventral colon turning upon itself at the **pelvic flexure** to form the left dorsal colon (Figs. 3-5 and 3-6). Notice particularly that the pelvic flexure usually extends over to the right side.

> You will see later that the left dorsal and ventral colon lie entirely free on the abdominal floor and thus can shift from the position in which they are normally found. They have been seen incarcerated in the narrow space between the dorsal end of the spleen and the left kidney, a condition known as *dorsal displacement of the left colon* or *nephrosplenic entrapment.*. This mobility allows the ascending colon also to twist around its longitudinal axis, which causes a severe, usually fatal, *colic.*

Trace the **left dorsal colon** to the diaphragm. Here it turns upon itself, forming the dorsal diaphragmatic flexure, to become the very large right dorsal colon. The **dorsal diaphragmatic**

flexure usually is in contact with the ventral body wall and the xiphoid cartilage cranial to the ventral diaphragmatic flexure (Fig. 3-11/3',4').

Trace the **right dorsal colon** by palpation as it passes first caudally and then caudomedially ventral to the duodenum. It rapidly narrows as it reaches the base of the cecum, turns medially, and crosses from right to left cranial to the root of the mesentery and the cranial mesenteric artery as the **transverse colon.** This diminution in size make the right dorsal colon particularly susceptible to impaction. Ventral to the left kidney the transverse colon is continued by the small colon. The **small colon** can be readily differentiated from the small intestine by its sacculations and longitudinal **bands** (teniae). The small colon and jejunum are intermingled in the dorsal half of the left side from the stomach to the pelvic inlet (Fig. 3-5).

By lifting the spleen and stomach and at the same time applying traction to the right dorsal colon and the small colon, the **transverse colon**

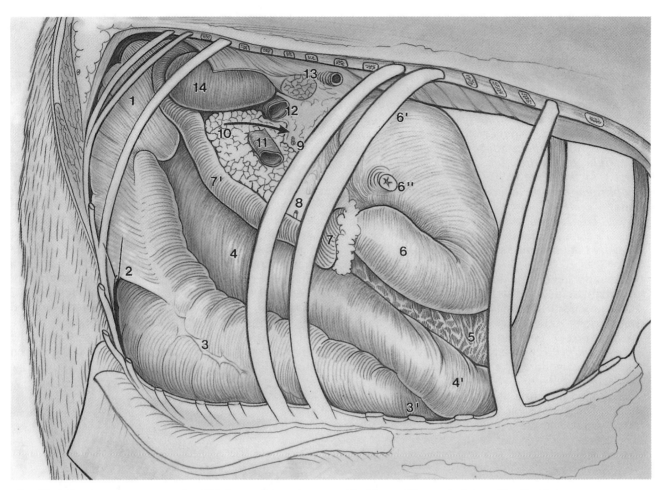

1.	Base of cecum	6.	Pyloric part of stomach (fundus at 6' esophagus at 6")	10.	Pancreas (the arrow points through the epiploic foramen)
2.	Cecocolic fold, elevated			11.	Portal vein
3.	Right ventral colon (ventral diaphragmatic flexure at 3')				
4.	Right dorsal colon (dorsal-diaphragmatic flexure at 4')	7.	Cranial part of duodenum (descending part at 7')		
5.	Greater omentum	8.	Bile duct		
		9.	Hepatic artery		

12. Caudal vena cava
13. Crus of diaphragm and aorta
14. Right kidney

FIGURE 3-11. Abdominal viscera after the removal of the diaphragm and liver; right craniolateral view.

can be demonstrated. It is fixed in position.

The large intestine of the horse evolved from the same primitive pattern seen in the dog. The entire large colon is a loop produced by elongation of the primitive ascending colon (Fig. 3-9). The loops of the small colon are produced by elongation of the primitive descending colon. If the small colon were shortened and straightened, and the right ventral colon were anastomosed with the transverse colon, the simple pattern would be restored.

Colic (pain in the abdomen) is a common and often fatal disease of horses that has many causes. One is obstruction to the flow of ingesta in the jejunum. The wide and long mesentery gives the jejunum much range, and this freedom of movement permits "intestinal accidents" to occur, such as twisting on itself or incarceration of a segment through a rent in the mesentery or in a natural opening such as the epiploic foramen or the vaginal ring of stallions.

Before the abdominal organs are removed, it is interesting to determine which of them you would reach if you could perform a rectal palpation on your specimen. (Unfortunately, anus and rectum cannot be dilated in embalmed subjects for such a procedure.) Stand behind your horse and hold your arm against the lateral surface of the pelvis so that the middle of your upper arm is opposite the anus. See how far cranially your fingertips reach in the median plane, how far in the flank (bend your arm at the elbow), and how far ventrally. Or, obtain the large plexiglass calipers from the demonstration tables and measure the distances between the anus and various organs (spleen, kidneys, ovaries, liver, root of mesentery, and so forth) and compare these distances with the distance between the middle of your upper arm and fingertips. Unless you are working on a pony (in which rectals are possible) you will be astonished how little of the abdominal cavity is within range (Fig. 3-20).

To remove the liver: Free the esophagus from the diaphragm and liver. Sever the sternal attachments of the diaphragm and the falciform ligament. Transect and free the left crus of the diaphragm just cranial to the dorsal attachment of the spleen. Separate the diaphragm from the aorta. On the right cut the lesser omentum and mesoduodenum, freeing the liver from the stomach and duodenum. Sever the right triangular ligament and the hepatorenal ligament between the right kidney and the caudate process of the liver. At this level transect the right crus of the diaphragm and the caudal vena cava and dissect bluntly ventrally along the visceral surface of the liver. Transect the portal vein, hepatic artery, and the bile duct as they are encountered. Remove the liver and the attached strip of diaphragm.

5
4
3
R

Identify the organs that were in contact with the **visceral surface of the liver** (Fig. 3-11). Some of them produced impressions on the liver. Find the impressions and correlate them with the organs left in the horse. You should be able to outline the areas where the esophagus, stomach, descending duodenum, right dorsal colon, and right kidney contacted the liver.

Examine the porta on the visceral surface of the liver. The portal vein and branches of the hepatic artery enter, and the bile duct leaves the liver here. There is no gall bladder in the horse. The hepatic lymph nodes surround the structures at the porta.

The fibrous tags seen occasionally on the parietal surface of the right lobe are not adhesions (to the diaphragm) but are possibly of parasitic origin.

Raise the stomach and identify the **greater omentum** attached to the greater curvature of that organ. The attachment then passes along the following organs: pylorus, along the descending duodenum, transverse colon, and about 25 cm along the small colon. Then it returns from the small colon passes to the base of the spleen, and via the hilus of that organ back to the stomach, forming the previously noted *gastrosplenic ligament.* We will trace these attachments when the stomach is being removed.

The **stomach** is located caudal to the diaphragm and liver in the dorsal part of the left half of the abdominal cavity. Its position is variable, depending on the degree of distension and the state of respiration—the stomach moves caudally a distance of one vertebra with each inspiration. Regardless of the amount of movement or distention, however, the stomach is always covered by the ribs and thus is inaccessible except with a nasogastric tube. In acute gastric dilatation the distention of the stomach may displace the spleen toward the pelvic inlet.

5
3
6
R

For the passage of a nasogastric tube it is important to know the position of the cardia (opposite the upper part of the (palpable) 11th rib) so the tube is not advanced any farther after it has entered the stomach.

Palpate the pylorus and note that the **cranial**

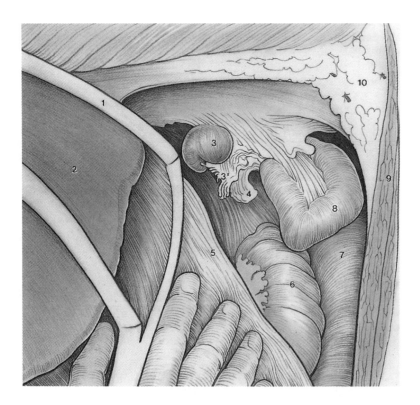

1. Last rib
2. Spleen
3. Left ovary (infundibulum at 3')
4. Epoöphoron
5. Descending mesocolon
6. Small colon
7. Left dorsal colon
8. Uterine horn
9. Cut surfaces of the abdominal muscles
10. Stumps of the branches of the deep circumflex iliac artery

FIGURE 3-12. The left ovary and uterine horn *in situ;* left craniolateral view. The coxal tuber is in the right upper corner.

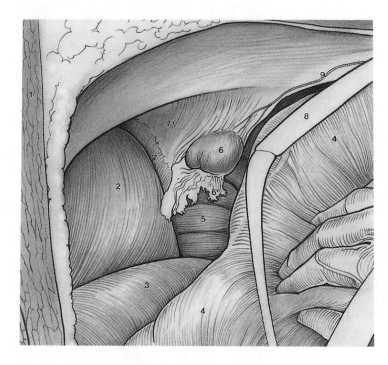

1. Cut surface of internal abdominal oblique muscle
2. Pelvic flexure
3. Jejunum
4. Base of cecum
5. Small colon
6. Right ovary (infundibulum at 6')
7. Uterine horn (broad ligament (mesometrium) at 7')
8. Last rib
9. Un-named artery—not ovarian

FIGURE 3-13. The right ovary and uterine horn *in situ*; right craniolateral view. The coxal tuber is in the left upper corner.

part of the duodenum forms an S-shaped flexure (ansa sigmoidea). The second bend of the S is the cranial flexure of the duodenum at which the descending part begins.

Now on the right locate the **descending duodenum** and follow it caudally and then medially over the top of the base of the cecum and caudal to the root of the mesentery. Here it forms the caudal flexure and continues cranially on the left of the root of the mesentery as the **ascending duodenum**. The caudal flexure (when distended) is palpable per rectum. The ascending duodenum is continuous with the jejunum at the duodenojejunal flexure ventral to the left kidney. Note the **duodenocolic fold** of peritoneum between the ascending duodenum ventrally and the small colon dorsally. The fold has a free caudal border.

Draw the **jejunum** out on the left side, beginning at the duodenojejunal flexure and working distally. The jejunum lies chiefly in the dorsal portion of the left side from the stomach to the pelvis. The last segment of the small intestine, the **ileum**, is usually tightly contracted (and hard to the touch) and is attached by the **ileocecal fold** to the dorsal band of the cecum (Fig. 3-16/9). Follow the ileum from left to right caudal to the root of the mesentery and ventral to the caudal flexure of the duodenum to its junction with the cecum. This junction is to the right of the median plane and at the level of the first or second lumbar vertebra, roughly opposite the middle of the 17th intercostal space.

The left horn of the uterus and the left ovary are visible on the left side dorsal to the mass of small colon (Fig. 3-12/8,3), while the right horn and the right ovary are visible medial to the base of the cecum (Fig. 3-13/7,6). It is important for their (rectal) palpation to remember that, in the live, nonpregnant mare, the ovaries are usually *in contact with the dorsal abdominal wall*. The position of the uterine horns varies depending on the stage of pregnancy and the number of foals carried in the past. Could you reach the ovaries rectally in your horse?

To remove the stomach and spleen: Cut the dorsal attachment of the spleen, the gastrophrenic ligament, and the gastrosplenic ligament which connects the greater curvature of the stomach to the hilus of the spleen.

The **omental bursa** is now open, and the attachment of the **greater omentum** may be followed from the inside of the bursa: along the greater curvature of the stomach to the ventral surface of the pylorus and medial side of the cranial part of the duodenum; then caudally following the descending duodenum; back to the left on the transverse colon, and then for about 25 cm on the small colon. The omentum then makes a sharp cranial turn, leaves the small colon and reaches the base of the spleen, then via the hilus of the spleen back to the greater curvature of the stomach.

Ligate the duodenum twice distal to the cranial flexure and transect between the ligatures. Bluntly free the duodenum and stomach from the pancreas and right dorsal colon. The branches of the celiac artery must be cut. Remove the stomach and spleen.

Separate the stomach from the spleen. Open the **STOMACH** along the greater curvature from the **blind sac** (saccus cecus) through the pylorus and out into the duodenum. The mucous membrane is clearly separated into two parts. White, nonglandular mucosa covered with stratified squamous epithelium lines the blind sac and a part of the body. A raised edge, the **margo plicatus**, separates the nonglandular mucosa from the glandular mucosa of the rest of the stomach. *Gastrophilus intestinalis* larvae (bots) or ulcerations caused by them may be found in the nonglandular and pyloric parts of the stomach. Demonstrate the thick **cardiac sphincter** surrounding the cardiac opening by incising the esophagus into the wall of the stomach. The **pyloric sphincter** has been exposed by the incision along the greater curvature.

Locate the **major duodenal papilla** and probe the openings of the **bile duct** and of the **pancreatic duct**. Probe also the small accessory pancreatic duct which opens on the **minor duodenal papilla** 4-5 cm and almost opposite the major papilla.

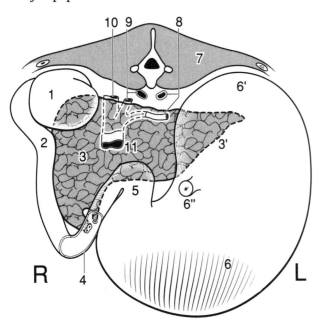

R   4   L

1. Right kidney
2. Descending duodenum
3. Pancreas, right lobe (left lobe at 3')
4. Cranial part of duodenum, opened to show major and minor duodenal papillae
5. Pylorus
6. Stomach (blind sac at 6', esophagus at 6")
7. Transverse section of back at level of T17
8. Splenic vein and aorta
9. Caudal mesenteric vein and caudal vena cava
10. Cranial mesenteric vein
11. Portal vein

FIGURE 3-14. The pancreas *in situ*, the *craniodorsal* surface of the gland faces the reader; schematic; cranial view.

Remember, the stomach, even when distended, lies entirely within the thoracic cage. The thick cardiac sphincter and the acute angle the esophagus forms with the stomach makes it practically impossible for stomach contents and gases to enter the esophagus; this is the reason why horses rarely vomit. The unfortunate inability to relieve a greatly distended stomach can lead to rupture followed by rapid death. *Enteritis* (inflammation of the intestines) may cause swelling and blockage of the orifices of the bile and pancreatic ducts in the duodenum, causing stasis and jaundice.

Return to the horse and note the position of the **pancreas** which is soft and gray and does not show up well in embalmed subjects. Most students have difficulty gaining a perception of its actual position in the body. It is a flat gland with dorsal and ventral surfaces, but positioned obliquely so that the dorsal surface faces dorsocranially and the ventral surface ventrocaudally (Fig. 3-11/10). It extends—high in the abdominal cavity—from the right kidney and descending duodenum on the right, across the median plane, to touch the spleen caudal to the blind sac of the stomach on the left (Fig. 3-14/3).

Separate the duodenum from the right dorsal colon and mesoduodenum to the duodenojejunal flexure. Cut the ileum 10 cm from the cecum. Grasp the root of the mesentery and cut it across. Remove the small intestine en masse and spread it out on the table as if the horse were lying on its right side.

The **jejunal lymph nodes** of the horse are situated near the root of the mesentery as in the dog. Examine the arcades of arteries and veins and the numerous lymphatics in the mesentery.

If your horse is younger than 2 years old, open the intestine at the ileal end and locate the raised **patches of aggregated lymph nodules** (formerly and still commonly called Peyer's patches). They cause the mucosa to take on an irregular, cribriform appearance and are scattered throughout the intestine but are most numerous in the ileum, and are larger in younger animals. (Lymphatic tissue generally tends to atrophy with age.) With some care the mucosa, submucosa, the muscular layer, and serosa may be identified and separated.

Ligate and transect the small colon at the junction with the transverse colon. Draw it out on the left side cutting it free from its mesentery, the descending mesocolon. At the pelvic inlet ligate and transect the small colon again, remove it from the horse, and place it on the table.

Examine the **small colon**. It is sacculated and has two bands, one of which is concealed in the mesocolic attachment. The small colon is the only part of the intestinal tract that contains fecal balls. Many small lymph nodes are scattered along the mesocolic attachment; compare this arrangement

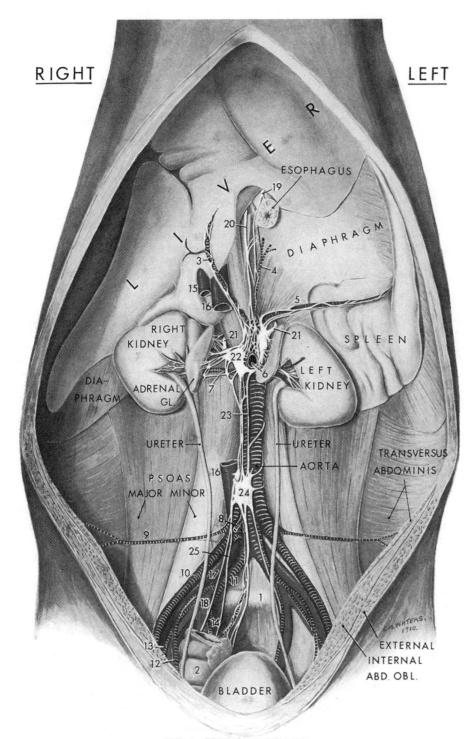

RIGHT   LEFT

ESOPHAGUS

VER
LI
L

DIAPHRAGM

RIGHT KIDNEY

SPLEEN

DIA-PHRAGM

ADRENAL GL.

LEFT KIDNEY

URETER

URETER

AORTA

TRANSVERSUS ABDOMINIS

PSOAS MAJOR MINOR

BLADDER

EXTERNAL INTERNAL ABD. OBL.

1. Sacral promontory
2. Small colon
3. Hepatic artery and plexus
4. Left gastric artery
5. Splenic artery and plexus
6. Cranial mesenteric artery, cut
7. Renal artery
8. Caudal mesenteric artery
9. Deep circumflex iliac artery
10. External iliac artery
11. Internal iliac artery
12. Umbilical artery
13. Internal pudendal artery
14. Obturator artery
15. Portal vein
16. Caudal vena cava
17. External iliac vein
18. Internal iliac vein
19. Ventral vagal trunk
20. Dorsal vagal trunk
21. Greater splanchnic nerves
22. Combined right celiac and cranial mesenteric ganglia
23. Aortic plexus
24. Caudal mesenteric ganglion
25. Hypogastric nerve

FIGURE 3-15. Roof of the abdominal cavity with liver, spleen, and kidneys *in situ*. (From Hopkins, 1937.)

with that seen in the small intestine.

In the horse find the previously exposed and transected cranial mesenteric artery. The **caudal mesenteric artery** is 12-15 cm farther caudally in the descending mesocolon; its branches supply most of the small colon you just removed (Fig. 3-15/8).

The mesenteric arteries are vulnerable to damage by *Strongylus vulgaris* larvae that migrate from the intestine to the aorta in the walls of the arteries supplying the gut. The larvae concentrate at the origin of the intestinal vessels where they damage the arterial wall causing enlargement, bulges, or other irregularities (*verminous arteritis*). Parts of the deformed and irregular intimal surface can break off and be carried downstream where they may block blood vessels and cause patchy necrosis of the bowel wall (thromboembolic colic). Fortunately, good deworming programs are available that control both the larval and adult forms of this parasite.

Locate the area of adhesion between the base of the cecum and the right dorsal colon. Find the

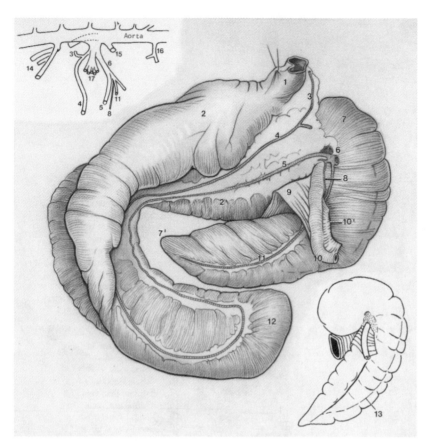

1. Transverse colon, reflected dorsally
2. Right dorsal colon (right ventral colon at 2')
3. Middle colic artery
4. Right colic artery
5. Colic branch of ileocolic artery
6. Stumps of ileocolic artery and vein
7. Base of cecum (apex at 7')
8. Ileal artery
9. Ileocecal fold
10. Ileum (stump of mesentery at 10')
11. Medial cecal artery on medial band
12. Pelvic flexure
13. Ventral band
14. Branches of the celiac artery
15. Left renal artery
16. Caudal mesenteric artery
17. Jejunal arteries

FIGURE 3-16. Cecum and great colon arranged as they are *in situ*. Cranial is to the left, left lateral view. The transverse colon (1) has been reflected dorsally. The lower inset shows the full medial surface of the cecum, and the ventral band (13) joining the medial band. The ventral band was poorly developed in the specimen of the main Figure. The upper inset shows the origin (from the cranial mesenteric artery) of the arteries shown in the main Figure.

 Cran.

cecocolic fold connecting the lateral band of the cecum to the lateral free band of the right ventral colon. Trace out again the course and flexures of the large colon. You should be able to trace the path of ingesta from the stomach to the rectum and to point out the possible sites of impaction.

You will be asked to remove the **cecum** and **large colon**. In the process you will realize that they are attached to the abdominal wall *only* via the kidneys, the cecocolic artery (branch of cranial mesenteric), and via the right and cranial aspects of the root of the mesentery. Thus, most of these large intestinal segments rest on the abdominal floor and, especially those on the left, can shift freely.

Carefully free the cecum and transverse colon from the kidneys and adjacent sublumbar area, cut the cecocolic artery, and remove the remaining intestine en masse. Orient the structures on the table as they were in situ (Fig. 3-16).

The bands and sacculations of the **large intestine** are characteristic of the different parts and are aids in the identification of its parts per rectum, at autopsy, or during surgery:

1. Cecum—sacculated and has four bands.
2. Right and left ventral colon—sacculated and has four bands, the dorsal pair of which is concealed in the ascending mesocolon.
3. Left dorsal colon—no sacculations and has only one band which is concealed in the mesocolic attachment.
4. Right dorsal colon—has two distinct bands and one concealed in the mesocolic attachment.
5. Small colon—sacculated and has two bands, one of which is concealed in the mesocolic attachment.

Examine the **BASE OF THE CECUM**. It is strongly curved forming a dorsal greater curvature and a ventral lesser curvature. The ileum enters, and the right ventral colon leaves the cecum at the lesser curvature roughly opposite the 17th intercostal space. Open the base of the cecum from the lateral side and remove the ingesta. The **ileal papilla**, bearing the **ileal orifice**, is on the medial side of the lesser curvature. Its prominence is caused by the intruding ileal musculature and a submucosal venous plexus. The erectile properties of the plexus and the thick circular muscle of the terminal ileum regulate the flow of ingesta. The **cecocolic orifice** is more lateral and separated from the ileal orifice by a large fold; the orifice faces *caudally* into the narrow initial part of the right ventral colon. This forms a tight bend that nestles in the lesser cecal curvature. The right ventral colon then gains rapidly in diameter and passes cranioventrally toward the diaphragm.

Open the initial part of the right ventral colon and trace the passage of ingesta from the cecocolic orifice caudally, then ventrally, and finally cranioventrally.

The round *blind end* of the base of the cecum lies cranial to these orifices and is directed ventrally. This part of the base is embryologically the first part of the colon. As in other species, the ileocecal junction marks the morphologic division between cecum and colon, but in the horse, the first curvature of the colon appears externally to be a part of the cecum.

Wherever the large intestine is sharply flexed and/or rapidly decreases in diameter there is danger of impaction. Three prominent sites are: the cecocolic junction, the pelvic flexure, and the junction between right dorsal and transverse colon. Impaction of ingesta is also a common cause of colic in the horse.

It is remarkable that as much bulk as 95% of the large colon can be removed surgically without ill effects—not a routine operation, of course.

The large cecum permits up to 4 m(!) of ileum and jejunum to enter its lumen by intussusception (one segment of intestine telescoping into an adjacent segment), yet another cause of colic.

Locate the stump of the **ileocolic artery** on the craniomedial aspect of the cecal base. Trace its branches to the medial and lateral surfaces of the body of the cecum (medial and lateral *cecal arteries*) and to the right ventral colon (*colic branch*; Fig. 3-16/6,11,5). The latter artery runs to the pelvic flexure where it anastomoses with the *right colic artery* (/4) that takes a similar course on the right and left dorsal colon; the origin of the right colic artery from the cranial mesenteric is often destroyed when the jejunum is removed.

The origin of the cranial mesenteric artery, the parent artery of the ileocolic, is enclosed on three sides by the U-shaped mass of the combined right and left **celiac and cranial mesenteric ganglia** which connect caudal to the

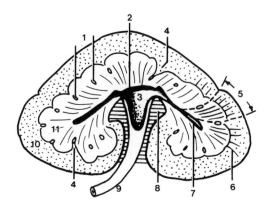

1. Interlobar vessels	7. Terminal recess
2. Renal crest	8. Renal sinus
3. Renal pelvis	9. Ureter
4. Renal column	10. Cortex
5. Renal pyramid	11. Medulla
6. Medullary rays	

FIGURE 3-17. Opened left kidney; the renal artery and vein have been removed; schematic.

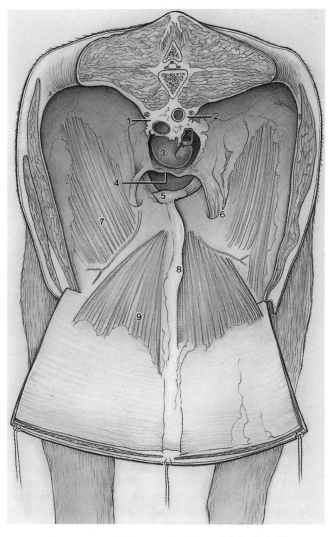

1. Caudal vena cava and right ureter	7. Internal abdominal oblique
2. Aorta and left ureter	8. Median lig. of bladder
3. Rectum	9. Rectus abdominis, cranially
4. Genital fold	covered by fat but visible
5. Empty bladder	again at the cut surface of
6. Vaginal ring	the abdominal floor

FIGURE 3-18. Appearance of specimen after the removal of the thorax; cranial view.

artery (Fig. 3-15/22). Autonomic nerve plexuses from the ganglia accompany the arteries to the intestines. Palpate the ganglia in the horse; the nerve plexuses can only be demonstrated by meticulous dissection.

Kidney, Uterus, Ovary

The **right kidney** is located in the retroperitoneal fat ventral to the last two or three ribs and the first lumbar transverse process (Fig. 3-7). It has a strong peritoneal attachment to the caudate process of the liver (hepatorenal ligament). Incise the peritoneum over the lateral edge of the right kidney and reflect it ventromedially. Expose the

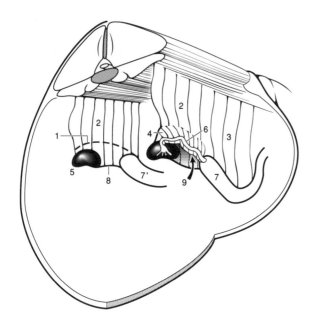

1. Attachment of mesosalpinx
2. Mesovarium
3. Mesometrium
4. Mesosalpinx, arising from the *lateral* surface of the mesovarium
5. Ovary
6. Uterine tube
7, 7' Left and right uterine horns
8. Proper ligament of ovary
9. Arrow into ovarian bursa

FIGURE 3-19. The suspension of the reproductive organs in the caudal part of the abdominal cavity; craniolateral view; schematic.

hilus of the kidney by blunt dissection in the perineal fat. Locate the renal artery and vein. Trace the **ureter** medial to the caudal extremity (pole) of the kidney; cut it and tag the distal end. Several small renal lymph nodes are scattered in the hilar region. The **right adrenal gland** lies on the medial surface of the cranial extremity (Fig. 3-15).

The **left kidney** is more elongate than the right, placed closer to the median plane and is relatively loosely attached. It is located ventral to the last rib and the first two or three lumbar transverse processes. Expose the hilus, vessels, and renal lymph nodes as was done on the right. Trace the **ureter** medial to the caudal extremity; cut and tag. The **left adrenal gland** lies between the medial surface of the cranial extremity and the cranial mesenteric artery.

Remove the kidney and, with a large knife, cut through hilus and poles, dividing it into dorsal and ventral halves as in Fig. 3-17; do not use your scalpel for this.

STRUCTURE OF THE KIDNEY. Find the small **renal pelvis** in the center of the opened kidney (Fig. 3-17/3). Urine produced in this area enters the renal pelvis through tiny foramina in the equally small **renal crest**. Urine from the poles enters tubular extensions (**terminal recesses** /7) of

the renal pelvis. Because the recesses lack walls, they are difficult to find. The renal pelvis is the dilated origin of the ureter and contains numerous mucus-secreting glands and goblet cells which contribute to the peculiar, viscid character of horse urine. The renal pelvis, artery and vein lie, imbedded in fat, within the renal sinus (/8). Note the striated appearance (collecting ducts) of the medulla and the granular look (renal corpuscles) of the cortex. Strip the **capsule** from the kidney. Generally, the capsule of a healthy kidney strips easily because it does not adhere to the parenchyma.

Section the **adrenal gland** and examine its capsule, cortex, medulla, and medullary veins.

To remove the thorax: With a large knife cut along the costal arch toward the xiphoid cartilage, separating the abdominal wall from the thorax. Saw through the back muscles and vertebral column just caudal to the last rib so that the cut is completed about 15 cm, i.e., about 6 inches, cranial to the coxal tuber. Divide the detached thorax into two manageable pieces by cutting all ribs at about their middle, and discard it. With a large knife cut the abdominal wall transversely, 25 cm—about 10 inches—cranial to the umbilicus. Trim the sides of the remaining abdominal wall so that your specimen looks like Fig. 3-18. Loop three pieces of string through holes cut into the skin as shown in the same Figure. The pelvic cavity dries out quickly and should be carefully covered with moist cloth, and the flap of abdominal wall tied up to the loin and to the hook to close the front end of the specimen at the end of the laboratory period.

Examine the cut surface of the ventral abdominal wall. Right and left **rectus abdominis** muscles are joined at the midline by the tough, white fibrous **linea alba**. The **internal lamina of the rectus sheath** is formed by the aponeurosis of the transversus abdominis, and caudal to the aponeurosis, by the transverse fascia. The **external lamina of the rectus sheath** is formed by the fused aponeuroses of the internal and external oblique muscles.

In the following dissection particular attention should be paid to the structures encountered in rectal palpation.

The **broad ligaments** are the "mesenteries" of the female reproductive tract. They contain a large amount of smooth muscle and are given different names according to the portion of the tract they suspend:

1. **Mesometrium**—suspends the body and horns of the uterus.
2. **Mesosalpinx**—suspends the uterine tubes.
3. **Mesovarium**—suspends the ovary (Fig. 3-19).

Generally speaking, the **OVARIES** are located midway between the last rib and the coxal tuber and a few cm lateral to the median plane. They are about 50 cm from the anus. (Measure 50 cm (20 inches) on your arm to see that they are within easy reach.) The ovaries are attached to the sublumbar region by the **mesovarium** which ends in a free border cranially and is continuous caudally with the mesosalpinx and mesometrium. The free cranial border of the mesovarium is homologous to the suspensory ligament you have seen in the dog. The **ovarian bursa**, wide open ventrally, lies mainly caudal to the ovary. The **proper ligament of the ovary** (/8)is medial to the opening of the bursa, running in the free edge of the broad ligament from the uterine end of the ovary to the cranial end of the uterine horn. The **mesosalpinx** (/4) forms the *lateral* wall of the bursa. The **uterine tube** is flexuous and has a length of about 20 cm. It extends in the mesosalpinx from the tip of the uterine horn to the tubal end of the ovary where it terminates as the fimbriated **infundibulum**. Notice that the infundibulum turns back and overlaps the ventral surface of the ovary. By gentle palpation through the infundibulum the concave **ovulation fossa** of the ovary may be identified. The ovulation fossa develops as the animal matures because the tubal and uterine ends grow faster than the middle of the ovary. The fossa is peculiar to the mare and ovulation invariably occurs through it. The ovarian and uterine arteries may be seen and palpated in the broad ligament. They will be traced in detail later.

Cystic structures of varying sizes are routinely found in the mesovarium close to the ovary (epoöphoron, paroöphoron). They are normal embryonic remnants and without pathological significance. In older mares grape-like clusters of cysts may also occlude the ovulation fossa.

The kidney-shaped ovaries are relatively large (about 7 cm long; Figs. 3-12/3 and 3-13/6). Normal follicles often reach a diameter equal to that of the ovary itself. The corpora lutea are deeply imbedded in the ovary, not projecting from the surface as in the cow and sow.

The horns of the **uterus** are about 25 cm long and diverge at right angles from an equally long body. The gravid uterus usually lies on the ventral abdominal wall to the left of the median plane. The lateral surface of the broad ligament gives off the round ligament of the uterus, which has a blunt pendulous tip and can be traced to the vicinity of the deep inguinal ring.

Ultrasound examination for pregnancy diagnosis is commonly used for early detection of the amniotic vesicle and embryo. It is a particularly useful technique for detecting the presence of twin embryos at an early stage when the condition can be readily managed. Twinning is considered undesirable in the mare because twin foals are often born stunted or weak.

The more caudal portions of the pelvic viscera are retroperitoneal. The reflections of the peritoneum from the pelvic walls on these organs and from one organ to another form pouches or excavations of clinical importance.

The **retrogenital pouch** is the space between the rectum and reproductive organs. The portions of the pouch on each side of the rectum and mesorectum and the **pararectal fossae**. In the female the pouch is bounded ventrally by the vagina (near the junction with the uterus) and laterally by the broad ligaments. In the male the

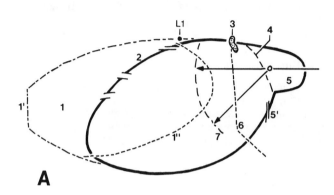

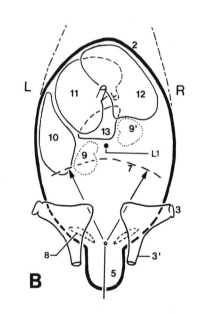

FIGURE 3-20. Abdominal and pelvic cavities in left lateral (A) and dorsal (B) outline. The dorsal outline (B) encloses a ring of the relatively fixed organs (9,10,11,12,9') with the pancreas (13) in the center.

1. Thoracic cavity, inlet at 1', costal arch at 1"
2. Diaphragm
3. Coxal tuber, shaft of ilium at 3'
4. Terminal line
5. Pelvic cavity, inguinal canal at 5'
6. Thigh and stifle
7. Approximate range in rectal palpation in the median plane (A) and directly ventral to the kidneys (B)
8. Deep inguinal ring
9. Left kidney, right kidney at 9'
10. Spleen
11. Stomach
12. Liver
13. Pancreas

uterus and vagina are replaced by the **genital fold** containing the ends of the deferent ducts, the cranial ends of the vesicular gland, the ureters, and the vestigial uterus masculinus (to be seen later). The genital fold, the homologue of the broad ligament, is continued cranioventrolaterally on each side as the narrow mesoductus deferens and enters the inguinal canal with the deferent duct.

The **vesicogenital pouch** lies between the uterus and vagina (or genital fold) dorsally, the bladder ventrally and the **lateral ligaments of the bladder** laterally. In the free edge of each lateral ligament is the **round ligament of the bladder**, a remnant of the fetal umbilical artery.

The **pubovesical pouch** lies between the bladder and the pubis and is divided into two halves by the **median ligament of the bladder**.

These pouches may be collapsed or contain loops of bowel in the intact animal. Notice particularly the caudal extent of the rectogenital pouch; vaginal ovariectomy may be performed by perforating the dorsal wall of the vagina and entering this pouch—an approach that avoids incising the abdominal wall.

Exercises on the Live Animal

Students at Cornell might find it helpful to view the videotape on the ABDOMEN in the series <u>Equine Anatomy Reviewed on the Live Animal</u> before attempting these palpations.

1---Visualize and outline the abdominal muscles on the surface of the horse. Test yourself by determining how many layers of muscle or aponeurosis an incision would encounter in different regions.

2---Palpate the coxal tuber, the cranial border of the thigh (tensor fasciae latae), the subiliac lymph nodes, and the fold of the flank. The caudal part of the abdominal cavity is medial to the thigh (Fig. 3-20/A).

3---Visualize the slope of the diaphragm in the median plane.

4---Visualize the position of the spleen, stomach, and liver on the left, and the liver on the right side of the horse and relate this to the basal border of the lungs.

5---Taking into account that abdominal organs (particularly the intestines) can shift, you should have a fair idea of what organs lie against any point of the abdominal wall.

6---Simulate rectal palpation by holding your extended arm horizontally against the lateral surface of the horse's pelvis, with the bulge of your deltoideus opposite the horse's anus. Estimate the lumbar vertebra opposite your fingertips. This would be your cranialmost rectal reach in *this* horse, but only in the median plane and with your hand close to the sublumbar muscles (Fig. 3-20/A,7).

PELVIS

Purpose and Plan of the Dissection

1---To see the vessels that leave the caudal segment of the abdominal aorta and go to the testes, ovaries, descending colon, and flank.
2---To see the break-up of the aorta and the lymph nodes in this area.
3---To study the inguinal canal and the structures that pass through it in both sexes.
4---To see the udder and the structure of the teat, and in the male the prepuce and structure of the glans and free part of the penis, and in both sexes the adjacent supf. inguinal lymph nodes.
5---To see the sacral plexus of nerves and the arteries of the pelvic wall on both sides of the sacrosciatic ligament.
6---To study the muscles and supplying structures of the perineum in both sexes.
7---To see the muscles and blood vessels in the tail (optional).
8---To explore the parts and structures of the isolated reproductive organs and the tissues between the anal canal and the vulva.

Plan.   After reflection of the peritoneum that lines the caudal abdominal wall, the internal abdominal oblique is transected to expose the inguinal canal. In the female the canal is opened fully to see the dorsal surface of the udder and the mammary vessels. Working in the groin, the teats are opened and in the male the tissues adjacent to the penis are exposed and the penis is transected several times. Then the muscles of the croup are reflected to expose the sacrosciatic ligament, and the anal canal and reproductive tract caudal to it. The tail is transected a short distance caudal to the anus. Finally, the pelvic viscera are removed and the tracts opened for study on the table. The rectum of the male is removed from the pelvic urethra. In the female, the perineum is sectioned midsagittally to expose the perineal body.

Pelvic Inlet

Time saver: During the dissection of the PELVIC INLET two students of each group can begin the dissection of the PELVIC WALL AND PERINEUM on page 61. It is imperative that all students remain informed of what is going on in the two simultaneous dissections by demonstrating important steps to each other periodically. If you do not elect simultaneous dissection, it is advantageous for studying the pelvic inlet to lower the hindquarters a little and to place the feet of the horse on two stools.

Identify and preserve the ureters in the following dissection, which will consist mainly of removing the peritoneum and fat covering the structures described. Students should remember throughout the dissection of the pelvis that they are responsible for the anatomy of both the male and female.

In the male (next paragraph for mare): Locate the **testicular artery** in the mesorchium and trace it from its origin on the aorta caudoventrally to the vaginal ring (Figs. 4-1/5 and 4-2). Note: In the gelding the testicular artery may have retracted away from the ring after castration.

In the mare: Locate the **ovarian artery** in the mesovarium and trace it to its origin on the aorta and to the ovary (Fig. 4-3/4).

The testicular and ovarian arteries are the only arteries in this area that cross ventral to the ureter.

Just as the nerve plexuses that arose from the cranial mesenteric ganglion followed the arteries to the intestines, the **testicular and ovarian nerve plexuses** arise from the caudal mesenteric ganglion and follow their respective arteries to the organs they supply. Do not attempt to trace these nerves.

Pick up the **caudal mesenteric artery** in the descending mesocolon and trace it to its origin on the aorta next to the testicular and ovarian arteries you have just seen.

Clean the ventral surface of the **aorta** caudally to the origins of the large, paired external iliac arteries. Just caudal to the origin of the external iliacs, the aorta ends by bifurcating into the internal iliac arteries, don't look for them now (Fig. 4-2). The aortic bifurcation is located a few cm cranial to the **sacral promontory** formed by the midventral prominence of the first sacral segment at the lumbosacral articulation. It is palpable per rectum—find it on your specimen (Fig. 3-15/1). The **external iliac artery** courses caudoventrally over the lateral side of the pelvic inlet. The first branch, the **deep circumflex iliac artery,** may be seen without dissection passing laterally to its bifurcation ventromedial to the coxal tuber. The distribution of its branches has been noted in the dissection of the flank (p. **34**), but follow its caudal branch ventrally to the subiliac lymph nodes.

The **lumbar lymph nodes** are scattered along the course of the aorta and the caudal vena cava. Their efferents pass cranially into the thoracic duct. They drain the abdominal wall, nearby viscera, and the iliac lymph nodes. The **medial iliac lymph nodes** (palpate) are grouped about the

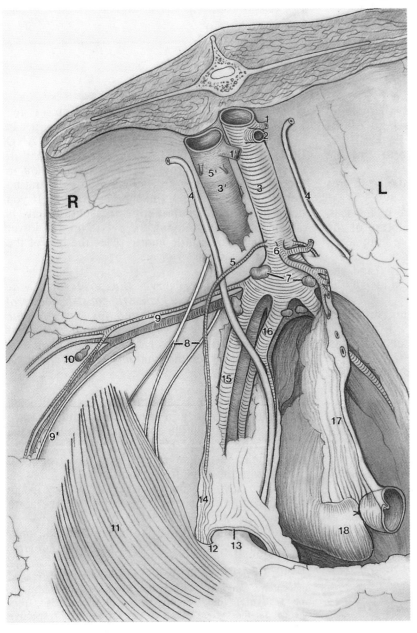

1, 1' Left renal artery and vein
2. Cranial mesenteric artery
3. Aorta, caudal vena cava at 3'
4. Ureters
5. Testicular artery, testicular veins at 5'
6. Caudal mesenteric artery
7. Medial iliac lymph nodes
8. Genitofemoral nerves
9. Deep circumflex iliac vessels, their caudal branches and the lateral cutaneous femoral nerve at 9'
10. Lateral iliac lymph node
11. Internal abdominal oblique muscle
12. Vaginal ring
13. Deferent duct
14. Mesorchium
15, 16 External and internal iliac arteries
17. Descending mesocolon
18. Small (descending) colon entering pelvic cavity

FIGURE 4-1. Vessels and nerves in the vicinity of the break-up of the aorta; gelding; looking caudally and dorsally.

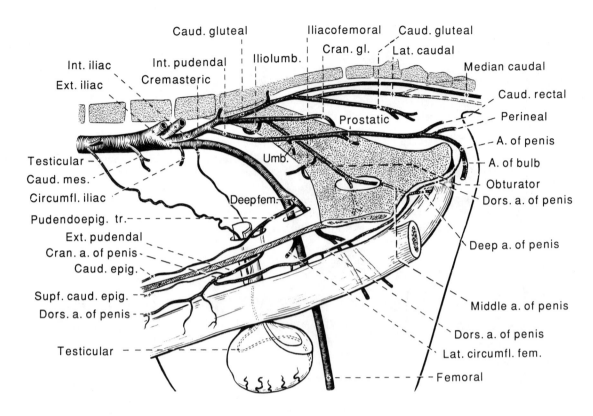

FIGURE 4-2. Arteries associated with the right side of the pelvis and with the reproductive organs of the stallion; medial view; schematic.

termination of the aorta (Fig. 4-1/7). They drain the pelvis, pelvic viscera and testes, and receive lymph from the lateral iliac and deep inguinal nodes. The **lateral iliac lymph nodes** (/10) lie in bifurcation of the deep circumflex iliac artery. They drain the flank, lateral surface of the thigh, and the subiliac nodes.

The **genitofemoral nerves** (/8), derived principally from L3 are seen running across the dorsal and ventral surfaces of the deep circumflex iliac, lateral and parallel to the external iliac artery. They disappear behind the caudal border of the internal oblique and will be traced farther later.

The **uterine artery** (Fig. 4-3/8) arises from the external iliac near the origin of the deep circumflex iliac; find it in the broad ligament

Next we expose the deep inguinal ring and the inguinal ligament. *Incise the peritoneum ONLY, beginning at the terminal branching of the deep circumflex iliac, and cutting to the origin of the artery from the external iliac. In the mare, cut along the attachment of the broad ligament. In both sexes, cut ventrally along the lateral side of the pelvic inlet following the external iliac artery. Follow the curve of the pelvis to the median plane, then make a right angle turn and carry the incision cranially along the linea alba to the umbilicus. In the male, make appropriate incisions so that the mesoductus deferens and the mesorchium are left in place, and make an* *elliptical incision around the vaginal ring to preserve it. Now free all the cut edges and, by blunt dissection, reflect the entire flap of peritoneum cranially off the internal oblique, rectus, nerves, vessels, etc.*

With a stiff probe isolate the external iliac artery and vein to the point where they disappear into the vascular lacuna caudal to the inguinal ligament (Fig. 4-4). The vascular lacuna is the base of the narrow femoral triangle whose apex points ventrally. The femoral triangle contains the femoral vessels (continuations of the external iliacs) and the deep inguinal lymph nodes; it will be opened later. The **inguinal ligament** is the strengthened caudal edge of the aponeurosis of the external oblique. Free the caudal edge of the internal oblique and draw it cranially *just a little*. The ligament may be seen now sweeping from the prepubic tendon (p. 84) dorsolaterally toward the coxal tuber (Fig. 4-5/9).

The deep femoral artery is given off the mediocaudal surface of the external iliac caudal to the inguinal ligament and essentially passes away from you into the muscles ventral to the pelvic floor. Isolate the origin of the artery by blunt dissection. The deep femoral artery gives off the short **pudendoepigastric trunk** which runs ventrocranially over the inguinal ligament and divides into the small caudal epigastric artery and the **external pudendal artery** (Fig. 4-4). The

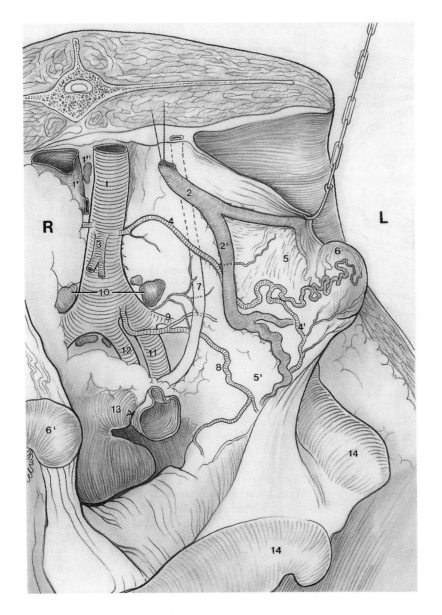

1,1',1" Aorta, caudal vena cava, and a
   lumbar lymph node
2. Ovarian vein, detached from 1' and
   reflected, its uterine branch at 2'
3. Caudal mesenteric artery
4. Ovarian artery, its uterine branch at 4'
5, 5' Mesovarium and mesometrium
   reflected laterally by the hook
6. Left ovary, right ovary at 6'
7. Left ureter, supplied by ureteric artery
8. Uterine artery
9. Deep circumflex iliac artery
10. Medial iliac lymph nodes
11,12 External and internal iliac arteries
13. Small colon entering pelvic cavity
14. Uterine horns

FIGURE 4-3. Blood vessels in the
vicinity of the break-up of the aorta; mare;
looking caudally and dorsally.

epigastric follows the lateral border of the rectus
abdominis. Cut the artery and reflect it cranially
(Fig. 4-5/11).

The external pudendal artery and the
genitofemoral nerve may now be seen passing
over the inguinal ligament and caudal to the free
border of the internal oblique as they enter the
deep inguinal ring. The ring is bounded cranially
by the internal oblique, caudally by the external
abdominal oblique aponeurosis, medially by the
prepubic tendon, and laterally by the origin of the
fibers of the internal oblique from the inguinal
ligament. In short, the deep ring is the space
caudal to and along the *free* border of the internal
oblique. It is about 15 cm long. Structures
passing through the ring enter the inguinal canal.

Structures (such as the femoral vessels)
disappearing *caudal* to the inguinal ligament enter
the vascular lacuna. The inguinal ligament,
therefore, separates the vascular lacuna from the
inguinal canal. Structures in the former enter the
thigh, those in the latter enter the subcutaneous
tissues of the groin.

The external pudendal artery, genitofemoral
nerve, and lymphatic vessels are the only structures
passing through the inguinal ring of the female.
In the male, however, the parietal peritoneum is
evaginated down through the ring to form the
VAGINAL TUNIC (Fig. 4-6/6) composed of
visceral and parietal layers. The deferent duct with
its mesoductus and the testicular vessels and nerves
in the mesorchium come together at the deep

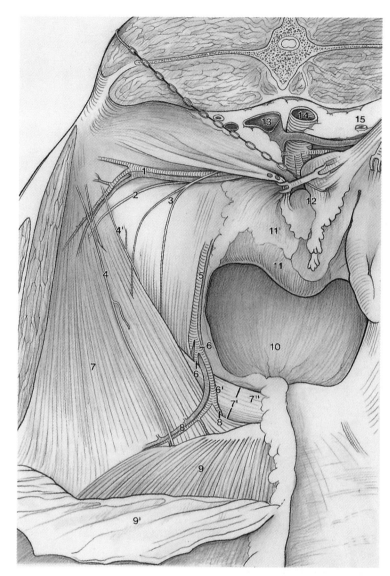

1. Deep circumflex iliac vessels
2. Lateral cutaneous femoral nerve
3. Genitofemoral nerve
4. Ventral branch L1, ventral branch L2 at 4'
5. External iliac vessels
6. Deep femoral artery, pudendoepigastric trunk at 6'
7. Internal abdominal oblique, deep inguinal ring at 7', inguinal ligament at 7"
8. External pudendal artery, caudal epigastric at 8'
9. Rectus abdominis, reflected peritoneum at 9'
10. Vesicogenital pouch (contained pelvic flexure in this horse)
11. Uterine horn, broad lig. at 11'
12. Ovaries, hooked together
13. Caudal vena cava
14. Aorta
15. Left ureter

FIGURE 4-4. Vessels and nerves exposed by the reflection of the peritoneum on the right side of the caudal abdominal cavity; mare; cranial view.

inguinal ring and pass down through inguinal canal as the **spermatic cord**. Their serous coats (visceral tunic) are united in a continuous covering which is joined to the parietal tunic along its caudal wall (Fig. 4-7). Distally the serous coat of the cord is continuous with the serous coat of the epididymis and testis.

The **cavity of the vaginal tunic** is the diverticulum formed by the evagination of the parietal peritoneum through the inguinal canal. The **vaginal ring** lies at the beginning of the evagination and forms the communication between the general peritoneal cavity and the cavity of the vaginal tunic. There is no vaginal ring in the mare.

Separate the cremaster from the caudal border of the internal oblique, using the fine tendinous slip on the edge of the oblique as a guide. The cremaster is closely applied to the caudolateral surface of the vaginal tunic and serves to elevate the testis.

The **SPERMATIC CORD** will be considered further with the isolated genitalia. The following facts are important:
1. The external pudendal artery and the branches of the genitofemoral nerve are separate from and independent of the spermatic cord.
2. The cremaster closely adheres to the outside of the parietal tunic and causes strong elevation of the testis.
3. The testicular and deferential arteries lie within the spermatic cord. The testicular artery is the important source of hemorrhage after castration if not properly crushed.
4. The cavity of the vaginal tunic communicates directly with the peritoneal cavity.
5. While the spermatic cord consists only of the deferent duct, its mesoductus, and the testicular vessels and nerves (in the mesorchium), surgeons generally include also the parietal tunic and the cremaster (Fig. 4-7).

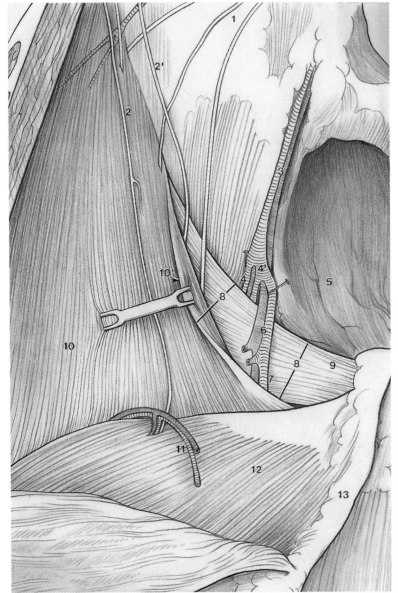

1. Genitofemoral nerve
2. Ventral branch L1, ventral branch L2 at 2'
3. External iliac vessels
4. Femoral artery, deep femoral at 4'
5. Vesicogenital pouch (contained pelvic flexure in this horse)
6. Pudendoepigastric trunk
7. External pudendal artery
8. Deep inguinal ring
9. Inguinal ligament
10. Internal abdominal oblique, its free border reflected at 10'
11. Caudal epigastric vessels, cut
12. Rectus abdominis
13. Fat-filled median lig. of bladder

FIGURE 4-5. The right deep inguinal ring (8) and surrounding vessels and nerves exposed by the reflection of the peritoneum; mare, cranial view; 13 indicates the median plane. This is an enlarged portion of Fig. 4-4.

By scraping away the fat, expose the fleshy end of the rectus abdominis. Transect the muscle 5 cm cranial to its end and reflect the cranial stump toward you. Transect the internal abdominal oblique opposite the external iliac artery and reflect the stumps dorsally and ventrally.

This exposes the aponeurotic caudal end of the external oblique, and a slit in the aponeurosis, the **supf. inguinal ring**, through which the ventral branch of L2, the genitofemoral nerve (from L3 mainly), the external pudendal artery, and in the male the spermatic cord descend (Fig. 4-8). The supf. inguinal ring is about 10 cm long and directed craniolaterally, from the edge of the prepubic tendon. It divides the large expanse of the external oblique aponeurosis into abdominal and pelvic tendons; the abdominal tendon ends at the linea alba, the pelvic tendon ends as the inguinal ligament which stretches between prepubuc tendon and coxal tuber. The medial edge (crus) of the supf. inguinal ring is free; the lateral edge (crus) is continuous with a lamina that is detached from the aponeurosis of the external oblique to the femoral fascia on the medial surface of the thigh. When the hindlimbs are abducted this lamina moves laterally with the thigh and causes the supf. ring to gape. This may be of significance in the development of inguinal hernia in the stallion at the time of service.

Reconstruct the internal oblique and identify again the boundaries of the deep inguinal ring. The **INGUINAL CANAL** is the space between the internal and external oblique muscles extending from the deep to the supf. inguinal ring. The canal can be entered from the abdominal cavity

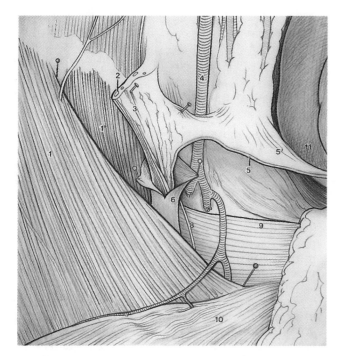

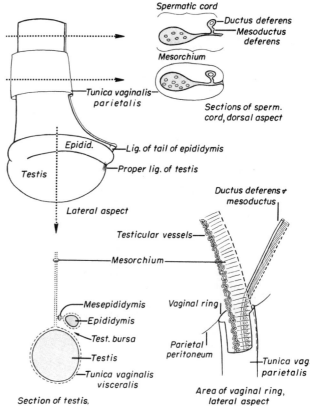

1. Internal abdominal oblique, cremaster at 1'
2. Testicular vessels
3. Mesorchium
4. External iliac artery
5. Deferent duct, genital fold at 5'
6. Vaginal tunic, opened at vaginal ring
7. Femoral artery, deep femoral at 7'
8. Genitofemoral nerve
9. Inguinal ligament
10. Rectus abdominis
11. Rectum

FIGURE 4-6. Cranial view of right deep inguinal ring of a gelding. The peritoneum has been removed.

FIGURE 4-7. Left testis, spermatic cord, and vaginal tunic; schematic.

through the deep inguinal ring, and from the subcutaneous tissue between udder or penis and the thigh through the supf. inguinal ring.

Make a 10 cm long skin incision along the line where the skin is reflected from udder or penis to the thigh and forcefully push your hand dorsally through the superficial inguinal ring and

inguinal canal until your fingers can be palpated within the boundaries of the deep inguinal ring.

Most male horses are castrated when they are young. Castrations may be performed on a standing, sedated horse using local anesthesia or on an anesthetized recumbent patient. Generally, two incisions are made, both parallel to the median raphe and through the scrotum over each testis. The exposed testis is retracted and the spermatic cord isolated

1. Internal abdominal oblique, transected and reflected dorsally and ventrally
2. Ext. abd. oblique aponeurosis, inguinal lig. at 2'
3. Ventral branch L1, ventral branch L2 at 3'
4. Genitofemoral nerve
5. Supf. inguinal ring between pins
6. External pudendal artery
7. Caudal stump of rectus abdominis, external rectus sheath at 7
8. Median lig. of bladder, indicating median plane
9. Uterine horn

FIGURE 4-8. Cranial view of right supf. inguinal ring of a mare.

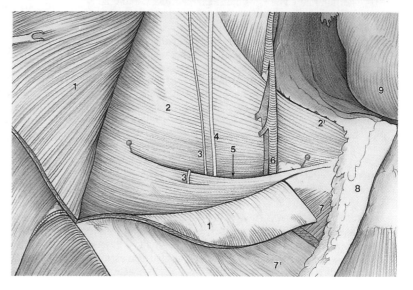

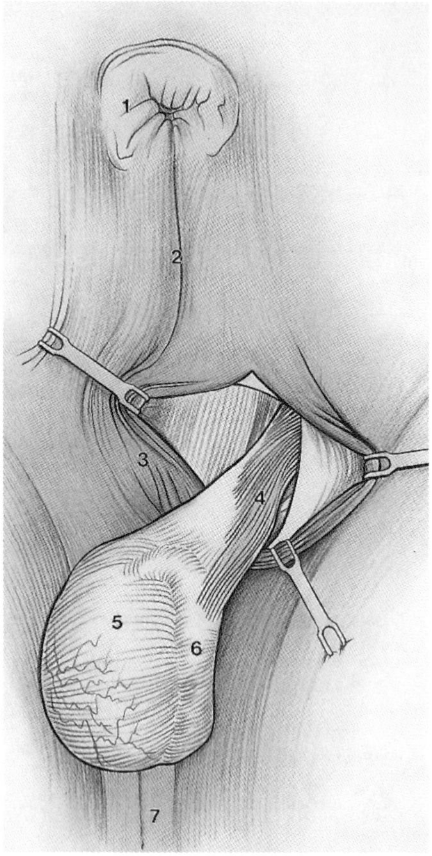

1. Prepuce
2. Preputial raphe
3. Scrotum, incised
4. Cremaster
5. Left testis, inside vaginal tunic
6. Epididymis
7. Perineal region between the swell of the thighs

FIGURE 4-9. Left testis inside vaginal tunic exposed by incising scrotal wall. Cranial is at the top.

so that it may be crushed and cut using an emasculator. The actual procedure takes only a few minutes. The testicular artery is the important source of post-operative hemorrhage if it was not properly crushed or ligated.

The inguinal canal is of considerable clinical importance because of the prevalence of cryptorchidism in colts. Undescended testes are infertile (they produce no sperm), but they will produce hormones in the abdominal environment and they have a relatively higher incidence of neoplasia. A retained testis may be removed through the inguinal canal after an incision over the palpable superficial inguinal ring, a more time consuming and technically demanding procedure than a routine castration. Laparoscopic cryptorchidectomy is an option for removal of an abdominal testis as the equipment becomes more widely available.

It is considered unprofessional to remove only the scrotal testis in a unilateral cryptorchid. Testicular agenesis has been reported in the horse, but it is very uncommon.

Inguinal hernias are relatively common in colts (congenital) and stallions (acquired). In this condition, an abdominal organ – most commonly a loop of the small intestine – passes through the vaginal ring and comes to lie in the vaginal cavity adjacent to the spermatic cord. A short herniated segment may remain within the confines of the inguinal canal and is diagnosed using an internal examination per rectum. A longer herniated segment will descend into the scrotum (a scrotal hernia) and can be diagnosed with an external examination. Standardbred foals are particularly prone to congenital inguinal hernia. Acquired inguinal hernias in adults are usually associated with sexual activity (service) or strenuous exercise.

Examine the **external rectus sheath** that was exposed by the reflection of the rectus abdominis. Note that it is formed by the fused aponeuroses of the internal and external oblique muscles, and that it is thick and strong close to the brim of the pubis.

000000000—From here to the next row of zeros the dissection and description refer only to the **mare**. Students working on a gelding or stallion proceed to the next row of zeros.

Transect the free edge of the supf. inguinal ring at its middle and extend the cut in a cranioventral direction to the midline so that it reaches the linea alba about 25 cm cranial to the pubis. Reflect the triangular flaps.

By doing this you have cut the external rectus sheath and exposed the base of the mammary gland. Trace the branches of the **external pudendal artery** through the fat and the supf. inguinal lymph nodes dorsal to the gland. The branches are the caudal supf. epigastric and the **mammary arteries** (to the udder). The genitofemoral nerve (also visible) supplies the gland and the skin of the inguinal region and adjacent thigh. The **supf. inguinal lymph nodes** drain the mammary gland and adjacent superficial region.

The mare's **UDDER** comprises two mammary glands, right and left, separated by the intermammary groove. Each gland has one teat. Remove the left half of the udder, cutting close to the abdominal wall (leave the right half for review). Probe the two **teat canals** in the tip of the teat. Each canal drains a separate **lactiferous sinus** which in turn receives a separate system of **lactiferous ducts** from the glandular tissue. The part of the lactiferous sinus contained in the teat is the **teat sinus,** and the part contained in the bottom of the gland is the **gland sinus**.

Split the **teat** by a sagittal cut through the teat canals and note the septum dividing the two teat sinuses. The two duct systems they drain also remain separate.

With a sharp scalpel cut off the tip of the right teat, through the **teat canals,** and note their folded mucosa and the pale smooth muscle sphincters surrounding them. There is a concentration of sebaceous glands cranial to the cranial and caudal to the caudal teat canal. Yellowish-green material may be found congealed in the ducts or sinuses; this is the secretion of the normal dry mammary gland.

The udder of the pregnant mare usually develops noticeably in the few weeks prior to parturition. Following glandular development, the udder then distends with colostrum several days prior to foaling. Many mares will exude some of this colostrum as a covering to the teat ("waxing") indicating that foaling is imminent.

0000000000—From here to the next row of zeros the dissection and description refer only to the **male**. Students working on a mare proceed to the next row of zeros, but should periodically observe the dissection on the male.

For the dissection of the external male genitalia it is best to lay the hindquarters on the floor (or on a table if you are working on a pony)—right limb down—pry the hindlimbs apart as far as possible and push the left abdominal wall craniodorsally to expose the left side of the penis. The dissection is done only on the left side. The dissection of the thighs will be temporarily interrupted.

If you have a stallion (next paragraph for gelding): Identify the left testis by pulling it down into the **scrotum**, tense the scrotal skin over it and make a generous longitudinal skin incision along the ventral surface of the testis. **Note:** it is important to incise only the skin, which is thin. Bluntly isolate the testis, enclosed in the parietal tunic, from the wall of the scrotum by peeling back the scrotal skin and underlying dartos. This blunt separation goes fairly easily and is done within the loose supf. spermatic fascia deep to the dartos. Isolate testis and vaginal tunic fully from the scrotum by ventral traction with one hand and by pushing the fascia up along the vaginal tunic toward the supf. inguinal ring with the other (Fig. 4-9). If your horse were alive, and you crushed and cut the spermatic cord enclosed in the tunic now, you would have performed a *closed* castration; closed, because the vaginal cavity (peritoneal cavity) would not have been opened. When removing the testis by *open* castration the incision through the scrotal wall is made deeper so that the parietal tunic is also cut, i.e. the vaginal cavity is opened (Fig. 4-10). Don't do either. Instead, pin the testis to the abdominal wall and proceed with the next paragraph. *Since stallions are rare in dissection rooms, be prepared to share your specimen with others.*

Extend the previously made 10 cm skin incision (where thigh meets abdomen) cranially to the level of the preputial orifice. Make a second longitudinal skin incision along the lateral aspect of the penis, also to the preputial orifice. Connect the two incisions caudally where thigh and penis are in contact and reflect the triangular skin flap cranially.

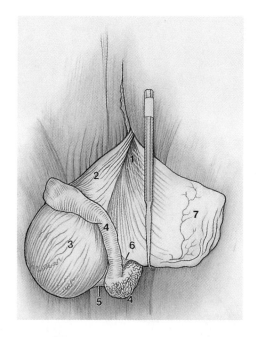

1. Cremaster shining through parietal vaginal tunic
2. Spermatic cord
3. Left testis
4. Body of epididymis, tail at 4'
5. Proper lig. of testis
6. Lig. of tail of epididymis
7. Parietal vaginal tunic incised and reflected

FIGURE 4-10. Left testis exposed by incising scrotal wall and parietal vaginal tunic. Cranial is at the top.

Blunt dissection in the fat and supf. fascia dorsolateral to the penis exposes the **supf. inguinal lymph nodes.** They drain the sheath (prepuce), penis, scrotum, and adjacent regions of the abdominal wall and thigh. The testis and epididymis drain directly into the lumbar lymph nodes by way of lymphatics in the spermatic cord. Swelling of the supf. inguinal nodes, therefore, does not indicate orchitis.

Search by blunt dissection among the lymph nodes until you find an artery. Trace it caudally by sharp dissection to the **external pudendal artery.** When all the branches of the latter are exposed you will note that it breaks up to form the **caudal supf. epigastric,** which sends branches to the prepuce, and the **cranial artery of the penis** (Fig.4-11/b,a'). This supplies the thin **dorsal artery of the penis** (/c).

Follow the cranial artery of the penis into the extensive plexus of large veins covering the dorsal and lateral surfaces of the penis. This necessitates cutting through a layer of elastic tissue derived from the abdominal tunic and acting as a suspensory ligament for the prepuce. The veins drain into the **accessory external pudendal vein.** The latter does not accompany its satellite external pudendal artery but perforates the cranial part of the tendon of origin of the gracilis and joins the deep femoral vein. It anastomoses with the obturator vein and its fellow of the opposite side. By careful dissection and separation of the venous plexus trace the dorsal artery of the penis (/c) cranially for a short distance, on the dorsolateral surface of the penis, and locate also the

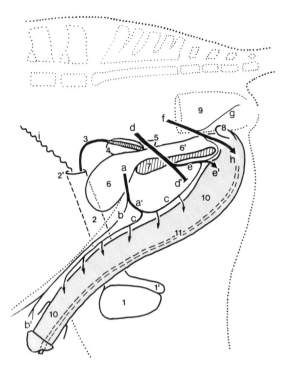

a. Ext pudendal a., cranial a.
   of penis at a'
b. Supf. caudal epigastric a.,
   branches to prepuce at b'
c. Dorsal a. of penis
d. Obturator a., into thigh
   muscles at d'
e. Middle a. of penis, deep a. of
   penis at e'
f. Internal pudendal a., becomes
   a. of penis and then h
g. Caudal rectal a.
h. A. of bulb of penis
i. Testicular a.

i. Testis, epididymis at 1'
2. Vaginal tunic, vaginal ring at 2'
3. Deferent duct
4. Vesicular gland
5. Prostate
6. Bladder, pelvic urethra
   at 6'
7. Pelvic symphysis
8. Bulbourethral gland
9. Rectum
10. Penis
11. Urethra

FIGURE 4-11. The triple blood supply of the penis; schematic.

dorsal nerve of the penis (from the pudendal to be seen later). The artery gives off short branches to the corpus cavernosum, and longer ones to the supf. inguinal lymph nodes, scrotum, and prepuce. It ends at the glans. The segment of the dorsal artery of the penis that links up with the middle artery of the penis (/e) is difficult to demonstrate. It passes caudally on the penis, also giving off branches to the corpus cavernosum. Remember that the arteries and nerves of the penis are paired.

Examine the **PREPUCE**, commonly referred to as the sheath in the horse. When the penis is retracted, the prepuce is telescoped, thereby forming two folds (Fig. 4-12/3,4). The outer fold corresponds to the simple prepuce of other animals—its opening is called the **preputial orifice**. The outer surface (external lamina) of the outer fold is continuous with the haired skin of the abdomen. At the preputial orifice, the external lamina reflects upon itself and is continuous with the unhaired skin of the internal lamina. At the deepest part of the **preputial cavity**, the internal lamina reflects upon itself, giving rise to an inner fold, the cylindrical **preputial fold** (/4). The

cranially directed free opening (free edge) of the preputial fold lies within the prepuce and is called the **preputial ring**. The internal lamina of the preputial fold is continuous with the skin that covers the free part of the penis.

The musculocavernous penis of the horse undergoes considerable enlargement when it is engorged. The arrangement of redundant skin folds provides a reserve of skin which is easily drawn out and applied to the surface of the penis when it is extended during erection.

The secretion of the sebaceous glands present in the prepuce mixed with desquamated epithelial cells forms the fatty **smegma** which in life may accumulate to require removal.

PENIS: Examine the **glans**. The glans is a soft erectile cushion attached to the tip of the very much firmer (when erect) corpus cavernosum which forms the bulk of the penis. It has a long flat dorsal process that extends caudally on the dorsal surface of the corpus and is exposed on transverse sections of the penis near the glans. The urethra protrudes into the **fossa glandis** as the free **urethral process**. Dorsal to the urethral process the fossa forms a diverticulum, the **urethral sinus**, which occasionally becomes packed with smegma. This localized accumulation of smegma, when hardened into a pellet, is known as the "bean of the penis".

Pull the penis from the prepuce and make several transverse sections as far caudally as possible. The large **corpus cavernosum** is surrounded by the thick, fibroelastic **tunica albuginea**. Numerous trabeculae pass from the tunica albuginea and interlace through the cavernous tissue of the corpus. The urethra lies in the **urethral groove** on the ventral surface of the

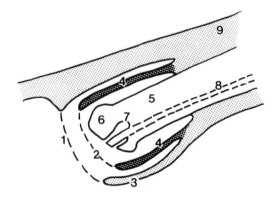

1. Preputial orifice
2. Preputial ring
3. Prepuce proper
4. Preputial fold
5. Free part of penis
6. Glans
7. Urethral sinus, caudal part of fossa glandis
8. Urethra
9. Body wall

FIGURE 4-12. Median section of penis within prepuce; schematic.

corpus cavernosum, surrounded by the **corpus spongiosum** and the **bulbospongiosus muscle**. The origins of these structures in the perineal region will be seen later. Study the triple blood supply of the horse's penis on Figure 4-11 and look for the cranial and middle arteries of the penis (and the nerves of the penis—from pudendal) on the transverse sections.

0000000000—The following applies to both male and female horses.

The **umbilical artery** arises from the internal pudendal artery, the first branch of the internal iliac, 2-3 cm from its origin (Fig. 4-13/6). The umbilical supplies the ureter and deferent duct before it is gradually reduced to a thick-walled fibrous vessel with a very small lumen. It passes caudoventrally in the free edge of the lateral ligament of the bladder as the round ligament of the bladder (seen earlier) and may still supply part of the bladder. Transect the artery to see its tiny lumen. This is a good time to review fetal circulation.

Trace the **ureter** by probing the lumen. It passes caudally in the attached border of the broad ligament, turns medioventrally into the attached border of the lateral ligament of the bladder and enters the neck of the bladder.

Pelvic Wall and Perineum

Identify on the skeleton and by palpation of your specimen the **coxal tuber** and the **ischial tuber** (Fig. 3-1). These two bony prominences indicate the **slope of the pelvis**. The **sacral tuber** is important in the diagnosis of sacroiliac luxation, but is difficult or impossible to palpate in well muscled subjects. The **greater trochanter** of the femur marks the position of the hip joint. Note that the greater trochanter has low cranial and high caudal parts, both of which are easily palpable. The hip joint that lies medial and ventral to the greater trochanter is too deeply positioned to be palpable externally. The high caudal part of the greater trochanter lies on the line that marks the slope of the pelvis.

Asymmetry or excessive prominence of the sacral tubers (hunter's bumps) indicates sacroiliac subluxation. Tearing and strain of the complex ligaments that normally maintain the stability of the sacroiliac articulation allows the tuber sacrale to displace upward relative to the sacrum. This displacement may be more obvious when the horse bears weight on the affected limb if the joint is unstable. This condition is caused by trauma – either a single traumatic incident such as a slip or fall, or repetitive trauma, such as

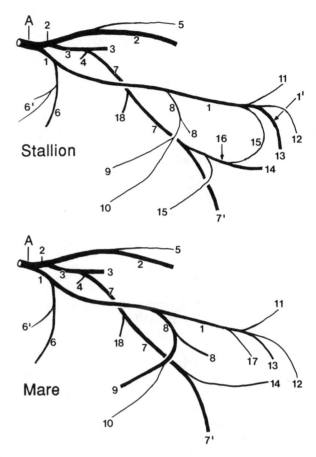

FIGURE 4-13. Branches of the right internal iliac artery in both sexes, medial view.

A	Internal iliac	10.	Caudal vesical
		11.	Caudal rectal
1.	Int. pudendal, a. of penis at 1'	12.	Perineal
2.	Caudal gluteal	13.	A. of bulb of penis,
3.	Cranial gluteal		a. of vestibular bulb
4.	Iliolumbar	14.	Deep a. of penis,
5.	Into tail		a. of clitoris
6.	Umbilical, ureteric at 6'	15.	Dorsal a. of penis
7.	Obturator, into thigh muscles	16.	Middle a. of penis
	at 7'	17.	Vestibular branch
8.	Prostatic, vaginal	18.	Iliacofemoral
9.	Deferential, uterine branch		

might occur in a jumping horse or harness race horse.

The greater trochanter plays a role in the diagnosis of luxation of the hip in the horse (a rare condition). In hip luxation, the high part of the greater trochanter is displaced from the line that marks the slope of the pelvis.

Make a midline incision over the croup to the tail (Fig. 4-14). Circle the root of the tail and continue ventrally as shown in the Figure, not more than a cm away from the anal and vulvar openings and returning to the midline ventral to these. Reflect the skin off the croup to about the level of the flank fold, carefully removing the skin also from the anal and vulvar elevations. The hairs of the tail may be in the way during the subsequent dissections. Saw the tail off short (6 - 8 cm caudal to the anus) and trim the hair that remains with scissors.

There are five pairs of **sacral nerves** in the horse. The medial branches of the dorsal branches are muscular and are not visible. The lateral branches become the **dorsal cutaneous branches** and ramify over the croup and thigh as far ventrally as the stifle joint (Fig. 2-14). They cannot be traced that far grossly. A small area over the proximal portion of the semitendinosus and semimembranosus is innervated by the first caudal nerve. The *ventral branches* of the sacral nerves contribute to the lumbosacral plexus and the pudendal and caudal rectal nerves.

The **caudal cutaneous femoral nerve** (derived from the sciatic to be seen later) may be seen emerging from the caudal edge of the biceps and ramifying over the caudal surface of the thigh below the ischial tuber. The lateral surface of the hip and thigh is innervated cranially by dorsal cutaneous branches of the lumbar nerves (Fig. 2-14).

The purpose of the following dissection is to demonstrate the intermuscular septa between the large muscles of the croup and thigh and to use the septa for an orderly reflection of these muscles to expose the hip joint and the vessels and nerves in the lateral wall of the pelvis.

Remove the fat from the muscles if you are working on a horse in good condition. In many subjects it is possible at this stage to determine the (vertical) boundaries between the tensor fasciae latae, superficial gluteal, biceps, semitendinosus, and semimembranosus muscles (from cranial to caudal) as shown in Figs. 5-1 and 4-17; ask an instructor if you are not certain. Push a finger (through a short incision) between each of these muscles until you feel smooth muscle surfaces on each side of your finger. The bottom of Figure 4-15 gives the directions of the septa separating these muscles. By following the fascial planes, extend the intermuscular incisions dorsally and ventrally to fully separate these five muscles from close to the dorsal midline (coxal tuber for the tensor) to the skin reflection. With this

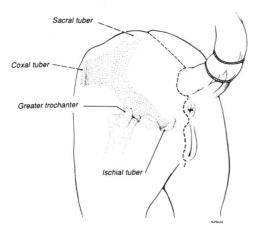

FIGURE 4-14. Skin incisions on the hindquarters.

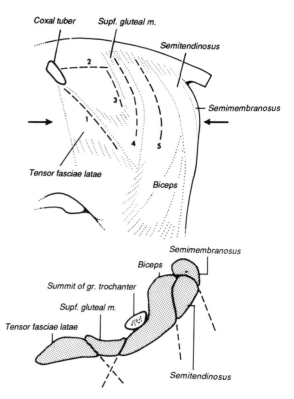

FIGURE 4-15. *Top:* The five fascial incisions (1-5), identified in the text, on the lateral surface of the hindquarters. *Bottom:* Dorsal view of a section taken at the level of the arrows in the top drawing, to indicate the direction (broken lines) of the intermuscular septa. (After Barone.)

accomplished, continue at the next row of zeros.

For further definition of the fascial sheaths that cover and separate these large muscles, the following optional dissection may be done. Make an incision (Fig. 4-15/1) through the deep fascia close to the caudal edge of the **tensor fasciae latae** from the coxal tuber to the skin reflection. Reflect the flap of fascia caudally, off the tightly adhering muscle fibers, to the intermuscular septum between the tensor and the cranial head of the V-shaped **gluteus superficialis** (Fig. 4-16). The septum attaches deeply to the coxal tuber and the lateral edge of the ilium. Locate these points on the skeleton. The tensor arises largely from the coxal tuber, but many fibers take origin from this septum. The fleshy part of the cranial head of the gluteus superficialis does not extend to the coxal tuber; it originates from the intermuscular septum.

Make a longitudinal incision (Fig. 4-15/2) through the deep gluteal fascia over the **gluteus medius**, carrying it from the level of the coxal tuber to the cranial edge of the caudal head of the superficial gluteal. Make a perpendicular incision (/3) along the cranial edge of the caudal head of the gluteus superficialis. Reflect the fascial flaps thus formed by scraping the fibers of the gluteus medius off the deep surface of the fascia.

Now make a vertical incision (/4) over the caudal head of the superficial gluteal and reflect the flaps to the septa that bound the muscle. The cranial and caudal heads are connected by gluteal fascia (Fig. 5-1).

The next muscle caudal to the gluteus superficialis is the **biceps femoris**. Make a vertical incision (Fig. 4-15/5) over the biceps from the dorsal midline to the skin reflection and reflect the fascial flaps to the intermuscular septa. Caudal to the biceps is the **semitendinosus.** Make a similar incision and reflection to demonstrate the fascial sheath of this muscle.

0000000000—*Incise the deep fascia over the triangular vertebral head of the semimembranosus (Fig. 4-17/2) from the side of the tail head ventrally to the skin reflection, and medially and laterally along the skin reflection for a short distance. Beginning ventrally, reflect the lateral flap of fascia to the intermuscular septum between the semimembranosus and semitendinosus. Then make a horizontal fascial incision from the first incision toward the space between the tail head and the anus, and reflect the medial flap as far as possible into the deep groove between the semimembranosus and the external genitalia. The flap attaches cranially to the*

caudal border of the sacrosciatic ligament (Fig. 4-20/A).

Caution: In performing the following dissection always stay lateral to this flap of fascia to avoid mutilating the vessels and nerves around the external genitalia (Fig. 4-18).

Transect the semimembranosus at the level of the ischial arch and again just ventral to the root of the tail. Free the lateral border from the semitendinosus. Now, exerting traction on the lateral border, free the isolated portion of the muscle by sharp dissection from the ischial tuber. Working from this tuber toward the root of the tail, draw this portion of the muscle strongly dorsally and caudally, severing its deep attachments to the sacrosciatic ligament, and remove it (Fig. 4-18).

Free the cranial border of the tensor fasciae latae from the aponeurosis of the external oblique

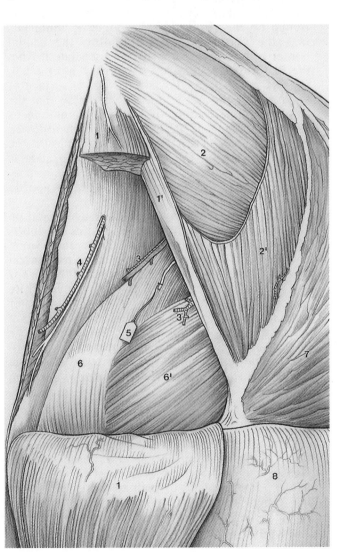

1. Tensor fasciae latae, cut and reflected ventrally, intermuscular septum at 1'
2. Gluteus medius, gluteus supf. at 2'
3. Branches of iliacofemoral artery
4. Caudal br. of deep circumflex iliac artery, and lateral cutaneous femoral nerve
5. Branch of cranial gluteal nerve, tagged
6. Rectus femoris, vastus lateralis at 6'
7. Biceps femoris
8. Reflected skin

FIGURE 4-16. Lateral view of left thigh after reflection of tensor fasciae latae. Cranial is to the left.

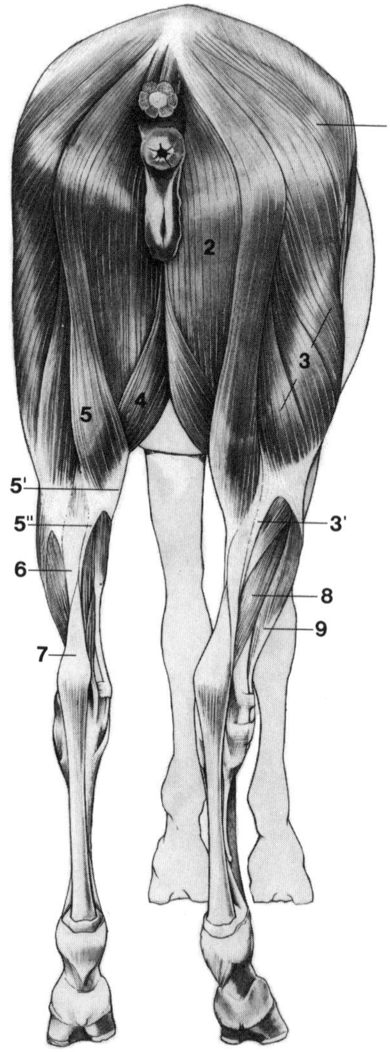

1. Gluteus supf.
2. Semimembranosus
3. Biceps femoris, its tarsal tendon at 3'
4. Gracilis
5. Semitendinosus, its tibial tendon at 5', its tarsal tendon at 5"
6. Gastrocnemius
7. Supf. digital flexor, passing over point of hock
8. Deep digital flexor
9. Lat. digital extensor

FIGURE 4-17. Superficial muscles of the hindlimb of a mare, caudal view. (From Ellenberger-Dittrich-Baum by Horowitz/Geary.)

muscle. Free the caudal border from the cranial head of the gluteus superficialis, working proximally from the skin reflection, scraping the muscle from the intermuscular septum. Transect the tensor fasciae latae at its origin from the coxal tuber and reflect it ventrally.

A nerve (a branch of the cranial gluteal) and branches of the iliacofemoral artery enter the deep

surface of the muscle. Cut them close to the muscle so as to leave long stumps. Tag the nerve (Fig. 4-16/5); it will be needed shortly.

Parts of the rectus femoris and vastus lateralis, the cranial and lateral heads respectively of the **quadriceps femoris**, are exposed.

Free the long caudal head of the superficial gluteal from the septum between it and the biceps. Cut its dorsal origin from the deep surface of the deep gluteal fascia. Reflect the muscle ventrally off the mass of the gluteus medius. Isolate the cranial head and sever its origins from the intermuscular septum. Reflect it ventrally also. The entire muscle should now hang freely from its insertion on the third trochanter which is easily palpated on your specimen.

The **semitendinosus** arises on the first two caudal vertebrae and the ventral surface of the ischial tuber. (Both dog and domestic ruminants lack the vertebral origin.) Follow the caudal border of the muscle dorsally and separate it from the sacrocaudales muscles which pass into the tail. Clean the sacrocaudales and the lateral surface of the root of the tail of fat and fascia so that the small proximal stump of the semimembranosus can be isolated and its tendinous origin followed dorsally to the sacrosciatic ligament. Transect the semitendinosus at the level of the sacrocaudales and reflect it ventrally, cutting the many attachments to the intermuscular septa as you do so.

The **biceps femoris** has an extensive origin on the sacrum, sacrosciatic ligament, and ischial tuber. (The domestic ruminants have the same arrangement, but the dog lacks the direct sacral origin.) Sever the sacral attachment of the biceps and reflect it ventrally off the shiny, white sacrosciatic ligament to the level of the greater trochanter. Carefully preserve the underlying caudal gluteal vessels and nerve. Sever them close to the muscle, leaving long stumps (Fig. 4-19). The ischial lymph nodes are distributed along the course of the vessels. They drain adjacent structures.

The **sacrosciatic ligament**, present in the ungulates, is a sheet of strong connective tissue that completes the wall of the pelvis laterally. It arises dorsally from the lateral border of the sacrum and transverse processes of the first two caudal vertebrae, and extends to the ischial spine and tuber (Fig. 4-20). The opening it leaves between the latter two points is the **lesser sciatic foramen; the greater sciatic foramen** is a similar opening between the ligament and the ilium cranial to the ischial spine. The caudal border of the sacrosciatic ligament is free and corresponds to the sacrotuberous ligament of the dog. Examine its features on a dried demo specimen.

With the reflection of the biceps and semitendinosus and the partial removal of the semimembranosus, portions of the perineum have come into view. The **perineum** is the body wall that closes the pelvic cavity caudally. Since it must, by necessity, include and surround the urogenital tract and the anal canal, it is rather more complicated than ordinary body wall like that of the flank, for example. Still, it has the same components, which are from inside-out: peritoneum, fascia, a muscle layer, fascia again, and skin. The perineum has deep and supf. boundaries. The deep are: dorsally the sacrum and the beginning of the tail, laterally the sacrosciatic ligaments, and ventrally the floor of the bony pelvis (Fig. 4-20/B). The supf. boundaries, those on the surface of the animal, are quite different. They are: dorsally the base of the tail, laterally the semimembranosus muscles, and

ventrally the scrotum or the udder. While the deep boundaries are triangular in caudal view, the superficial form a narrow strip between the buttocks that extends cranially between the thighs (Fig. 4-17).

Before reflecting the very large **gluteus medius** you have to have some idea of its origins on the bony pelvis—it is inserted of course on the greater trochanter. The muscle originates from the entire gluteal (dorsal) surface of the ilium and from the sacroiliac ligaments that cover the lateral aspect of the sacrum (see skeleton). (There is also an origin from the dorsal surface of the longissimus *cranial* to the pelvis (Fig. 3-3/1), but we can disregard this for the moment.)

Palpate the dorsalmost part of the coxal tuber and determine from a skeleton the position of the sacral tuber—near the midline but a little caudal to the level of the coxal tuber. With a post mortem

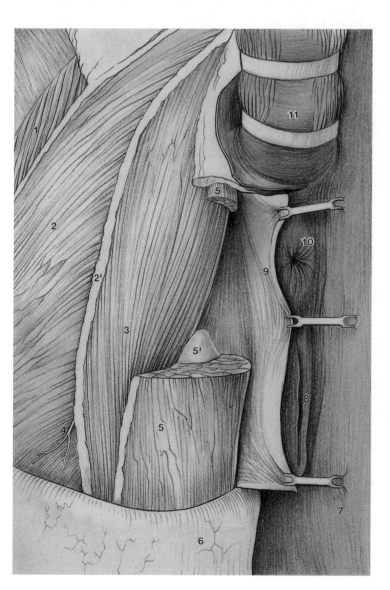

1. Gluteus superficialis
2. Biceps femoris, fat-filled edge of intermuscular septum at 2'
3. Semitendinosus
4. Caudal cutaneous femoral nerve
5. Semimembranosus, resected; ischial tuber at 5'
6. Reflected skin
7. Right thigh
8. Vulva
9. Fascial flap between semimembranosus and external genitalia
10. Anus
11. Underside of tail

FIGURE 4-18. Left thigh muscles after resection of the semimembranosus, caudolateral view.

knife held vertically, transect the gluteus medius along the line joining these two points, i.e., along the iliac crest which connects the two tubers. Feel the iliac crest with your fingers at the depth of the transection and, by pulling the caudal stump of the gluteus medius caudally, scrape the muscle off the dorsal surface of the wing of the ilium. Cut the muscle off the caudal part of the coxal tuber and medially off the sacroiliac ligaments covering the spinous processes of the sacrum.

Continue scraping the muscle off the wing of the ilium until the **cranial gluteal vessels and nerve** are encountered at the greater sciatic foramen (Fig. 4-21/3). These must be transected, but leave long stumps on the pelvis. Work along the medial and caudal borders of the muscle, retracting them laterally and ventrally. The **caudal gluteal vessels and nerve** emerge separately through the sacrosciatic ligament and are coming now into view. Using the tagged nerve to the tensor fasciae latae as a guide, work along the lateral border of the gluteus medius, reflecting it medially and caudally off the **gluteus profundus**. The latter may be recognized by its numerous tendinous bands (Fig. 4-21).

Reflect the entire muscle to its insertions on the greater trochanter and the crest below the trochanter. See skeleton. A smaller portion with a straplike tendon, the gluteus accessorius, can be demonstrated by blunt dissection on the deep surface of the gluteus medius. The tendon of the gluteus accessorius curves over the lower cranial part of the trochanter to be inserted on the lateral surface. The **trochanteric bursa** lies between the tendon and the cranial part of the trochanter (Fig. 4-21/5'). It is occasionally the site of a bursitis producing the syndrome of trochanteric lameness. Remove the great mass of the gluteus medius by

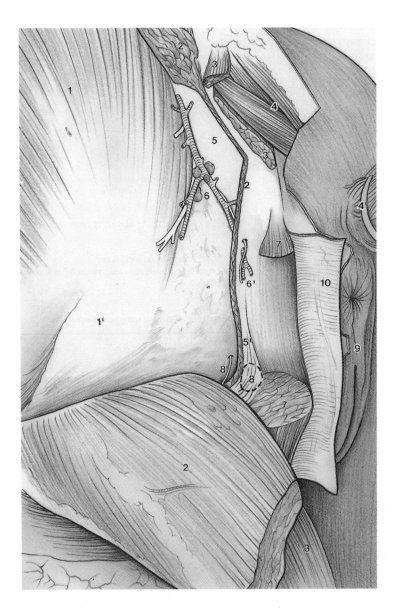

1. Gluteus medius, attaching on greater trochanter at 1'
2. Stumps of reflected biceps
3. Stumps of reflected semitendinosus
4. Tail muscles, tailhead at 4'
5. Sacrosciatic lig., its caudal (sacrotuberous) part at 5'
6. Caudal gluteal artery and nerve and ischial lymph nodes, semitendinosus branches at 6'
7. Stumps of resected semimembranosus
8. Ischial tuber, caudal cutaneous femoral nerve at 8'
9. Vulva and anus
10. Fascial flap between semimembranosus and external genitalia

FIGURE 4-19. Caudal part of left thigh after reflection of semitendinosus and biceps, caudolateral view.

cutting it close to the insertions on the greater trochanter. The entire wing and and shaft of the ilium, and the sacroiliac and sacrosciatic ligaments (and the lateral border of the sacrum between these) should now be clearly visible and free of remnants of the middle gluteal muscle you have just removed.

Branches of the **iliolumbar** and **iliacofemoral arteries** can be seen emerging below the lateral border of the ilium. The iliolumbar emerges just caudal to the coxal tuber and the larger iliacofemoral emerges more caudally. Both are branches of the obturator artery, itself a branch off the cranial gluteal artery (Fig. 4-13/3,7,4,18). Branches of the iliacofemoral artery lie on the quadriceps (which they supply) and were seen before when the tensor fasciae latae was reflected (Fig. 4-21/4).

Nerves of the **SACRAL PLEXUS**, i.e., the ventral branches of the sacral nerves, lie on both surfaces of the sacrosciatic ligament; those on the supf. surface of the ligament are exposed now. The large **sciatic nerve** passes caudoventrally over the gluteus profundus to disappear caudal to the hip joint (Figs. 4-21/6 and 4-22). The **caudal gluteal nerve** arises with the smaller **caudal cutaneous femoral nerve** from the dorsal border of the sciatic and supplies the gluteus superficialis and medius and the proximal part of the biceps. The caudal cutaneous femoral nerve passes caudoventrally, sends a branch to the semi-tendinosus, and continues to the caudal surface of the thigh where its stump may have been seen earlier (Fig. 4-23/8). *Clean and free these nerves and the caudal gluteal vessels and preserve them. Transect the sciatic nerve at the greater sciatic foramen and reflect it distally.*

Muscles, Vessels, and Nerves of the Perineum

Remove all fascia and tags of muscle from the surface of the sacrosciatic ligament. Palpate the lateral border of the sacrum that provides the (dorsal) origin of the sacrosciatic ligament. With a shallow cut (so as not to transect the pudendal nerve; Fig. 4-20/A), sever the sacral origin of the ligament beginning at the greater sciatic foramen and ending at the point of emergence of the caudal gluteal vessels. This exposes the caudal gluteal vessels; you may have even opened the large caudal gluteal vein. Free the caudal gluteal artery and pin it to the side of the sacrum.

The pudendal nerve (cranially) and the caudal rectal nerve (caudally) are now seen passing caudoventrally (Fig. 4-24/4,5); they represent a commingling of the ventral branches of sacral nerves 3 & 4 which emerge from foramina on the ventral surface of the sacrum. With the two nerves identified, reflect the sacrosciatic ligament ventrally; it is thin cranially and should be cut

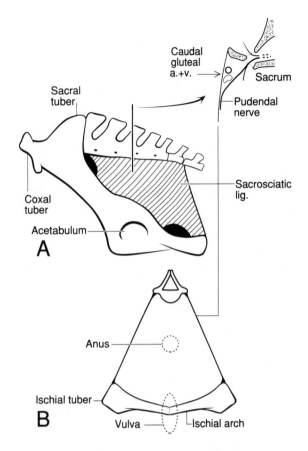

FIGURE 4-20. A: Left lateral view of bony pelvis with sacrosciatic ligament, and transverse section of sacrum to show the relationship of the sacrosciatic ligament to the pudendal nerve. B: Caudal view of pelvis and sacrosciatic ligament and relationship to anus and vulva.

from around the roots of the sciatic nerve.

The **pudendal nerve** is partially embedded in the sacrosciatic ligament so that tracing the nerve and reflecting the ligament ventrally will have to be done simultaneously. Trace the nerve to where it joins the internal pudendal artery, and continue to cut the sacral and caudal attachments of the ligament, leaving a narrow strip of the caudal border (sacrotuberous part) in place for a landmark. After the pudendal nerve is exposed, reflect the ligament fully to the level of the ischial spine, sparing the **coccygeus** which arises from the ischial spine and passes to the tail. The **caudal rectal nerve** should now also be visible (Fig. 4-24/5).

Where the pudendal nerve joins the internal pudendal artery it gives off the **deep perineal nerve** which passes caudally, communicates with the branches of the caudal rectal nerve, and with that nerve innervates the muscles and skin of the perineum (Fig. 4-22).

The **caudal rectal nerve,** after giving branches to the coccygeus, levator ani, and the anal sphincters, supplies the **superficial perineal nerves.** These emerge lateroventral to the anus. In the female, one branch runs ventrally on the semimembranosus, and other branches—the labial nerves—pass ventrally on the labium (Fig. 4-23/5,6). In the male, the corresponding caudal scrotal nerves course ventrally on the bulbospongiosus to the scrotum, one nerve covered by superficial fascia, the other by deep fascia.

The continuation of the **pudendal nerve**, the dorsal nerve of the penis or the nerve of the clitoris, will be exposed shortly.

The **anorectal lymph nodes** are exposed in the area between the anus and the root of the tail (Fig. 4-24/11). They drain the anal canal, perineum, and tail. Surgical removal of malignant tumors in this region should include the anorectal lymph nodes.

Melanomas are clinically important tumors in horses. They are very common in horses over 15 years of age with gray or white coat colors. Melanomas are frequently found in the perineal region and at the root of the tail although they may also be found at other sites, such as head, prepuce and limbs. Most often, melanomas grow slowly and are locally invasive and do not metastasize to distant locations. Occasionally, melanomas show more aggressive growth characteristics typical of a malignant neoplasm. Surgical reduction of melanomas in the perineal region is sometimes possible, but complete excision is difficult because of the tendency of the melanoma to grow cranially deep into the perineum where the mass can interfere with urination or defecation by virtue of its size and location.

Pick up the **internal pudendal artery** ventral to the stumps of the cranial gluteal vessels and follow it caudally (Fig. 4-24/7). A little cranial to the level of the hip joint it gives off the small **prostatic** (male) or medium-sized **vaginal** (female) **artery** which supplies the pelvic viscera and will be traced on the isolated genitalia.

In the gelding or stallion (next paragraph for mare): After giving off the prostatic, the **internal pudendal artery** (Fig. 4-13) continues caudally deep to the pudendal and deep perineal nerves and gives off the small caudal rectal artery which passes over the levator ani to the anal canal. At the

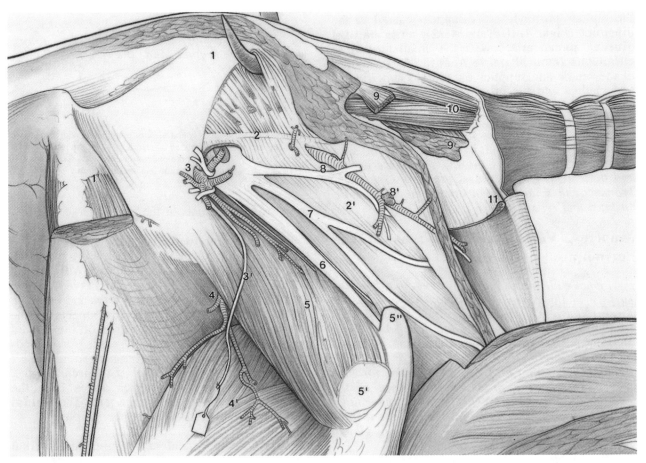

1.	Sacral tuber, stump of tensor fasciae latae arising from coxal tuber at 1'	7.	Caudal cutaneous femoral n.
2	Lateral border of sacrum, sacrosciatic lig. at 2'	8.	Caudal gluteal a. & n., ischial lymph nodes at 8'
3.	Cranial gluteal a & n., branch to tensor fasciae latae at 3'		
4.	Iliacofemoral a., quadriceps at 4'	9.	Stumps of semitendinosus
5.	Gluteus profundus, trochanteric bursa at 5', high part of gr. trochanter at 5"	10.	Tail muscles
		11.	Stump of semimembranosus
6	Sciatic nerve		

FIGURE 4-21. Nerves and arteries on the sacrosciatic ligament after reflection of gluteus medius and biceps femoris, lateral view.

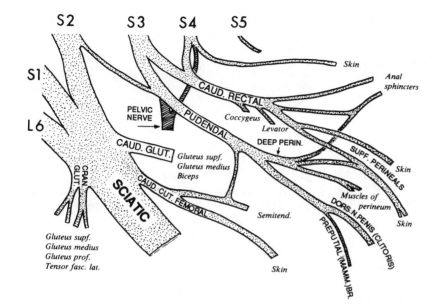

FIGURE 4-22. Left sacral plexus, lateral view. (After Habel.)

level of the ischial arch the pudendal gives off one or two perineal arteries for the region ventral to the anus. The continuation of the internal pudendal, the **artery of the penis**, may give off a small dorsal artery of the penis that passes around the ischial arch (Fig. 4-2). The artery of the penis then becomes the **artery of the bulb of the penis** which dips under the bulbospongiosus to enter the corpus spongiosum.

In the mare: After giving off the vaginal, the **internal pudendal artery** continues caudally deep to the pudendal nerve and gives off the vestibular branch which extends to the region of the ventral commissure of the vulva. The next branch is the caudal rectal artery which passes over the levator ani to the anal canal, as in the male. Then follows the large **perineal artery**; trace it to the anus and labia. The continuation of the internal pudendal is the **artery of the vestibular bulb**. It ramifies on the lateral surface of the vestibule and supplies the erectile tissue of the **vestibular bulb** (Fig. 4-31/8').

Remove the caudal part of the sacrosciatic ligament and the fascia from the lateral surface of the coccygeus and levator ani. The **coccygeus** arises aponeurotically from the ischial spine and inserts on the first few caudal vertebrae and the deep caudal fascia (Fig. 4-24/9). The caudal edge of the muscle may be demonstrated on the live horse by raising the tail.

The **levator ani** lies ventral to the coccygeus. It arises in similar fashion as the coccygeus and inserts on and around the anal canal as shown in Fig. 4-25.

The dorsal part of the **levator ani** inserts on the lateral wall of the anus between the external anal sphincter caudally and the retractor clitoridis (penis) cranially. Some bundles may pass over the dorsal surface of the anus, covered by the sphincter, to meet those of the other side (Fig. 4-25). The middle part of the levator runs around the ventral surface of the anus, joining the muscle of the other side to form a continuous fleshy subanal loop, which is closely associated with the cranial part of the external anal sphincter. The

ventral part inserts mainly on the fascia (perineal septum) between the anus and the vestibule.

Transect the coccygeus and levator and reflect the stumps cranially and caudally. The lateral wall of the rectum and the retractor penis (clitoridis) are now exposed (Fig. 4-26/6',6).

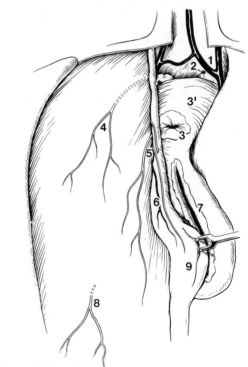

1.	Veins draining the tail	5.	Supf. perineal nerves
2.	Caudal rectal artery and anorectal lymph node	6.	Labial branch of perineal artery
3.	Anus, external anal sphincter at 3'	7.	Vulva
4.	Cutaneous nerve from ventral branch of S4	8.	Caudal cutaneous femoral nerve
		9.	Supf. fascia, reflected

FIGURE 4-23. Perineal vessels and nerves of the mare.

The **retractor penis** (clitoridis) is a band of smooth muscle that originates from the first and second caudal vertebrae and passes ventrally between the terminal part of the rectum and the levator ani.

It is a peculiarity of the horse that the greater part of the **retractor**, the rectal part, passes under the rectum to become continuous with the rectal part of the opposite muscle. Right and left retractor muscles also give off fibers that cross in the connective tissue between the anal canal and the male urethra or vestibule. From this decussation in the male the retractor passes ventrally to become incorporated in the penis. In the mare, the retractor passes around the ventral border of the levator ani and runs caudoventrally on the vestibule into the labium. It does not reach the clitoris.

With reference to Fig. 4-27 identify the four sacrocaudales and the small intertransversarii muscles on the transverse section of the tail. A double band of smooth muscle fibers, the **rectococcygeus**, derived from the longitudinal muscle coat of the rectum, lies ventral to the vertebra and extends as

far caudally as the fifth vertebra. The **median caudal artery** (from the caudal gluteal) lies also ventral to the vertebra.

It is possible, though not customary, to take the pulse on the median caudal artery. This artery can be used for measuring indirect blood pressure using a commercial cuff system. The skin and subcutis on the dorsal surface of the tail is much thicker than that on the ventral surface.

The sacrocaudalis dorsalis medialis muscle is surgically accessible for biopsy. This muscle is composed predominantly of slow-twitch fibers and has been used to confirm the diagnosis of equine motor neuron disease (EMND). EMND is a lower motor neuron disease that disproportionately affects type 1 muscle fibers.

0000000000—From here to the next row of zeros the dissection and description refer only to the **male**. Students working on a mare proceed to the next row of zeros, but should view the male

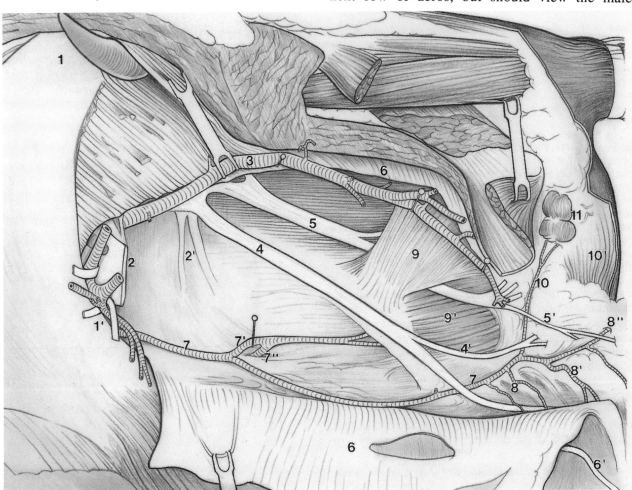

1.	Sacral tuber, cranial gluteal a. & n. at 1'	5.	Caudal rectal nerve, supf. perineal nerve at 5'	8.	Vestibular br., artery of vestibular bulb at 8', perineal artery at 8"
2.	Stump of sciatic nerve, pelvic nerve at 2'	6.	Sacrosciatic lig., cut and reflected, caudal cutaneous femoral nerve at 6'	9.	Coccygeus, levator ani at 9'
3.	Caudal gluteal artery, elevated	7.	Int. pudendal artery, vaginal artery at 7', uterine br. at 7"	10.	Caudal rectal artery, ext. anal sphincter at 10'
4.	Pudendal nerve, deep perineal nerve at 4'			11.	Anorectal lymph nodes

FIGURE 4-24. Left nerves and arteries after reflection of the sacrosciatic ligament in a mare, lateral view. Cranial is to the left.

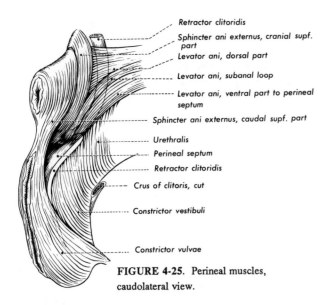

Retractor clitoridis
Sphincter ani externus, cranial supf. part
Levator ani, dorsal part
Levator ani, subanal loop
Levator ani, ventral part to perineal septum
Sphincter ani externus, caudal supf. part
Urethralis
Perineal septum
Retractor clitoridis
Crus of clitoris, cut
Constrictor vestibuli
Constrictor vulvae

FIGURE 4-25. Perineal muscles, caudolateral view.

dissection on a neighboring specimen.

In the male, remove the fascia from the ventral surface of the anal sphincter and distally as far as the line of skin reflection. The circular fibers of the bulbospongiosus are now exposed. The **bulbospongiosus** is the continuation of the urethralis and covers the corpus spongiosum. It is closely attached to the caudal and ventral surfaces of the corpus cavernosum. Contraction of the muscle aids in emptying the extrapelvic portion of the urethra.

Dissect between the anal sphincter and the proximal edge of the bulbospongiosus at the same time tensing the proximal end the **retractor penis**. Clean the loop formed by the rectal parts of right and left retractor muscles and trace the continuation of this muscle through the proximal part of the bulbospongiosus and out on the ventral surface of the penis (Fig. 4-28/6,7).

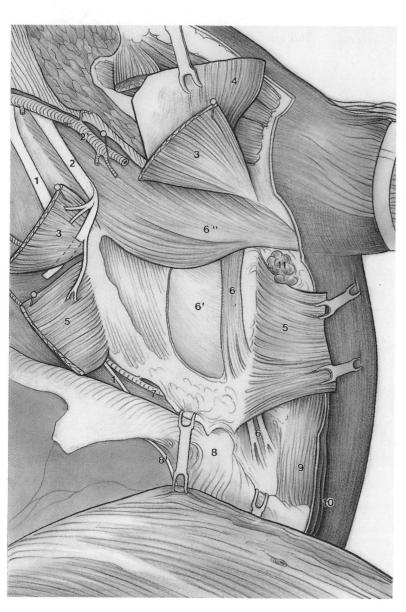

1. Pudendal nerve
2. Caudal rectal nerve, caudal gluteal artery at 2'
3. Coccygeus transected and reflected
4. Stump of semimembranosus, elevated
5. Levator ani transected and reflected
6. Retractor clitoridis, rectum at 6', 6" tail muscle
7. Internal pudendal artery
8. Ischial tuber, caudal cutaneous femoral nerve at 8'
9. Constrictor vulvae
10. Vulva
11. Anorectal lymph nodes

FIGURE 4-26. Structures lateral to the rectum in the mare, lateral view. Cranial is to the left.

From here to the next row of zeros the dissection is done only on the left side. There is not enough room for two students working so close together.

Remove the fascia between the bulbospongiosus and the semimembranosus, exposing the **ischiocavernosus**. This short, strong muscle, situated in a depression on the deep surface of the semimembranosus, passes from the ischial tuber to the crus and adjacent part of the body of the penis. Transect the ischiocavernosus and reflect the stumps to expose the cavernous **crus of the penis** in its center (Fig. 4-28/1'). The two crura unite below the ischial arch to form the corpus cavernosum.

Cut the left crus of the penis from the ischial arch and reflect it caudally. This exposes the deep artery of the penis (from the obturator) as its branches enter the deep (cranial) surface of the crus (Fig. 4-11/e').

Pick up the left **pudendal nerve** where it was last seen and, by displacing the pelvic viscera dorsomedially, trace it caudally. Note that it turns around the ischial arch close to the midline (Fig. 4-29/4). From here it is continued forward as the **dorsal nerve of the penis;** it may have been seen already in the transverse sections you made of the penis. The nerve supplies the ischiocavernosus, the corpus cavernosum and corpus spongiosum, and terminates in the prepuce and glans.

With the viscera and penis displaced, the **artery of the bulb** can be seen entering the bulbous beginning of the corpus spongiosum 2 to 3 cm dorsal to where the pudendal nerve winds around the ischial arch (Fig. 4-29/6').

It may be well before the male reproductive organs are removed to summarize the **blood supply of the penis** which is derived from three sources as shown in Figure 4-11:

1. The *cranial artery of the penis* (/a'; from the external pudendal) supplies the glans, prepuce, and cranial part of the corpus cavernosum.

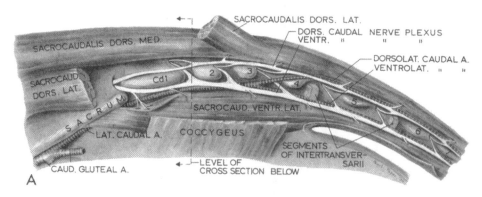

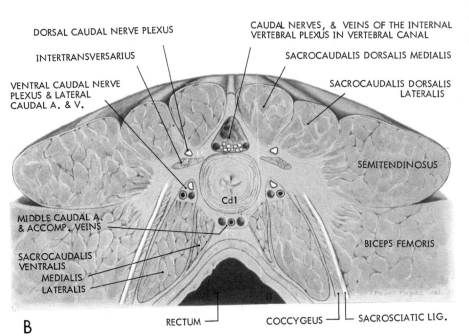

FIGURE 4-27. *A:* Dorsal and ventral nerve plexuses in the left half of the tail; lateral view. Cd 1-7, Transverse processes of caudal vertebrae. *B:* Transverse section between first and second caudal vertebrae, looking cranially. (From Hopkins, 1935.)

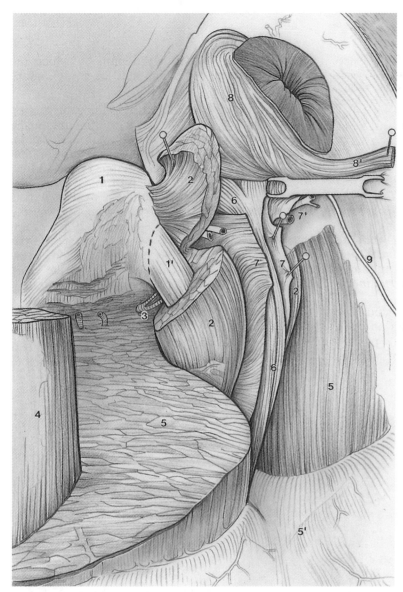

1. Ischial tuber, crus of penis at 1'
2. Ischiocavernosus, the left muscle transected and reflected
3. Deep artery of penis (from obturator)
4. Semitendinosus
5. Semimembranosus, the left muscle resected; reflected skin at 5'
6. Retractor penis
7. Bulbospongiosus, split where it covered the retractor penis; perineal a. & v. at 7'
8. External anal sphincter, median slip to the undersurface of the perineal skin at 8'
9. A supf. perineal nerve

FIGURE 4-28. The root of the penis with the left crus of the penis exposed, left caudolateral view.

2. The *artery of the bulb* (/h; from internal pudendal) enters the corpus spongiosum (as just seen).

3. The *deep artery of the penis* (/e';from the obturator) enters the crus and thus the corpus cavernosum with several branches. There is an inconstant proximal connection around the ischial arch to the internal pudendal artery, and a constant distal one (/c) to link up with the cranial artery of the penis.

0000000000—From here to the next row of zeros the dissection and description refer only to the **mare**. The dissection should be done only on the left.

Pick up the pudendal nerve where it was last seen giving off the deep perineal nerve. Cut the deep perineal fascia (urogenital diaphragm) which anchors the genital tract to the ischial tuber and arch. Displace the genital tract, rectum, and the coccygeus and levator muscles dorsomedially. The continuation of the pudendal nerve, the dorsal nerve of the clitoris, may now be exposed. It passes caudally ventral to the vestibule, crossing the ischial arch close to the contralateral nerve, and terminates in the clitoris as its sole sensory nerve (Fig. 4-31/1).

0000000000

Isolated Male Reproductive Organs

If your specimen is a mare, turn to "Isolated Female Reproductive Organs" farther on. Remember that you are responsible for both male and female anatomy.

To remove the pelvic viscera of the male: With a horizontal cut, transect the penis at the ischial arch. Beginning caudally, cut the rectum free from the roof of the pelvic cavity. Cut the genital fold and the mesorectum at their parietal attachments. Remove the pelvic viscera through the pelvic inlet, bluntly freeing the rectum and urethra from the surrounding connective tissue.

In urethrotomy the urethra is entered by making a median incision at the ischial arch between the retractor penis muscles and through the bulbospongiosus, corpus spongiosum, and urethral mucous membrane. See these structures on the horizontal transection of the peinis left on the horse and imagine that only skin covered its caudal surface.

If your specimen is a stallion the already isolated left testis should be removed with the rest of the reproductive organs as follows: Follow the left deferent duct from the urethra to where it enters the vaginal tunic at the vaginal ring. Free the tubelike vaginal tunic and pull it and the enclosed testis up through the supf. inguinal ring, widening the latter if necessary. Cut the right duct at its vaginal ring, and leave the right testis in the scrotum.

While the isolated (stallion) organs are studied on the table, two students could perform an open castration (p.59) on the right testis, paying particular attention to the disposition of vaginal tunic, ligaments, and mesorchium by which the testis is attached, and which must be cut to remove it.

Orient the pelvic viscera of gelding or stallion on the table and find (but do not trace) the **prostatic artery** and its cranial and caudal branches, which supply bladder, ureter, deferent duct, and a portion of the rectum (Fig. 4-13/8). More caudally, find the stump of the large (5 mm diameter) **artery of the bulb of the penis** and trace it to where it enters the corpus spongiosum at the caudal end of your specimen (Fig. 4-29/6'). Turn the specimen over and see the artery in the transverse section of the penis you made a few minutes ago at the ischial arch. It is the most caudal of the three arteries supplying the horse's penis (Fig. 4-11/f,h).

Dissect the rectum free and remove it from the urethra and incise the rectum in the middorsal line. The **internal anal sphincter** is the terminal thickening of the circular muscle of the rectum. It

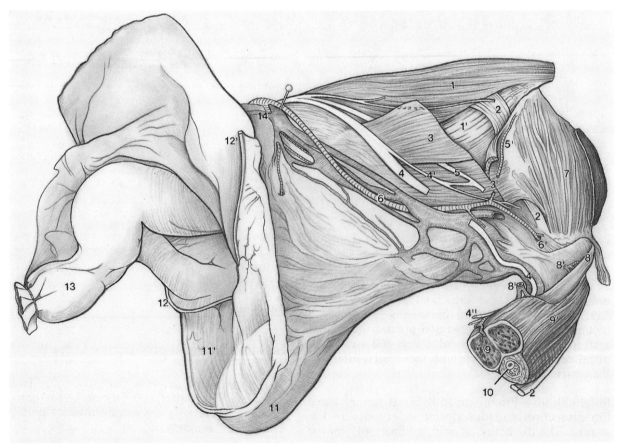

1. Tail muscle, recto-coccygeus at 1'
2. Retractor penis
3. Coccygeus, levator ani transected at 3'
4. Pudendal nerve, deep perineal nerve at 4', dorsal nerves of penis at 4"
5. Caudal rectal nerve, caudal rectal artery at 5'
6. Internal pudendal artery, a. of bulb of penis at 6'
7. Ext. anal sphincter
8. Crus of penis, deep a. of penis at 8'
9. Corpus cavernosum, ischiocavernosus at 9'
10. Urethra and corpus spongiosum, surrounded by bulbospongiosus
11. Bladder, right lateral lig. of bladder at 11'
12. Right deferent duct, left at 12'
13. Descending colon
14. Prostatic artery

FIGURE 4-29. Isolated rectum and male genitalia of a gelding, with penis transected close to its root; lateral view.

is thick and pale (smooth muscle) and lies between the external sphincter and the anal mucosa. The **external anal sphincter** is darker because it is striated voluntary muscle.

On the **PELVIC URETHRA** locate the genital fold and trace the two deferent ducts caudally through the fold. The elongated **vesicular glands** lie lateral to the ducts; their cranial extremities are covered by the peritoneum of the genital fold. They are 15-20 cm long in the stallion but are considerably reduced in the gelding. (You may hear them referred to as seminal vesicles occasionally.)

The insignificant **uterus masculinus** lies between the deferent ducts. It is a remnant of the paramesonephric ducts and is the homologue of the female uterus.

The deferent ducts and vesicular glands converge caudally and disappear beneath the isthmus of the **prostate**. Remove the fascia from its surface; it is composed of two lateral lobes and a connecting isthmus (Fig. 4-30/4).

Caudal to the prostate the urethra is covered by the circular fibers of the striated **urethralis**. At the level of the ischial arch incise the dorsal surface of this muscle sagittally and carefully reflect it laterally to expose the paired **bulbourethral gland**. This is small in the gelding but about 4 cm long in the stallion. The urethralis is continued on the extrapelvic portion of the urethra as the bulbospongiosus.

Open the **bladder** along the midventral line. Locate the cut ends of the ureters and probe the lumina caudally into the bladder. At the internal urethral orifice the mucosa of the bladder forms many small longitudinal fold. In the triangle formed by the ureteric and urethral orifices the mucosa is closely attached to the submucosa and does not form folds. This is the **trigone of the bladder**.

Continue the midventral incision caudally, opening the **pelvic urethra**. Locate the **colliculus seminalis** on the dorsal surface of the urethra. The vesicular glands and deferent ducts open side by side into a common **ejaculatory orifice** on each side of the colliculus. Probe the openings. Numerous small prostatic ductules open into the urethra craniolateral to the colliculus. Farther caudally the ducts of the bulbourethral glands open in two parallel rows on each side of the dorsal midline.

As the urethra turns around the ischial arch it joins the corpus cavernosum (derived from the crura) and the corpus spongiosum of the penis. The latter begins as an enlargement, the **bulb of the penis**, and more distally surrounds the urethra. The corpus spongiosum is covered by the bulbospongiosus. The structures, except for the bulb, were seen on the transverse sections you made of the penis (Fig. 4-30/13,14).

0000000000—The section from here to the next row of zeros refers to the stallion. If there is no stallion in the dissection room, study stock specimens. Consult your instructor. Students at Cornell should view the videotape "Genitalia of the Stallion," correlating it with this section.

The **scrotal wall** consists of two layers, the skin and tunica dartos. The skin is thin and oily and contains numerous sweat and sebaceous glands. It is marked by a median raphe which is continued cranially on the prepuce and caudally on the perineal region. The **dartos** is a layer of smooth muscle and connective tissue closely adherent to the skin. It forms the median **scrotal septum** which divides the scrotum into the two compartments for the testes.

The **spermatic fascia** lies between the dartos and the parietal vaginal tunic, is loosely attached to these structures, and contributes to the ease with which the testes slide along the scrotal wall. The **cremaster** inserts on the caudolateral surface of the vaginal tunic (Fig. 4-9/4). The tunic is invaginated along its caudal wall to provide the spermatic cord, testis, and epididymis with their serous covering, the visceral vaginal tunic (Fig. 4-7).

The **testis** of the horse lies in the scrotum with its long axis nearly in craniocaudal direction. The **epididymis** is attached to the dorsal border and overlaps the lateral surface of the testis. The enlarged head of the epididymis is attached to the cranial end of the testis where it receives the efferent ductules (Fig. 4-10/4). The body is narrow and connected to the testis by membrane which, together with the testis and epididymis, forms the testicular bursa. The bursa opens to the lateral side of the testis. The fold of visceral vaginal tunic between the enlarged tail of the epididymis and the caudal end of the testis is the proper ligament of the testis. The serous fold between the tail of the epididymis and the parietal vaginal tunic is the ligament of the tail of the epididymis. The two ligaments are remnants of the gubernaculum (/ 5, 6).

The deferent duct arises from the tail of the epididymis and, enclosed in a narrow serosal fold (mesoductus), passes dorsally into the inguinal canal. Note that the duct lies on the medial side of the spermatic cord.

In summary, the structures in the **spermatic cord** are:

1. The deferent duct has just been noted. It is suspended by the mesoductus deferens (Fig. 4-7).

2. The testicular artery passes to the testis in the cranial border of the cord. On the testis it runs close to the tunica albuginea from where it sends branches into the interior (Fig. 4-2).

3. The testicular veins form the pampiniform plexus around the .rtery.

4. The lymphatics of the testis and epididymis accompany the veins and ascend directly to the lumbar and medial iliac lymph nodes.

5. The testicular plexus of nerves accompanies the vessels. The nerves carry general visceral afferent fibers that are sensory to the testis and epididymis, and general visceral efferent fibers that are motor to the blood vessels.

6. Testicular vessels and nerves are enclosed by the mesorchium, a fold of serous membrane that attaches caudally to the parietal vaginal tunic and ends distally by forming the ligament of the tail of the epididymis (along with the mesoductus deferens).

565R

000000000000000

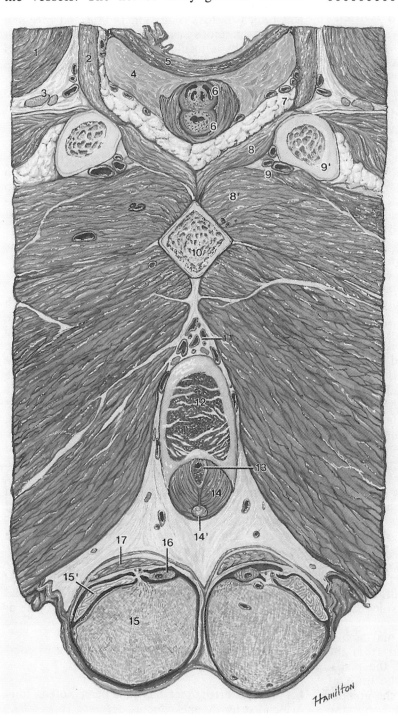

1. Gluteus medius
2. Levator ani
3. Sciatic nerve
4. Lobe of prostate
5. Wall of rectum
6. Pelvic urethra; deferent ducts and vesicular glands joining it at 6'
7. Internal pudendal vessels
8. Internal obturator muscle, external obturator at 8'
9. Obturator vessels; ischium just caudal to acetabulum at 9'
10. Caudal branches of pubic bones fused in the pelvic symphysis
11. Venous plexus and dorsal arteries and nerves of penis
12. Corpus cavernosum enclosed by tunica albuginea
13. Penile urethra within corpus spongiosum
14. Bulbospongiosus; retractor penis at 14'
15. Testis; epididymis at 15'
16. Deferent duct
17. Cremaster

FIGURE 4-30. Transverse section of the stallion's scrotum and penis and of the lower part of the pelvis at the level of the obturator foramen (space between 9' and 10).

Isolated Female Reproductive Organs

To remove the pelvic viscera of the mare:
Beginning caudally, cut the rectum free from the
tail and the roof of the pelvic cavity. Cut the
mesorectum and the broad ligaments at their
parietal attachments. Cut the vaginal artery close
to its origin so that it remains on the viscera.
Return to the back of the specimen and free the
vulva from the ischial arch by cutting close to the
bone. By pushing your hand forward ventral to
the urethra free the viscera also ventrally and
remove them through the pelvic inlet.

When the vulva is cut from the ischial arch the
two crura of the **clitoris** are severed as they pass

ventrally from the arch. Find them on your
isolated specimen (Fig. 4-31/12). The crura join
to form the body of the clitoris which extends into
the ventral commissure of the vulva. Crura and
body constitute the erectile tissue of the corpus
cavernosum which is homologous to the corpus
cavernosum of the penis. Transect the body of the
clitoris midway and see its erectile tissue and heavy
tunica albuginea.

Orient the pelvic viscera on the table. Pick up
the **vaginal artery** and trace its branches. The
first and largest branch is the uterine which turns
cranially, gives off the caudal vesical, and passes
cranially on the uterus to anastomose with the
uterine artery (Fig. 4-13/9). The vaginal artery

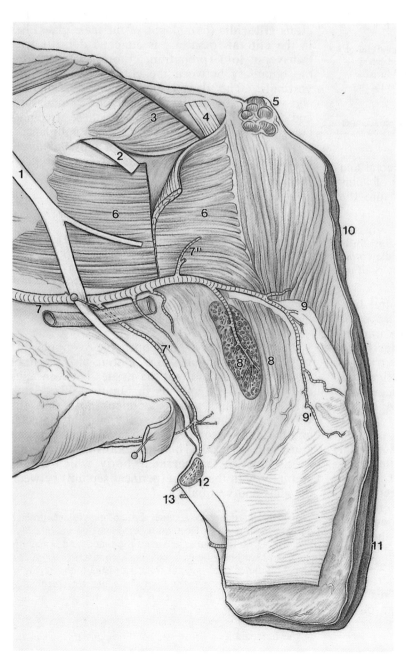

1. Pudendal nerve
2. Caudal rectal nerve
3. Proximal stump of coccygeus
4. Prox. part of retractor clitoridis
5. Anorectal lymph nodes
6. Levator ani, transected
7. Internal pudendal a. & v., vestibular brr. at 7',
   caudal rectal artery at 7"
8. Constrictor vestibuli, fenestrated to show
   vestibular bulb with its artery at 8'
9. Perineal arteries, labial branch at 9'
10. Anus
11. Vulva
12. Left crus of clitoris
13. Artery of clitoris (from obturator)

FIGURE 4-31. Caudal portion of isolated rectum and
genitalia of a mare, lateral view.

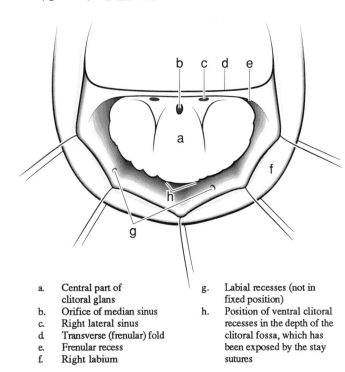

a. Central part of
   clitoral glans
b. Orifice of median sinus
c. Right lateral sinus
d. Transverse (frenular) fold
e. Frenular recess
f. Right labium
g. Labial recesses (not in
   fixed position)
h. Position of ventral clitoral
   recesses in the depth of the
   clitoral fossa, which has
   been exposed by the stay
   sutures

FIGURE 4-32. The glans of the clitoris exposed by the retraction of the ventral ends of the labia; schematic.

continues caudally, gives off the middle rectal and supplies the vagina. Note the rich plexus of veins in the wall of the vagina which drains into the internal pudendal veins.

Transect the **constrictor vestibuli** and reflect it dorsally and ventrally to expose the oval **vestibular bulb**. This is a patch of erectile tissue homologous to the corpus spongiosum of the male. It is supplied by the artery of the vestibular bulb (Fig. 4-31/8').

Open the **bladder** along the midventral line. Locate the cut ends of the ureters and probe the lumina caudally into the bladder. At the internal urethral orifice the mucosa of the bladder forms many small longitudinal folds. In the triangle formed by the ureteric and urethral orifices the mucosa is closely attached to the submucosa and does not form folds. This is the **trigone of the bladder**.

Determine the caudal extent of the **rectogenital pouch** between the rectum and the genital tract. Then transect the rectum (only) about 10 cm cranial to the anus and remove the segment of the rectum that is cranial to the transection, so that the anal canal alone remains on the specimen. Remove the feces from the anal canal. At the level of the caudal extent of the rectogenital pouch make a midline stab incision (with the scalpel) through the dorsal wall of the genital tract, large enough to admit one finger into the lumen of the tract. Did you gain access into the vagina or the cervix? You will know better when the tract is opened in a little while.

The length of the vagina that is covered dorsally with peritoneum depends on the fullness of the rectum. The fuller the rectum, the less vagina is covered with peritoneum. When the rectum is empty, usually the cranial 10 cm of the roof of the vagina are covered. This is of significance to surgeons who enter the peritoneal cavity through a similar, but reversed, stab incision such as you made on your specimen. This "bloodless" transvaginal approach (colpotomy) is used occasionally for the removal of the ovaries (ovariectomy).

Incise the attached anal canal in the middorsal line. The **internal anal sphincter** is the terminal thickening of the circular muscle of the rectum. It is thick and pale (smooth muscle) and lies between the external sphincter and the anal mucosa (Fig. 4-33/2). The **external anal sphincter** is darker because it is striated voluntary muscle.

Part the labia at the ventral commissure. The **glans clitoridis** (homologue of the male glans) lies in the clitoral fossa and is attached dorsally to a transverse fold (preputium clitoridis) that forms the boundary between the clitoral fossa and the vestibule. The glans is thus surrounded laterally and ventrally by the labia and ventral commissure, and dorsally by the transverse fold, these structures being known as the prepuce of the clitoral glans.

The glans is well developed in the mare. Probe the sinuses and recesses labeled in Fig. 4-32.

During estrus the clitoral glans may be alternately protruded and withdrawn between the labia ("winking").

The sinuses in the periphery of the glans harbor the organism responsible for contagious equine metritis (CEM). CEM was first diagnosed in the United States in 1978 and has since been eradicated from this country. Imported mares over 2 years of age that originate from countries in which CEM still exists must have repeated negative cultures of the clitoral sinuses in order to obtain an import permit.

Palpate the cervix and open the vestibule and vagina in the middorsal line, cutting also the floor of the anal canal so that the tissues between anus and vestibule are split as in Figure 4-33. Using this Figure and your specimen, note that the vertical fiber bundles of the external anal sphincter and the constrictor vulvae are continuous between anus and vulva. This musculofibrous column forms most of the **perineal body** which blends cranially with the fascia (perineal septum) between the anus and vestibule.

Birth in mares is a rather fast, often violent, process during which perineal lacerations sometimes occur. In severe lacerations, the tissues between the anus and vestibule (perineal body) may be torn, creating a common cavity. Fecal contamination of the genital tract necessitates the repair of this type of defect if the mare is to be sound for breeding. A common management approach is to allow the wound to heal followed in 4-6 weeks by surgical correction of the defect. Two horizontal shelves of tissue are fashioned from the edge of the retracted scar tissue and careful approximation of the shelves in two layers recreates walls to separate the digestive from the urogenital tract.

Repair of a laceration of the perineal body is often accomplished with the use of regional anesthesia to desensitize the area and control straining. Epidural anesthesia is administered through the interarcuate space between the first two caudal vertebrae. The dose of local anesthetic agent can be titrated to effect to achieve analgesia of the sensory nerves to the perineum (pudendal and caudal rectal)

The **external urethral orifice** is located on the floor of the vestibule about 12 cm from the ventral commissure of the vulva. The **vestibule** extends cranially from the labia of the vulva to the fleshy transverse flap that rises from the floor and overhangs the urethral orifice. In fillies the ends of the flap are continued on the lateral walls, constricting the entrance to the vagina and forming an incomplete hymen. The minute orifices of the **vestibular glands** may be seen in rows on the floor and roof of the vestibule.

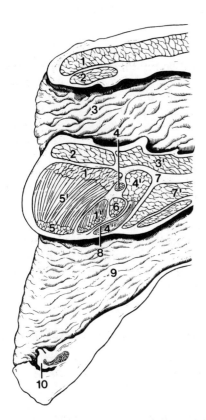

1. External anal sphincter, cran. supf. and deep parts at 1'	fibers continuous from ext. anal sphincter to constrictor vulvae at 5'
2. Internal anal sphincter	
3. Anal canal, rectal musculature at 3'	6. Subanal loop of levator ani
4. Clitoral part, 4' rectal part, 4" decussation of retractor clitoridis	7. Rectovaginal septum, vaginal musculature at 7'
	8. Perineal septum
	9. Vestibule
5. Constrictor vulvae, muscular	10. Glans of clitoris

FIGURE 4-33. Median section through the anus, perineal body, and vestibule.

Examine the part of the cervix (portio vaginalis) that projects into the **vagina**. In its center is the **external uterine orifice** surrounded by folds of cervical mucosa. The vagina is relatively long; its fornix projects farther forward dorsally than ventrally. The dorsal part of the fornix may be bisected by a substantial median fold. Now open the cervical canal, the body of the uterus, and one horn.

The **cervix** is about 6 cm long and tightly closed (except during parturition) by the thick spirally arranged muscle coats your longitudinal cut has exposed. The cervical epithelium secretes a tenacious mucous plug which closes the cervical canal during pregnancy. Grasp the vagina with one hand and then the cervix to notice the difference in consistency and thickness caused by the expanded cervical muscle coat.

The **body of the uterus** is about 20 cm long. The horns are slightly longer.

Did your stab incision from the caudalmost point in the rectogenital pouch enter the vagina?

Exercises on the Live Animal

Caution: If you are alone, do these exercises only if the horse is secured in stocks.

1---With reference to Fig. 4-14 palpate the coxal, sacral, and ischial tubers. The first lies under the skin—easily palpated; the second is just lateral to the dorsal midline a little caudal to the level of the first—difficult to palpate in well muscled horses; the third is covered by the semimembranosus—palpate deeply with the bottom of your palm lateral to the middle of the vulva. Palpate the spinous processes of the sacrum.
2---The line connecting coxal and ischial tubers on one side indicates the slope of the pelvis. Palpate the high caudal part of the greater trochanter of the femur on this line. It is covered by the biceps and requires deep palpation with the bottom of your palm. The greater trochanter is surprisingly close to the ischial tuber. Its lower cranial part is also palpable.
3---Raise the tail and see the narrow perineal region between the bulges of the semimembranosus muscles; it includes anus and vulva. With someone holding the tail, part the labia and observe the clitoral glans. In the male, palpate the rounded bulbospongiosus ventral to the anus. Do not attempt to palpate the prepuce and penis, or the udder.

5

HINDLIMB

Purpose and Plan of the Dissection

1---To see the distribution of the internal iliac artery on the inner aspect of the pelvic wall and the nerves vulnerable during parturition.

2---To follow the course of the (subcutaneous) saphenous veins and nerve in the limb and to explore their origin and the deep inguinal lymph nodes in the femoral triangle.

3---To see the break-up of the sciatic nerve deep to the biceps and to locate the resulting peroneal and tibial nerves in the leg (crus).

4---To study the components of the passive stay-apparatus that connect stifle and hock and cause these joints to move in unison.

5---To become familiar with the tendons and their tendon sheaths passing over the hock, with the tarsal bones, and with the joint capsules, bursae, ligaments, and retinacula associated with this important composite joint.

6---To know the bones in the metatarsus and the tendons and interosseus that accompany them to the fetlock (metatarsophalangeal) joint, and to locate the plantar and plantar metatarsal nerves.

7---To follow the principal arteries from the level of the hip joint to the fetlock.

8---To study the patellar, collateral, and cruciate ligaments, and the menisci and joint capsules of the stifle joint; and to see the resting surfaces on patella and femoral trochlea which together with the medial and intermediate patellar ligaments enable the horse to lock this joint.

Plan. The hindquarters are lowered to the floor and split in the median plane; the two hindlimbs are now light enough to be dissected on the table. The medial thigh muscles are reflected to expose the course of the femoral vessels. Next the muscles near the hip joint are dissected and cut, and the

joint disarticulated so the half-pelvis can be discarded. The crural fasciae are reflected to follow the peroneal nerve to the hock. While the muscles of the leg are individually transected and reflected to their attachments at the hock and beyond, the tendon sheaths and bursae they form, and the arteries passing to the hock are exposed. Then follows the dissection of the tendons, nerves, and blood vessels as they pass into the metatarsus, stopping at the fetlock joint since the digit is studied only on the forelimb (next chapter). With the tendons reflected off the hock, the joint capsules and articular surfaces are exposed for study. Similarly, removal of the thick fascia on the cranial surface of the stifle and of the vessels and the popliteus on the caudal surface exposes this joint for detailed study of its ligaments and joint capsules. Finally, the locking mechanism of the stifle and the remaining parts of the stay-ap—paratus are passively worked as far as that is possible with an embalmed specimen.

Thigh, Leg, Tarsus, and Metatarsus

(If a hindlimb, disarticulated at the hip joint, from the post mortem room is to be dissected, start at the row of zeroes on page 85.)

To split the specimen into right and left halves: *Lower the specimen to the floor so that it rests on the hocks and the ischial tubers, and remove the hook. With a large knife cut the abdominal wall along the ventral midline to the pubis, staying on one side of the prepuce. Insert a saw into the pelvic cavity and saw ventrally through the pelvic symphysis. Spread the limbs a little and with a large knife, cut the tissues and skin ventral to the symphysis, keeping the penis to one side, but caudally you better split the penis. Beginning*

80

cranially, split the lumbar vertebrae aiming the saw for the promontory so as to stay in the median plane. Split sacrum and tail in the same way. If, when the limbs drop apart, the vertebral canal has not been fully opened, open it with a second cut.

Remove the flap of abdominal wall close to the thigh, cutting the internal abdominal oblique in the process. Remove the previously reflected

large, lateral flap of skin from the thigh. Wash the cut surfaces with water and sponge and place the limb on the table medial side up. (End of instructions for splitting hind quarters)

Examine the opened vertebral canal. The spinal cord terminates in the second sacral vertebra.

The **INTERNAL ILIAC ARTERY** is very short and lies ventrolateral to the body of L5, where it bifurcates into internal pudendal and caudal gluteal arteries (Fig. 4-13). The **internal pudendal** passes caudally in the lateral wall of the pelvic cavity and gives origin to the previously seen umbilical artery. Trace these two vessels to where they were cut when the pelvic viscera were removed. The **caudal gluteal artery** passes caudally in the dorsolateral wall of the pelvic cavity deep to the dorsal attachment of the sacrosciatic ligament. At about the middle of the sacrum it pierces the ligament and sends several substantial branches into the biceps and semitendinosus which have been seen when these muscles were reflected. The caudal gluteal also gives rise to the arteries of the tail which have also been seen in transverse section when the tail was removed.

At its origin the caudal gluteal gives off the **cranial gluteal artery** which immediately gives rise to the iliolumbar (concealed, so don't look for it) and the large obturator artery. The cranial gluteal passes laterally through the greater sciatic foramen and was seen entering the gluteus medius when that muscle was removed from the lateral surface of the sacrosciatic ligament; it is accompanied by the cranial gluteal nerve. The **obturator artery** gives off the iliacofemoral which has already been seen on the lateral side on the vastus lateralis, after the reflection of the tensor fasciae latae. The obturator artery and nerve may be seen with little dissection passing caudoventrally on the shaft of the ilium to, and through, the obturator foramen which is covered by the internal obturator muscle. In the male the obturator artery supplies the adductors and gives rise to the middle and deep arteries of the penis (Figure 4-11/e,e'). In the mare the obturator artery supplies the adductors and gives off a caudal branch to the clitoris, the artery of the clitoris, which has been exposed.

The **thigh** is the part of the limb between the hip and stifle joints. The **leg** (crus) is the part of the limb between the stifle and hock joints. The hock joint is also known as the tarsus. The **metatarsus** is the part of the limb between the hock and fetlock (metatarsophalangeal) joints and contains the large metatarsal or cannon bone. The part distal to the cannon bone is the **digit** (Fig. 5-1).

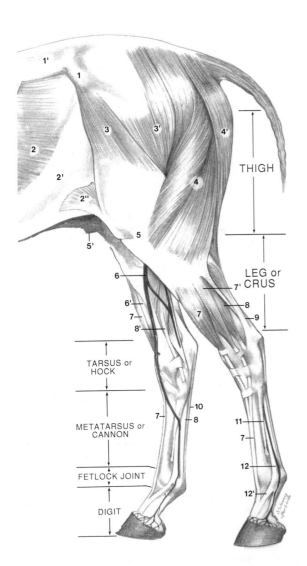

1. Coxal tuber, lumbar muscles at 1'
2. External abdominal oblique, its aponeurosis at 2'; 2" stump of cutaneous muscle of the trunk forming stifle fold
3. Tensor fasciae latae, supf. gluteal muscle at 3'
4. Biceps, semitendinosus at 4'
5. Stifle, sheath at 5'
6. Medial saphenous vein, tibialis cranialis at 6'
7. Long digital extensor, lat. dig. extensor at 7'
8. Deep digital flexor, its medial dig. flexor at 8'
9. Common calcanean tendon
10. Supf. digital flexor
11. Mt4, lateral splint bone
12. Interosseus, its extensor branch at 12'

FIGURE 5-1. Superficial structures and the common divisions of the hindlimbs. (From Ellenberger-Dittrich-Baum by Horowitz/Geary.)

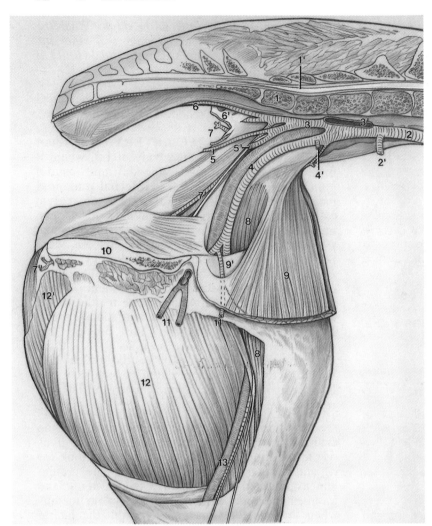

1. L6, Spinal cord at 1'
2. Aorta, caudal mesenteric a. at 2'
3. Internal iliac a., stump of right iliac arteries at 3'
4. Ext. iliac vessels, uterine a. at 4'
5. Int. pudendal a., umbilical a. at 5'
6. Caudal gluteal a., roots of sciatic nerve at 6'
7. Cranial gluteal a., obturator vessels and nerve at 7', a. of clitoris at 7"
8. Sartorius
9. Int. abdominal oblique, deep inguinal ring at 9'
10. Pelvic symphysis
11. Vessels for udder
12. Gracilis, semimembranosus at 12'
13. Medial saphenous v., saphenous a. and nerve

FIGURE 5-2. Left pelvis and thigh of a mare after removal of pelvic viscera and udder, medial view.

Examine the chestnut and ergot. The **chestnut** is a horny excrescence found on the medial surface proximal to the carpus and at the distal end of the tarsus. On the carpus it is regarded as a vestige of the carpal pad. (The dog has a carpal pad.) On the tarsus it is a vestige of the tarsal pad. (The dog has no tarsal pad, but the bear and other plantigrade animals do.) The **ergot** (French for spur) is located in a tuft of hair on the back of the fetlock joint and is a vestige of the metatarsal or metacarpal pad (present in the dog).

*During the dissection of the limb, refer to the skeleton whenever bony structures are mentioned. Make skin incisions along the cranial and caudal borders of the limb to the level of the chestnut and remove the skin from the medial surface of thigh, leg, and hock, preserving the superficial fascia. **Important:** Keep the parts of the limb not actually being dissected wrapped in cloth soaked in a mold-inhibiting solution and plastic.*

Both the cranial gluteal and obturator nerves lie on bones facing the birth canal which exposes them to injury during parturition (see skeleton). "Obturator" paralysis is an uncommon post-foaling complication in the mare; this type of injury is far more common in cows. Ipsilateral signs of nerve damage range from stiffness to paraplegia and may be accompanied by loss of muscle mass.

Look for an inconstant subcutaneous calcanean bursa in the superficial fascia over the point of the hock (calcanean tuber).

Enlarged inconstant bursae over the olecranon (point of elbow) and calcanean tubers (point of hock) are conditions known as capped elbow and capped hock, respectively.

On the medial surface of the thigh locate the **medial saphenous vein** as it emerges between the sartorius and gracilis muscles (Fig. 5-2/13). It is a branch of the femoral vein which lies deeper. Trace the medial saphenous over the stifle to the proximal part of the leg where it bifurcates (Fig. 5-1/6). The **caudal branch** passes caudodistally and runs in the depression between the common calcanean tendon and deep digital flexor to the hock. The **cranial branch** continues distally, crossing the medial surface of the tibia, and anastomoses with the cranial tibial vein at the hock. It ends on the dorsomedial surface of the hock by giving rise to the large **dorsal common digital vein II** and a smaller inconstant middle dorsal metatarsal vein. The dorsal common digital vein II passes obliquely distally over the medial surface of the metatarsus where it can be palpated.

Open the fascia over the medial saphenous vein and locate the small **saphenous artery** on its cranial border. The artery is distributed variously, but in most horses it passes to the plantaromedial surface of the hock where it gives rise to the medial and lateral plantar arteries (Fig. 5-14).

The **saphenous nerve** emerges between the sartorius and gracilis cranial to the artery (Fig. 5-2/13). It immediately breaks into cutaneous branches which ramify on the medial and cranial surfaces of the limb (Fig. 5-12/B).

One **branch of the saphenous nerve** accompanies the cranial branch of the medial saphenous vein over the hock and ramifies on the medial surface of the metatarsus as far distally as the fetlock. It cannot be traced that far grossly (Fig. 5-12/B).

Remove the remainder of the internal abdominal oblique, cutting it at the prepubic tendon and the coxal tuber. Then transect the inguinal ligament and aponeurosis of the external abdominal oblique midway between these two points and reflect the stumps medially and laterally. This exposes the upper part of the **femoral triangle,** a space between the sartorius cranially, the pectineus caudally, the external abdominal oblique aponeurosis medially, and the quadriceps laterally. The vascular lacuna, the (dorsal) base of the narrow femoral triangle, was seen when we traced the external iliac vessels to their disappearance caudal to the inguinal ligament. The triangle contains the femoral vessels and the **deep inguinal lymph nodes** which receive nearly all the lymph from the hindlimb.

Clean the sartorius, transect it at the level of the pubis, and reflect the stumps, completely opening the femoral triangle. Demonstrate the origin of the medial saphenous vein and accompanying artery from the femoral vessels by probing and sharp dissection, but be careful not to cut the saphenous nerve. The saphenous nerve is a branch of the large and important **femoral nerve** (L4-L6). The femoral nerve is seen passing between the rectus femoris and the vastus medialis, the cranial and medial heads, respectively, of the **quadriceps femoris** (Fig. 5-4/2,9). The extensor action of the quadriceps on the stifle is essential to the support of the limb. If the femoral nerve is damaged, this extensor action is lost and the whole limb collapses because the hock will not remain extended if the stifle is flexed. The reason for this will be demonstrated when we dissect the muscles of the leg(crus).

The wide **gracilis** lies caudal to the sartorius and covers the greater part of the medial surface of the thigh. Clean the boundaries of the muscle. Cut it free from its origin on the pelvic symphysis, pubis, and prepubic tendon and reflect it distally; the medial saphenous vein will have to be transected at its origin for this reflection (Fig. 5-4/8). Isolate the semimembranosus. Cut the muscle free from its ischial origin and reflect it distally. Transect the **adductor** just ventral to its origin on the pubis and ischium. Reflect it distally, cutting its insertions off the caudal surface of the femur. At the distal third of the femur the femoral vessels perforate the adductor and pass obliquely laterally on the caudal surface of the femur to disappear between the two heads of the gastrocnemius (Fig. 5-6/7',9).

Identify the **pectineus** and clean its origin on the pubis and accessory ligament (to be seen shortly); transect the muscle leaving a *short* (2cm) proximal stump.

Remove the deep inguinal lymph nodes to expose the femoral vessels more fully. Locate the cross section of the external pudendal vein at the cranial end of the pelvic symphysis. Just cranial to the vein and between it and the proximal stump of the pectineus palpate the round, thick **accessory**

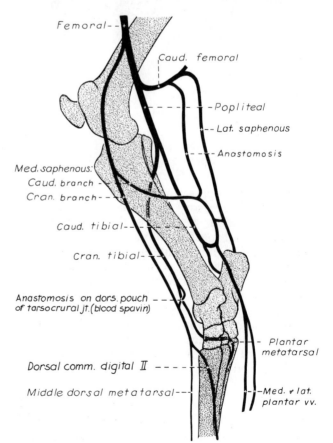

FIGURE 5-3. Veins of right hindlimb, medial view.

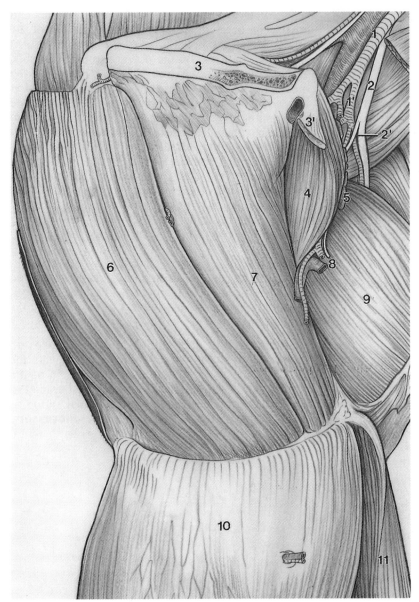

1. External iliac vessels, femoral artery at 1'
2. Femoral nerve, saphenous nerve at 2'
3. Pelvic symphysis, part of prepubic tendon at 3'
4. Pectineus
5. Deep inguinal lymph nodes
6. Semimembranosus
7. Adductor
8. Medial saphenous vein, and saphenous a. & n.
9. Vastus medialis
10. Gracilis, reflected
11. Sartorius, reflected

FIGURE 5-4. Medial view of left thigh after reflecting sartorius and gracilis.

ligament which passes away from you as the vein does. The accessory ligament arises from the prepubic tendon, perforates the origin of the pectineus and passes laterally on the ventral surface of the pubis, entering the acetabulum at the **acetabular notch** (see skeleton). It attaches on the head of the femur next to the ligament of the femoral head (Fig. 5-5). Of the domestic animals, only the Equidae possess an accessory ligament. It limits pronation (turning in) of the hindlimb. In addition it is thought to be a factor for the low incidence of hip joint dislocation in the horse. It will be traced into the hip joint later.

There are many paragraphs set in small print which could be left out. Ask an instructor which should be done and which not.

The **prepubic tendon,** which was bisected when the pelvis was split, is a mass of fibrous tissue that combines the tendinous attachments of the pectineus, rectus abdominis, and parts of the abdominal oblique and gracilis muscles on the pubic bones and the symphysial tendon below them (Fig. 5-5). It occasionally ruptures in late pregnancy.

Transect the femoral vessels and nerve at the level of the pubis and reflect the stumps. Clean the area exposed and locate the insertion of the **iliopsoas** (iliacus + psoas major) on the lesser trochanter of the femur.

The **iliopsoas** is an important locomotor muscle. After the completion of a stride, the iliopsoas draws the limb forward flexing it at the hip. The action of the quadriceps on the stifle causes the stifle and hock to be extended as the foot contacts the ground. Now the propulsion phase is initiated, and the caudal thigh muscles (biceps, semimembranosus, semitendinosus) together with the large mass of the gluteus medius drive the body forward over the limb. Then the cycle repeats with the iliopsoas returning the limb to the forward position. (Other muscles are involved in the stride; this description is greatly simplified.)

*We next separate the pelvis from the hindlimb by disarticulating the hip joint. This can be done in two ways: by radical cuts with a large knife or by a time-consuming step-by-step dissection. **Ask an instructor which to use.** The step-by-step dissection follows in small type; the radical separation follows the small type.*

Remove the deep femoral vessels which lie between the external obturator and the iliopsoas (Fig. 5-6/2",4,1'). Transect the iliopsoas at its insertion on the lesser trochanter of the femur and reflect the proximal stump dorsally, hooking it to the sublumbar muscles. This reflection usually opens the *hip joint* as its capsule adheres to the caudal surface of the muscle. Isolate and transect the medial tendon of origin of the rectus femoris on the ilium and clean the origin of the vastus medialis on the neck of the femur. Open the cranial aspect of the hip joint fully, and isolate the **transverse ligament** which bridges the acetabular notch on the medial surface of the joint.

The following structures can now be seen: The pyramidal external obturator passes laterally from its origin on the ventral surface of the pelvis to the trochanteric fossa on the femur (see skeleton); the **accessory ligament** passes into the hip joint dorsal to the transverse ligament; an extension of the hip joint capsule or a separate bursa lies between the accessory ligament and the ventral surface of the pubis; a small extension of the hip joint capsule lies between the accessory and transverse ligaments; and another large extension of the joint capsule lies between the femur and the external obturator, extending ventrally to the insertion of the quadratus femoris.

Isolate the external obturator by passing your finger around its caudal aspect, transect the muscle close to the femur, and remove the proximal stump piecemeal from the ventral surface of the pelvis. Isolate the slender quadratus femoris, transect it, and reflect the stumps dorsally and ventrally. It is now possible to open the caudomedial surface of the hip joint.

Roll the limb so that the caudal surface is up. Find the proximal end of the sciatic nerve on the surface of the gluteus profundus and avoid cutting it in the following dissection. Cut the **semitendinosus** (including the branches of the obturator vessels entering it) from the ventral surface of the pelvis. Cut the attachment of the *biceps* on the ischial tuber. Now transect both muscles at the level of the greater trochanter and discard their vertebral heads.

Roll the limb so that the lateral surface is up. The gluteus profundus arises from the ischial spine and adjacent shaft of the ilium and inserts on the cranial part of the greater trochanter. Transect the muscle near its origin and reflect it off the hip joint. (The gemellus and internal obturator are usually included in this reflection; do not identify them.) Transect the gluteus again close to the trochanter and remove it, including the sheet of fascia deep to it.

The fibrous layer of the capsule of the hip joint is heavy and modified to form strengthening, ligamentous bands. Open the joint and see the head of the femur already lifting away from the acetabulum. Identify and cut the insignificant articularis coxae muscle and the lateral tendon of origin of the rectus femoris.

Turn the limb again so that the medial surface is up and cut the accessory ligament and the ligament of the femoral head from the fovea on the head of the femur. The limb and pelvis should now be completely separated. Skip the next paragraph.

Locate the proximal end of the sciatic nerve and preserve it while transecting all the muscles in the vicinity of the hip joint with a large knife and disarticulating the joint in the acetabulum. After removal of the pelvis, the top end of the hindlimb should look like that in Fig. 5-7.

The fundamental difference between the equine **HIP JOINT** and that of the other domestic mammals is that the horse has an accessory ligament. Examine the **acetabulum**. The bony margin is supplemented by a fibrous rim. The sunken, nonarticular area in the acetabulum is the acetabular fossa. The articular surface of the acetabulum is interrupted ventrally by the **acetabular notch**. The notch is bridged by the **transverse ligament**, a continuation of the fibrous rim. The ligament of the femoral head and the accessory ligament pass through the notch dorsal to the transverse ligament. Note the location of the fovea capitis on the medial margin of the head of the femur (Fig. 5-5).

0000000000—(From here on, a fresh limb disarticulated at the hip joint can—with some adjustments—be used.)

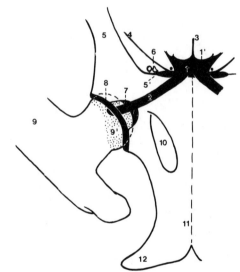

1. Prepubic tendon, insertion tendon of rectus abdominis at 1'
2. Accessory ligament
3. Linea alba
4. Inguinal ligament
5. Shaft of ilium, iliopubic eminence at 5'
6. Femoral artery and vein
7. Acetabular notch
8. Transverse ligament (of acetabulum)
9. Femur, head at 9'
10. Obturator foramen
11. Pelvic symphysis
12. Ischial tuber

FIGURE 5-5. A schematic ventral view of the prepubic tendon and accessory ligament. The two dots mark the medial extent of the inguinal canals. (After Preuss, Budras, and Traeder, 1972.)

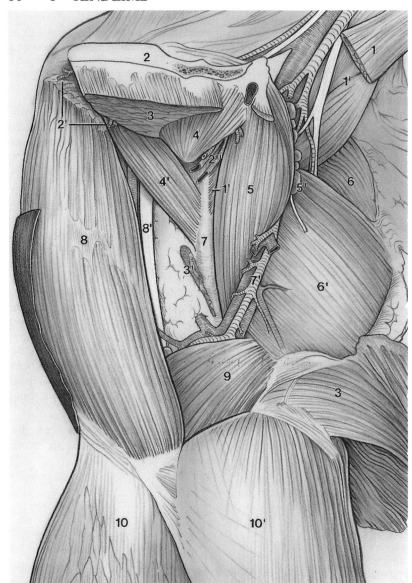

1. Sartorius, iliopsoas at 1'
2. Pelvic symphysis, obturator branches at 2', deep femoral branches at 2"
3. Stumps of adductor, intermediate insertion on femur at 3'
4. External obturator, quadratus femoris at 4'
5. Pectineus, deep inguinal lymph nodes at 5'
6. Rectus femoris, vastus medialis at 6'
7. Femur, femoral vessels at 7'
8. Semitendinosus, sciatic nerve at 8'
9. Medial head of gastrocnemius
10. Gracilis and 10' semimembranosus, reflected

FIGURE 5-6. Medial view of left thigh after reflecting semimembranosus and adductor.

Turn the limb so the lateral surface is up. Remove the skin from the lateral surface as far as was done on the medial surface (level of the chestnut). While this is being done, another student should make longitudinal skin incisions along the dorsal and plantar borders of the metatarsus and remove the skin on the lateral surface of the metatarsus to the middle of the fetlock joint.

Palpate, but do not dissect, the three distal divisions of the **biceps** (Fig. 5-7/4,4',4"). If overlying fascia and fat prevents you from determining the boundaries of the three divisions, remove the superficial fascia and fascia lata from the surface of the muscle, working from caudodorsal to cranioventral. The cranial division inserts on the lateral border of the patella (palpable). The middle division inserts by way of the middle layer of crural fascia on the lateral patellar ligament and the tibial crest (palpable).

The caudal division inserts by means of a thickened band of the middle crural fascia on the calcanean tuber, as will be seen later.

Palpate the insertion of the gluteus superficialis on the **third trochanter** (see skeleton), and remove the muscle leaving a small stump (Fig. 5-7/5'). Fractures with complete separation of the trochanter have occurred. Remove the tensor fasciae latae, cutting the fascia lata close to the stifle joint.

Separate the caudal border of the biceps from the semitendinosus and the cranial border from the vastus lateralis. (The ischial origin of the biceps has already been severed.) Preserving the sciatic nerve, reflect the biceps distally off the lateral head of the gastrocnemius. *Caution: Do not cut the common peroneal nerve in the process; it looks like a branch of the sciatic nerve into the biceps.*

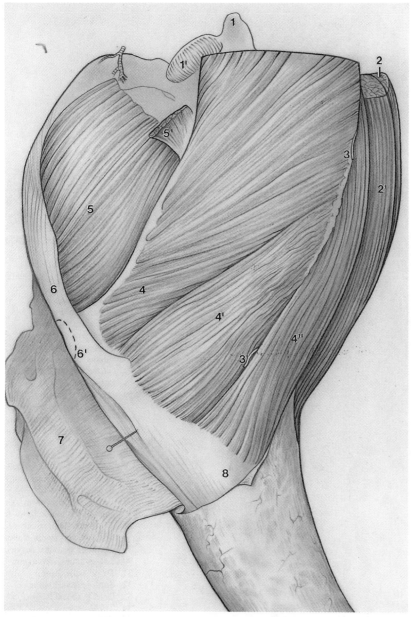

1. Caudal part of greater trochanter, trochanteric bursa at 1'
2. Semimembranosus, semitendinosus at 2'
3. Caudal cutaneous femoral nerve, lateral cutaneous sural nerve at 3'
4, 4', 4" Cranial, middle, and caudal divisions of biceps
5. Vastus lateralis, stump of gluteus supf. at 5'
6. Deep fascia (fascia lata), position of patella at 6'
7. Supf. fascia
8. Middle crural fascia

FIGURE 5-7. Muscles of the left thigh, lateral view.

The **common peroneal nerve,** passing craniodistally over the lateral head of the gastrocnemius, is derived from a band of nerve fibers running along the cranial border of the wide **SCIATIC NERVE** (Fig. 5-8/26). The **tibial nerve** comes from the middle band and dips in between the lateral and medial heads of the gastrocnemius. The large **muscular branches to the caudal thigh muscles** are given off the caudal border of the sciatic nerve at the level of the hip joint.

Examine the **popliteal lymph nodes** lying around the tibial nerve as it disappears between the heads of the gastrocnemius. These nodes receive the deep lymph vessels of the distal part of the limb.

The **caudal cutaneous sural nerve** arises from the tibial nerve and passes caudodistally on the caudal border of the lateral head of the gastrocnemius(Fig. 5-8/35). Trace the

nerve. It obliquely crosses the lateral surface of the common calcanean tendon and, accompanied by the lateral saphenous vein, passes distally to the hock. The nerve then passes over the lateral surface of the hock to innervate the skin of the plantarolateral surface of the metatarsus as far distally as the fetlock.

Turn the limb so that the medial surface is up. Pick up the caudal branch of the medical saphenous vein and trace it into the depression between the common calcanean tendon and the deep digital flexor. In this depression, find the large **tibial nerve** caudal to the vein and trace it proximally to its emergence from under the medial head of the gastrocnemius. At the hock the nerve splits to form the medial and lateral plantar nerves (Fig. 5-9/11,11'). Tag the nerves at the hock; they will be traced through the flexor canal to the metatarsus and digit later. Turn the limb again so that the lateral surface is up.

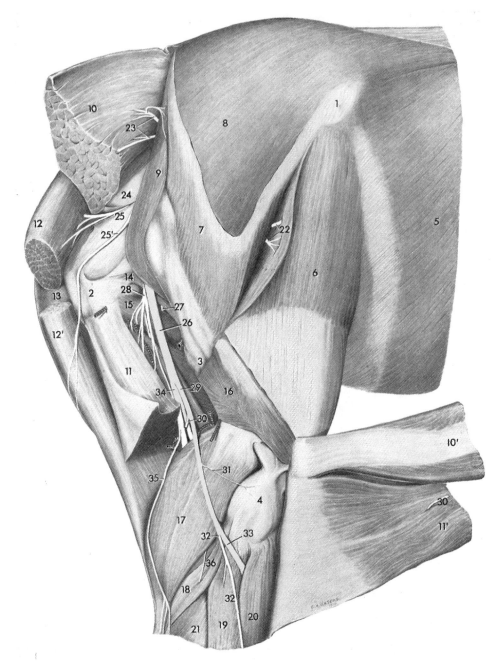

1. Coxal tuber
2. Ischial tuber
3. Third trochanter
4. Distal end of femur
5. External abdominal oblique
6. Tensor fasciae latae
7. Gluteus superficialis
8. Gluteus medius, its caudal part at 9
10, 10',11,11' Biceps
12, 12' Semitendinosus
13. Semimembranosus
14. Caud. part of gemellus
15. Quadratus femoris
16. Vastus lateralis
17. Gastrocnemius, lat. head
18. Soleus
19. Lat. digital extensor
20. Long digital extensor
21. Tibialis caud. (of deep dig. flexor)
22. Br. of cran.glut.n. to tensor
23. Br. of caud.glut.n. to biceps
24. Sacrosciatic lig.
25. Br. of caud.cut.fem.n. to semitendinosus, 25' caud.cut.fem.n.
26. Sciatic nerve
27. Br. of sciatic n. to int. obturator, gemellus, and quadratus femoris
28. Br. of sciatic n. to biceps, semitendinosus, and semimembranosus
29. Common peroneal nerve
30. Lat cut. sural nerve, cut
31. Br. to stifle joint
32. Supf. peroneal nerve
33. Deep peroneal nerve
34. Tibial nerve
35. Caud. cut. sural nerve
36. Br. of tibial n. to soleus

FIGURE 5-8. Deep dissection of right thigh, lateral view. (From Hopkins, 1937.)

The **fascia of the leg** (crural fascia) consists of three layers:

1. A loose supf. layer which continues the corresponding fascia of the thigh and fuses along the caudal border of the leg with

2. a shiny, fibrous middle layer which is continuous with the aponeuroses of the supf. muscles of the thigh (biceps, semitendinosus, sartorius, and gracilis), and

3. a deep layer of heavy fibrous tissue which closely invests the muscles of the crus. (Fig. 5-10/1,2,3).

Remove the supf. fascia from the lateral surface of the crus to where it blends with the middle crural fascia. Beginning between the middle and caudal divisions of the biceps, split the middle crural fascia (aponeurosis of biceps) down the middle of the leg to just beyond the hock, and reflect the flaps cranially and caudally. Detach the middle crural fascia from the middle division of the biceps, reflect it cranially, and clean the now exposed **common peroneal nerve** as it enters the muscles of the leg (Fig. 5-11/5,5').

Just above the hock find the **supf. peroneal**

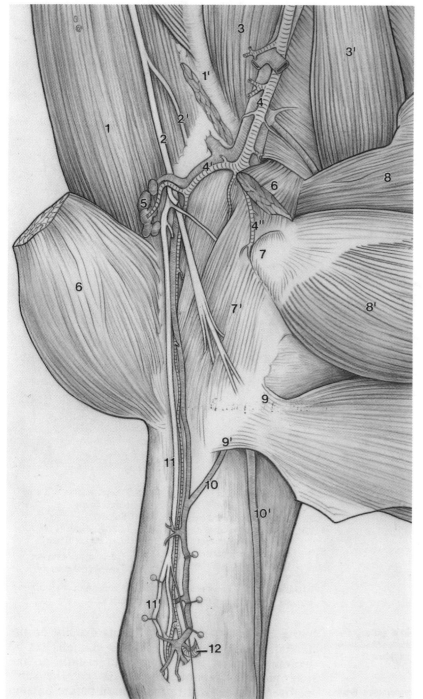

1. Biceps, femur at 1'
2. Tibial nerve, common peroneal nerve at 2'
3. Pectineus, sartorius at 3'
4, 4', 4" Femoral, caudal femoral, and popliteal vessels
5. Popliteal lymph nodes
6. Medial head of gastrocnemius, transected and reflected
7. Medial condyle of femur, popliteus at 7'
8. Adductor, 8' semimembranosus, both reflected
9. Tibial tendon, 9' tarsal tendon of semi-tendinosus
10, 10' Caudal and cranial branches of medial saphenous vein
11. Tibial nerve and anastomoses to caudal femoral vessels, medial plantar nerve at 11' (the lat. plant. n. is to the right of it)
12. S-shaped anastomosis between saphenous and caudal tibial arteries

FIGURE 5-9. Left thigh and leg after reflecting medial thigh muscles and medial head of gastrocnemius, medial view.

nerve in the groove between the long and lateral digital extensors. This groove marks the position of the intermuscular septum between these two muscles. Trace the nerve distally. It divides on the dorsal surface of the hock into two branches which pass distally on both sides of the extensor tendons (palpate) to innervate the skin of the lateral and dorsal surfaces of the metatarsus as far distally as the fetlock (Figs. 5-12 and 5-13).

Trace the nerve proximally to the point where it emerges through the deep layer of crural fascia. Incise the deep layer caudal and parallel to the intermuscular septum. Reflect the flap to the septum and continue tracing the nerve proximally (Fig. 5-11/5'). At the proximal end of the lateral extensor the supf. and **deep peroneal nerves** are seen originating from the common peroneal. A branch of the supf. peroneal supplies the lateral extensor, and the deep peroneal supplies the muscular branches to the other flexors of the hock and extensors of the digit.

Incise the deep layer of crural fascia cranial and parallel to the intermuscular septum. Reflect the flap to the septum and trace the deep peroneal

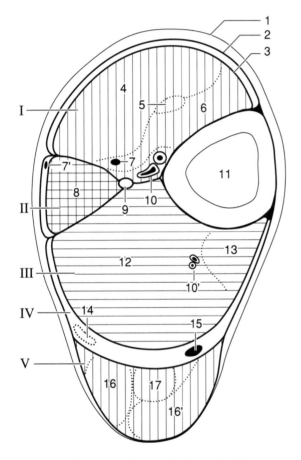

FIGURE 5-11. The break-up of the left common peroneal nerve exposed by reflection of the crural fasciae; lateral view.

1,1'	Middle and caudal division of biceps	5,5',5"	Supf., middle, and deep crural fasciae
2.	Lat. cutaneous sural nerve	6.	Soleus
3,3',3"	Common peroneal n., branch to lat. extensor, and supf. peroneal n.	7.	Tibialis caudalis (of deep digital flexor)
4.	Lateral head of gastrocnemius	8.	Lateral digital extensor
		9.	Long digital extensor

nerve as far as the hock. It runs distally on the lateral border of the flat tibialis cranialis (to be examined more fully later) and *cranial* to the intermuscular septum (Fig. 5-10/7). The supf. peroneal lies *caudal* to the septum before passing through the deep layer of the fascia. The deep peroneal nerve block 10 cm proximal to the hock may be combined with the tibial nerve block (at the same level) to anesthetize the deep structures of the hock, metatarsus, and the digit. Tag the deep peroneal nerve above the hock; your instructor may elect to have you trace it to the metatarsus and fetlock later.

Turn the limb over so the medial surface is up. Reflect the gracilis and its thin, wide tendon of insertion bluntly cranially. Then reflect the

FIGURE 5-10. Transverse section of the left leg (looking distally) to show the crural fasciae and osteofascial compartments (I-V). (After Updike, 1985.)

1,2,3	Supf., middle, and deep layers of crural fascia
4.	Long digital extensor
5.	Peroneus tertius
6.	Tibialis cranialis
7.	Deep peroneal nerve, supf. peroneal nerve at 7'
8.	Lateral digital extensor
9.	Fibula
10.	Cranial tibial vessels, caudal tibial vessels at 10'
11.	Tibia
12.	Deep digital flexor
13.	Popliteus
14.	Soleus (rudimentary)
15.	Tibial nerve
16.	Lateral head of gastrocnemius, medial head at 16'
17.	Supf. digital flexor
I.	Cranial compartment (vertically hatched)
II.	Lateral compartment (cross hatched)
III.	Caudal deep compartment (horizontally hatched)
IV.	Caudal intermediate compartment (blank)
V.	Caudal supf. compartment (vertically hatched again)

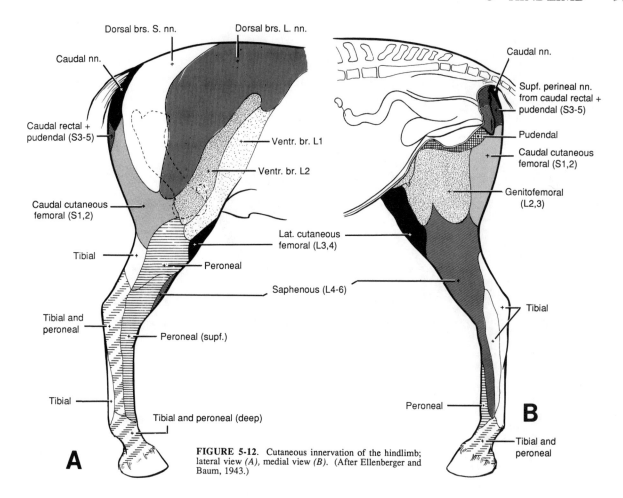

FIGURE 5-12. Cutaneous innervation of the hindlimb; lateral view *(A)*, medial view *(B)*. (After Ellenberger and Baum, 1943.)

semimembranosus in the same way so that it remains attached only by its tendon to the femur. Clean the surface of the **semitendinosus** and note its distinct tibial and tarsal tendons of insertion (Fig. 5-9/9,9'). The tibial tendon passes craniomedially to be inserted on the tibial crest. The tarsal tendon reaches the cranial surface of the common calcanean tendon and, fused with a similar (though less distinct) tendon derived from the caudal part of the biceps on the other side, passes distally to be inserted with the gastrocnemius on the calcanean tuber.

Cut the tarsal tendon of the semitendinosus and reflect the muscle cranially off the **gastrocnemius**. The lateral head of the latter muscle arises from the lateral supracondylar tuberosity (margin of the supracondylar fossa of the femur). The medial head arises from the medial supracondylar tuberosity. Locate these points on the skeleton. The **supf. digital flexor** takes origin from the supracondylar fossa. Both heads of the gastrocnemius terminate in a common tendon which passes from the supf. surface of the flexor tendon around the lateral side to reach the deep surface at the hock (Fig. 4-17/6,7). Palpate this relationship. It will be exposed later.

Separate the two heads of the gastrocnemius and transect the medial head 3 cm from its origin(Fig. 5-9/6). Reflect the distal stump. The course of the **tibial nerve** through the leg is now fully exposed; immediately after entering the space between the heads of the gastrocnemius large branches are detached to supply the muscles caudal to the tibia (extensors of the hock and flexors of the digit). The tibial nerve continues distally, medial to the common calcanean tendon where it has already been seen with the caudal branch of the medial saphenous vein.

Locate the femoral artery. The short **caudal femoral artery** arises from the femoral just proximal to the heads of the gastrocnemius and divides immediately into two branches. The ascending branch supplies the caudal thigh muscles; the descending branch supplies the more distal muscles. The femoral artery, after giving rise to the caudal femoral, becomes the popliteal artery which disappears deep to the popliteus. The popliteal artery then (as in the dog) divides into the cranial and caudal tibial arteries. It will be necessary to examine the muscles of the leg before these arteries can be exposed.

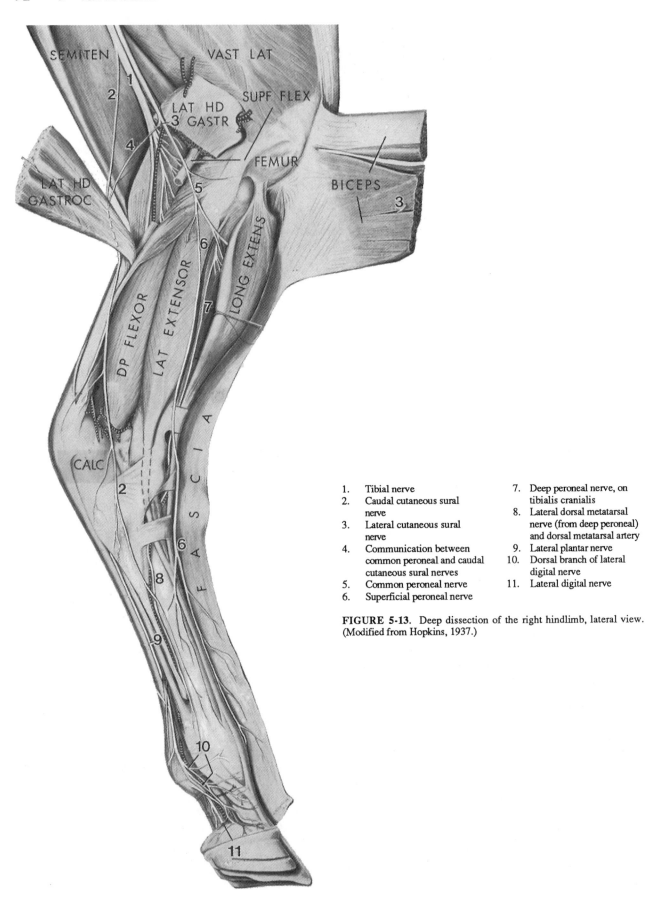

FIGURE 5-13. Deep dissection of the right hindlimb, lateral view. (Modified from Hopkins, 1937.)

1. Tibial nerve
2. Caudal cutaneous sural nerve
3. Lateral cutaneous sural nerve
4. Communication between common peroneal and caudal cutaneous sural nerves
5. Common peroneal nerve
6. Superficial peroneal nerve
7. Deep peroneal nerve, on tibialis cranialis
8. Lateral dorsal metatarsal nerve (from deep peroneal) and dorsal metatarsal artery
9. Lateral plantar nerve
10. Dorsal branch of lateral digital nerve
11. Lateral digital nerve

(At this point, students at Cornell should obtain the horse hindlimb skeleton from their course lockers and keep it, in the same orientation, next to the specimen.)

As the tendons of the muscles about to be described pass over the hock they are invested (and protected from friction) by **synovial sheaths** and held in place by five retinacula—bandlike thickenings of the deep fascia. The **retinacula** should be identified by palpation and preserved until you are directed to cut them. They are on the dorsal surface of hock:

1. Proximal extensor retinaculum—binds down the tendons of the long digital extensor, peroneus tertius, and tibialis cranialis on the distal end of the tibia (Figs. 5-13 and 5-15/10).

2. Middle extensor retinaculum—attached to the calcaneus and the (supf.) lateral tendon of the peroneus tertius, forming a loop around the tendon of the long digital extensor (Figs. 5-13 and 5-16/7').

3. Distal extensor retinaculum—extends across the proximal end of the large metatarsal bone and binds down the tendons of the long and lateral digital extensors (Fig 5-16/7").

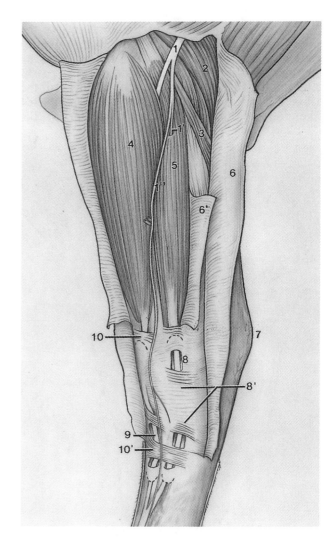

1,1',1" Common peroneal n., br. to lat. extensor, and supf. peroneal n.	extensor and extent of its tendon sheath, lat. extensor retinaculum at 8'
2. Lat. head of gastrocnemius	
3. Soleus	9. Tendon of long digital
4. Long digital extensor	extensor and extent
5. Lateral digital extensor	of its tendon sheath
6,6' Middle and deep crural fasciae	10,10' Proximal and distal
7. Point of hock	extensor retinacula
8. Tendon of lat. digital	

FIGURE 5-15. Left long and lateral digital extensors exposed by the reflection of the middle and deep crural fasciae; lateral view.

On the lateral surface of hock:

4. Lateral extensor retinaculum—blends with the lateral collateral ligament and binds down the tendon of the lateral extensor; its borders have to be fashioned, as shown in Fig. 5-13.

And on the plantar surface of hock:

5. Flexor retinaculum—blends with the medial collateral ligament and binds down the deep flexor tendon as it passes over the sustentaculum tali; it will be examined more fully later.

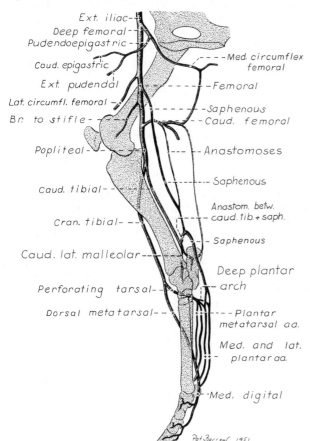

Ext. iliac-
Deep femoral -
Pudendoepigastric -
Caud. epigastric
Ext. pudendal
Lat. circumfl. femoral -
Br. to stifle -
Popliteal -
Caud. tibial - -
Cran. tibial - -
Caud. lat. malleolar - -
Perforating tarsal- -
Dorsal metatarsal - -

- Med. circumflex femoral
- Femoral
- Saphenous
- Caud. femoral
- Anastomoses
- Saphenous
Anastom. betw.
- caud. tib. + saph.
- Saphenous
Deep plantar
- arch
- - Plantar metatarsal aa.
Med. and lat.
- plantar aa.
- Med. digital

Pat Barrow, 1951

FIGURE 5-14: Arteries of the right hindlimb, medial view Schematic.

On the lateral surface of the limb reflect the deep crural fascia covering the **long digital extensor** and completely expose the belly of the muscle. Palpate the tendon of origin as it passes proximally through the extensor groove of the tibia to the extensor fossa of the femur (see skeleton). Separate the lateral border of the muscle from the lateral extensor and the medial border from the thin medial edge of the tibialis cranialis. The tendon distal to the muscle belly is bound down by the proximal extensor retinaculum which should be cleaned and isolated. Make a stab incision at the distal border of the retinaculum down to the tendon, opening the synovial sheath. Continue tracing the tendon distally, palpating, cleaning, and preserving the middle and distal extensor retinacula, until the tendon is joined by the lateral extensor tendon about 10 cm below the hock (Fig 5-15/9,8).

Explore the synovial sheath of the long extensor with a flexible probe. It extends proximally a little above the lateral malleous of the tibia and distally nearly to the palpable junction of the long and lateral extensor tendons.

Reflect the deep fascia off the surface of the **lateral digital extensor.** This muscle arises from the lateral collateral ligament of the stifle joint (palpable) and adjacent parts of the fibula and tibia. Do not attempt to isolate these origins. The tendon of the lateral extensor passes distally through the groove on the lateral malleolus of the tibia bound down by the most proximal part of the lateral extensor retinaculum. This retinaculum is extensive and blends with the lateral collateral ligament of the hock. Make a stab incision down to the tendon where it disappears behind the retinaculum, opening the synovial sheath. Clean the junction of the long and lateral extensor tendons but do not cut the distal extensor retinaculum, and then follow the combined tendon to the fetlock by palpation.

Probe the synovial sheath of the lateral extensor. It extends proximally a little above the lateral malleolus of the tibia and distally almost to the junction with the long extensor tendon.

The lateral digital extensor is sometimes resected to relieve the signs of stringhalt, an involuntary nervous flexion of the hock during progression. The musculotendinous junction is exposed, and the tendon is cut distal to the hock. Traction on the musculotendinous junction removes the tendon from its tendon sheath on the lateral aspect of the hock. The resection is completed by a second transection proximal to the musculotendinous junction.

At the proximal end of the lateral digital extensor find the rudimentary, fleshy **soleus.** It arises from the head of the fibula and eventually joins the tendon of the lateral gastrocnemius tendon (Fig. 5-15/3).

Transect the belly of the long digital extensor at its middle and reflect the stumps. Note the muscular branches of the deep peroneal nerve and the branches of the cranial tibial artery entering the deep face of the proximal stump. Deep to the long extensor and intimately adhered to the surface of the tibialis cranialis is the tendinous **peroneus tertius** (Fig. 5-16/4). The long extensor and the peroneus tertius arise by a common

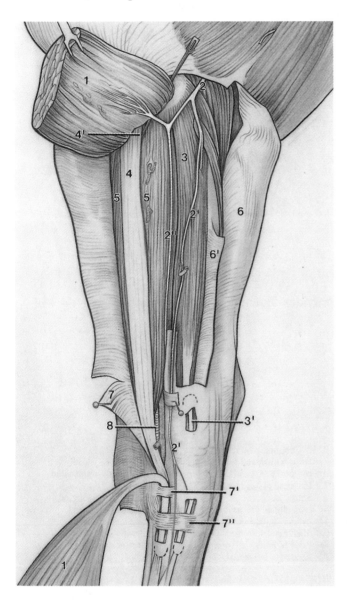

1. Long digital extensor, transected
2,2',2" Common, superficial, and deep peroneal nerves
3. Lat. digital extensor, its tendon and extent of tendon sheath at 3'
4. Peroneus tertius, the probe at 4' indicates the distal extent of the recess of the lat. femoroti-

bial joint capsule under the combined tendon of peroneus tertius and long dig. extensor
5. Tibialis cranialis
6, 6' Middle and deep crural fasciae
7,7',7" Proximal, middle, and distal extensor retinacula
8. Cranial tibial a. & v.

FIGURE 5-16. Left peroneus tertius and superficial and deep peroneal nerves exposed by the reflection of the long digital extensor muscle; lateral view.

tendon from the extensor fossa of the femur. The peroneus tertius mechanically opposes the action of the gastrocnemius and the tendinous supf. digital flexor. When the stifle is flexed, the peroneus tertius causes the hock to be flexed. When the stifle is extended, the gastrocnemius and supf. flexor cause the hock to be extended (reciprocal mechanism). Stifle and hock of your specimen cannot be flexed at this time. (A fresh limb from the post mortem room can be converted in about an hour to a movable specimen that demonstrates the reciprocal mechanism and indeed the entire stay-apparatus. See Appendix A, and consult your instructor about such a project.)

Separate the peroneus from the tibialis cranialis as far as the proximal extensor retinaculum. Transect the retinaculum. Carefully separate the tendon of the long digital extensor from the peroneus tertius and the underlying structures. Reflect it to one side and note its **mesotendon,** the fold of the synovial tendon sheath that carries vascular structures to the tendon.

The cranial tibial artery, the large cranial tibial vein, and the deep peroneal nerve are now exposed as they turn around the lateral borders of the tibialis cranialis and peroneus tertius (Fig. 5-16/8). Carefully preserve these structures as the dissection proceeds. They will be traced later.

Before continuing with the dissection, study the bones of the tarsus and metatarsus on an articulated specimen. The tarsus (or hock joint), clinically, is one of the important joints of the horse. It is also the most complex in terms of its construction and of the structures attaching to it or passing over it. No joint, except perhaps for the dog's stifle, better rewards anatomical study. The tarsus is composed of six **TARSAL BONES** arranged roughly in three transverse rows, (Fig. 5-17). The **talus** (T) is the medial bone of the proximal row and forms the trochlea that articulates with the distal end of the tibia. Note that the trochlea is obliquely oriented; this causes the distal end of the limb to be carried laterally as the joint is flexed while the limb is swung forward past the supporting contralateral limb. The medial surface of the talus presents proximal and distal tubercles for the attachment of parts of the medial collateral ligament. The lateral surface presents a roughened fossa in which part of the lateral collateral ligament attaches.

The **calcaneus** (C) is the largest bone of the hock. It is enlarged at its proximal end to form the calcanean tuber which provides insertion for the supf. flexor, gastrocnemius, and tarsal tendons of biceps and semitendinosus. The enlargement of the lower part of the medial surface of the calcaneus forms the sustentaculum tali on which a part of the medial collateral ligament attaches.

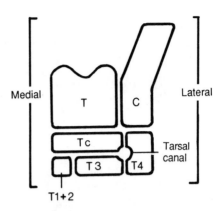

FIGURE 5-17: Schematic dorsal view of the left tarsal bones.

The plantar surface of the sustentaculum forms, with the smooth medial surface of the body, a groove for the passage of the deep flexor tendon. The lateral surface presents a rough distal prominence for the attachment of a part of the lateral collateral ligament. The plantar surface of the calcaneus is roughened for the attachment of the long plantar ligament.

The **central tarsal bone** (Tc) articulates proximally with the talus and distally with the fused **first** and **second** and **third tarsal bones** (T1+2, T3). The **fourth tarsal bone** (T4) provides attachment for the lateral collateral and long plantar ligaments and, with Tc and T3, forms the **tarsal canal** (Fig. 5-17). T1+2 gives attachment to the medial collateral ligament and to the medial branch of the tibialis cranialis tendon.

There are only three metatarsal bones in the horse. The **third metatarsal bone** (Mt3) is also called the large metatarsal or "cannon bone." The **second and fourth metatarsal bones**(Mt2, Mt4) are also known as the small metatarsal or "splint bones." Note particularly the small nodules on the distal ends of Mt2 and Mt4; they are palpable in the live horse. The ridge-like tuberosity on the proximal dorsal surface of Mt3 provides insertion for parts of the tibialis cranialis and peroneus tertius. The proximal ends of all three metatarsal bones receive numerous ligaments from the tarsal bones.

A reminder: Keep the articulated specimen from your course locker next to your dissection. Clean the peroneus tertius to its apparent bifurcation in the proximal part of the hock(Fig. 5-18/1,1',1"). The **tendon of the tibialis cranialis** emerges through the bifurcation (actually a ring-like tunnel), enveloped in a synovial sheath, and bifurcates also (/2,2',2"). (**Caution:** clean only the surfaces of the tendons mentioned and project them on the skeleton. Do not try to dissect the bony-tendinous junctions.) The dorsal branch of the tibialis cranialis tendon (/2") passes straight distally to insert on T3 and the ridge-like tuberosity at the proximal end of the large

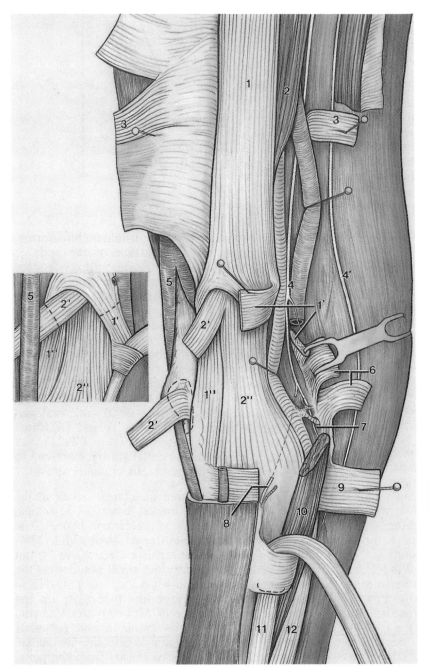

1. Peroneus tertius
1' (Supf.)lat. br. of peroneus tertius, transected
1" Dors. br. of peroneus tertius,
    much of the dors. br. is deep to 2"
2. Belly of tibialis cranialis
2' Med. br. of tibialis cranialis (cunean tendon,
    deep to it the cunean bursa)
2" Dorsal branch of tibialis cranialis
3. Proximal extensor retinaculum, transected
4. Cranial tibial a. and v., and deep peroneal
   nerve
4' Supf. peroneal nerve
5. Dorsal common dig. v. II (from cranial
   branch of medial saphenous)
6. Middle extensor retinaculum, transected
7. Perforating tarsal artery and lat. br. of deep
   peroneal nerve that becomes the lat. dors.
   metatarsal nerve.
8. Med. br. of deep peroneal nerve, becomes
   medial dorsal metatarsal nerve.
9. Distal extensor retinaculum, transected
10. Extensor brevis
11. Tendon of long digital extensor
12. Tendon of lateral digital extensor

FIGURE 5-18. Deep dissection of the left
hock joint, dorsolateral view. The insert shows
the med. br. of the tibialis cranialis, the supf. lat.
br. of the peroneus tertius, and the middle extensor
retinaculum before they were transected.

metatarsal bone. The medial branch (/2';also
known as the cunean tendon) curves medially to
insert on T1+2. Transect the medial branch 2 cm
from its origin and reflect the distal stump. This
opens the (cunean)bursa lying deep to the tendon.

Now reflect the proximal stump, exposing the
dorsal branch of the **peroneus tertius tendon** (/1").
It ends (together with the dorsal branch of the
tibialis cranialis tendon) on T3 and Mt3. The
(supf.) lateral branch of the peroneus (/1') blends
with the middle extensor retinaculum (/6) and
inserts on the calcaneus and T4.

A reinvestigation of the **peroneus tertius** and tibialis
cranialis (Updike, 1984) found that the peroneus actually

splits into four branches (Fig. 5-19). In addition to the
dorsal and (supf.) lateral branches (/1,2) we have just seen,
there is a medial branch (/4) that blends with the medial
collateral ligament in an attachment on Tc, T3, and Mt3; and
a (deep) lateral branch (/3) that passes distal to the medial
trochlear ridge to end where talus, calcaneus, Tc, and T4 come
together. The two lateral branches mediate attachment of the
loop-like middle extensor retinaculum to bone. The cranial
tibial artery passes between the two lateral branches as it
crosses the front of the hock. The ring-like tunnel (/5)
formed by the peroneus acts like a retinaculum for the tibialis
cranialis tendon It is said that the attachments of the dorsal
and medial branches of the peroneus coincide with the sites
that frequently develop osseous changes in the osteo-
arthropathies that befall this complex joint.

Transect the middle extensor retinaculum and the (supf.) lateral branch of the peroneus tertius. Transect the distal extensor retinaculum and reflect the long digital extensor out of the way (Fig. 5-18/9,11).

Trace the **cranial tibial artery** and the deep peroneal nerve distally on the dorsal surface of the hock(Fig. 5-18/4). The artery gives rise to the perforating tarsal artery at the level of the middle extensor retinaculum and continues distally under the small extensor digitalis brevis and the tendon of the lateral extensor to reach the metatarsus as the **dorsal metatarsal artery.** The perforating tarsal artery enters the tarsal canal formed between Tc, T3, and T4(Fig. 5-17).

The deep peroneal nerve (find it but do not trace its branches) innervates the tarsal joint capsules and bifurcates at the hock to form the medial and lateral dorsal metatarsal nerves. These thin nerves (because of drying) are difficult to trace; they are shown in Fig. 5-25 reaching the hoof; Fig. 5-24 shows them in a transverse section of the metatarsus.

Transect the lateral digital extensor just below the lateral collateral ligament of the stifle and reflect it distally. It will be necessary to scrape its fibers free from the fibula and from deeper structures. Draw the lateral border of the tibialis cranialis strongly cranially and trace the **cranial tibial artery** and vein proximally on its deep surface. The vein may be very large or replaced by a plexus of smaller veins. The artery passes between tibia and fibula (palpate the bones) to gain the caudal aspect of the proximal tibia where it arises (together with the caudal tibial artery) from the **popliteal artery.** In order to expose the caudal tibial artery, it is necessary first to examine the caudal muscles of the leg.

For the next few minutes it is best to hold the limb with the patella on the table and the distal part of the limb protruding over the edge of the table. Transect the tendons of the gastrocnemius and supf. flexor distal to the musculotendinous junction of the gastrocnemius.

Isolate the supf. flexor tendon and reflect it distally. This will open the large subtendinous **calcanean bursa** which is bounded superficially by the flexor tendon and deeply by the insertion of the gastrocnemius and the calcanean tuber. Note that at the point of the hock the supf. flexor tendon widens, forming a cap over the calcanean tuber. The lateral and medial borders of this cap blend with the tarsal tendon of biceps and semitendinosus (see further on) and insert on the sides of the tuber. Sever the medial insertion and reflect the tendon to expose the bursa to its full extent, 7-10 cm above and below the point of the hock (Fig. 5-20/5).

A smaller bursa lies between the combined gastrocnemius and tarsal tendons and the calcanean tuber and communicates with the large (calcanean) bursa across the lateral surface of the gastrocnemius tendon. You already determined whether your horse has a subcutaneous bursa ("capped hock"). Any or all of these bursae may be the site of inflammatory change and enlargement.

The tendons you have just dissected in the caudal part of the leg (gastrocnemius, supf. flexor, tarsal tendons of biceps and semitendinosus—plus a fascial band from the lateral side of the femur that was not dissected) form the **common calcanean tendon** (Fig. 5-21) which is easily identified in the live animal. All parts of this composite structure attach on the calcanean tuber and (with the exception of the supf. digital flexor) end there; the supf. digital flexor continues of course to the digit.

The **common calcanean tendon** is actually more complex than the brief description (above) suggests. To reduce the complexity, the tarsal tendons of biceps and semitendinosus have been referred to as a uniform "plate" on the cranial surface of the more salient components of the common tendon. In reality, the plate has supf. and deep parts (Fig. 5-20/4,4') which receive contributions also from the gracilis, the femoral fascia, and the fascial band that comes down from the femur. The supf. part of the plate consists of the fascial band, receives contributions from the biceps

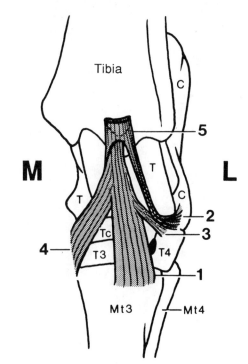

1. Dorsal branch	by the peroneus tertius
2. Supf. lateral branch	for passage of the tibialis
3. Deep lateral branch	cranialis tendon that is not
4. Medial branch	shown.
5. Ring-like tunnel formed	

FIGURE 5-19. Dorsolateral view of the hock showing the insertion branches of the peroneus tertius. (After Updike, 1984.)

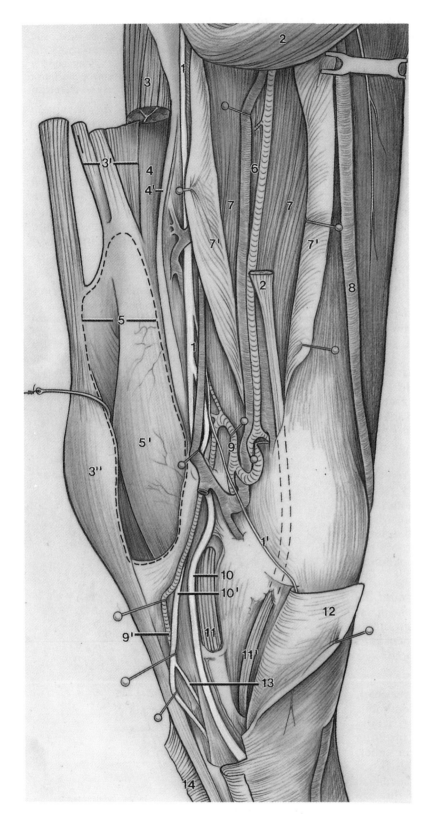

1. Tibial n. and caudal br. of med. saphenous v.
1' Cutaneous br. of tibial nerve
2. Stumps of medial (deep) digital flexor
3. Prox. stump of gastrocnemius and supf. dig. flexor
3' Distal stump of gastrocnemius
3" Cap of supf. digital flexor
4,4' Supf. and deep parts of the "plate" formed by the tarsal tendons of biceps and semitendinosus
5. Subtendinous calcanean bursa
5' Calcanean tuber
6. Caudal tibial artery and vein
7. Lateral (deep) digital flexor
7' Deep crural fascia, opened to expose 2, 6, and 7
8. Cranial br. of med. saphenous vein
9. S-shaped anastomosis, distal segment of saphenous artery at 9'
10,10' Med. and lat. plantar nerves
11,11' Tendons of deep flexors (lat. and med.)
12. Flexor retinaculum, reflected
13. Deep br. of lat. plantar nerve
14. Deep fascia, cut to expose supf. dig. flexor tendon

FIGURE 5-20. Dissection of left hock joint, medial view. The gastrocnemius and supf. digital flexor have been transected and the subtendinous calcanean bursa exposed. The break-up of the tibial nerve is also shown.

(mainly), semitendinosus, and gracilis, incorporates the rudimentary soleus tendon and joins the medial border of the gastrocnemius tendon at the calcanean tuber. The deep part is formed by the semitendinosus and gracilis (mainly), with contributions from the biceps; as it approaches the calcanean tuber it splits into medial and lateral branches that join the medial and lateral attachments of the supf. digital flexor on the tuber.

Turn the limb so that the medial surface is up. During the dissection that follows, one student should remove the skin from the medial surface of metatarsus and fetlock.

Remove the supf. fascia from between the cranial and caudal branches of the medial saphenous vein. The thin white tendon of the **medial (deep) digital flexor** is visible through the deep fascia. Open the deep fascia over the tendon and muscle from a few cm proximal to the medial malleolus of the tibia, proximally to the bifurcation of the medial saphenous vein. Isolate the muscle by reflecting the flaps of fascia. Transect it at the musculotendinous junction and reflect the proximal stump to see the **caudal tibial artery** which need not be traced(Fig. 5-20/2,6). This vessel arises together with the cranial tibial artery from the popliteal just distal to the stifle. It descends to the hock where (in most horses) it anastomoses with the saphenous artery and supplies the lateral surface of this joint (Fig. 5-14). The saphenous artery then receives the perforating tarsal artery and gives rise to several small vessels in the metatarsus. The **principal artery to the digit**, however, is the cranial tibial in the front of the limb; we already traced it to the dorsal aspect of the hock.

Find the S-shaped anastomosis between the caudal tibial and saphenous arteries just above the hock (Fig. 5-20/9) and trace it under the tendon you just transected to the **caudal tibial artery.** The latter continues distally to the lateral surface of the hock as the small caudal lateral malleolar artery. Trace the anastomosis the other way and note that it reinforces the saphenous artery (Fig. 5-14) which was seen earlier accompanying the caudal branch of the medial saphenous vein. After receiving the anastomosis, the saphenous artery (now much larger) passes distally with the flexor tendons and gives rise to the medial and lateral plantar arteries. In some horses the saphenous artery does not reach the hock. When this is the case the anastomosis is larger and supplies all the blood to the plantar arteries. (Why is this anastomosis so typically S-shaped?)

Incise the deep metatarsal fascia over the plantar surface of the supf. flexor tendon from the tarsus to the fetlock and expose the tendon. Do not cut the communicating branch connecting the plantar nerves (Fig. 5-22/10). Note that the fascia is thickest proximally, forming a strong sheath for the tendon.

Remove the loose supf. fascia from the plantaromedial surface of the hock. Using the tagged medial plantar nerve as a guide, cut the flexor retinaculum (down to the nerve) from the point where the nerve disappears under the retinaculum to below the hock, joining this cut with the one of the preceding paragraph that exposed the supf. flexor tendon. (Briefly, the retinaculum forms a canal for the large deep flexor tendon by bridging the space between the calcanean tuber and the sustentaculum tali [Fig. 5-27/11].) Remove the opened retinaculum from the tuber and from the medial aspect of the hock until the small tendon of the medial digital flexor is exposed (Fig. 5-20/11'). Remove also the fascial

flap between the supf. and deep flexor tendons created by the incision that earlier exposed the supf. flexor tendon. (The flexor retinaculum will be explained more fully later. It is unfortunately not as distinct as the three extensor retinacula on the front, but it forms the important flexor canal for the passage of the large deep flexor tendon over the hock.)

Trace the medial and lateral plantar nerves distally. The **medial plantar nerve** inclines from the plantar surface of the deep flexor tendon to the groove between the flexor tendons and the interosseus (Fig. 5-24) and descends to the fetlock.

The **lateral plantar nerve** passes laterally between the supf. and deep flexor tendons, reaches

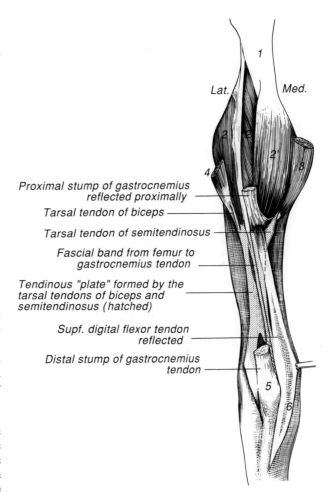

Lat.   Med.

Proximal stump of gastrocnemius reflected proximally

Tarsal tendon of biceps

Tarsal tendon of semitendinosus

Fascial band from femur to gastrocnemius tendon

Tendinous "plate" formed by the tarsal tendons of biceps and semitendinosus (hatched)

Supf. digital flexor tendon reflected

Distal stump of gastrocnemius tendon

1.	Femur	3.	Semitendinosus
2.	Lat. head of	4.	Biceps, caudal division
	gastrocnemius	5.	Calcanean tuber
2'	Med. head of	6.	Cap of supf. digital
	gastrocnemius		flexor, reflected

FIGURE 5-21. The components of the left common calcanean tendon, caudal view. The tendon of the gastocnemius has been resected and the supf. digital flexor has been reflected medially off the calcanean tuber. The labels to the left of the drawing list the components of the common calcanean tendon. (From EllenbergerBaum, 1943, by Horowitz/ Geary.)

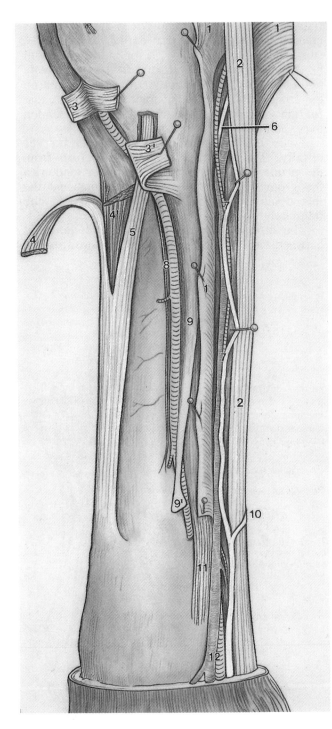

1. Deep fascia, reflected to expose supf. dig. flexor and plantar vessels and nerves
2. Supf. digital flexor
3,3' Middle and distal extensor retinacula
4,4' Long and short (brevis) dig. extensors
5. Lat. digital extensor
6. Deep br. of lat. plantar nerve
7. Lat. plantar a. v. & n.
8. Dorsal metatarsal a. and lat. dors. metatarsal n. (lat. br. of deep peroneal n.)
9. Lat. splint bone, its palpable end at 9'
10. Communicating br. between med. and lat. plantar nerves
11. Interosseus
12. Lat. digital a. v. & n.

FIGURE 5-22. Left metatarsus, lateral view. The deep fascia (1) has been reflected to expose the lateral plantar vessels and nerve.

the groove between the flexors and the interosseus on the lateral side, gives off a deep branch, and descends to the fetlock (Fig. 5-22/7). Near the middle of the metatarsus a communicating branch from the medial plantar nerve winds obliquely over the flexor tendons to join the lateral plantar nerve. It is occasionally absent. The deep branch of the lateral plantar nerve (do not trace) penetrates to the proximal end of the interosseus, supplies this structure, and bifurcates to form the **medial and lateral plantar metatarsal nerves.** These descend on the axial surface of the splint bones, emerge at the splint bones' distal end, and distribute themselves as shown in Fig. 5-25.

The **saphenous artery,** which has been seen earlier accompanying the plantar nerves, bifurcates in the flexor canal to form the *medial and lateral plantar arteries.* These small vessels anastomose at the proximal end of the large metatarsal bone with the perforating tarsal artery to form the deep plantar arch where four arteries arise that pass down the metatarsus (Fig. 5-23). Only the medial and lateral plantar arteries should be traced; they accompany the like-named nerves. The deep plantar arch, the anastomoses, and the medial and lateral plantar metatarsal arteries lie deep to the flexor tendons and are not of sufficient importance to be dissected.

Open the synovial **tarsal sheath** of the deep flexor tendon if this was not done when you traced the plantar nerves over the back of the hock. Probe the proximal and distal extent of the sheath and relate your findings to your articulated specimen.

The tendon of the medial digital flexor does not pass through the flexor canal. Provided with a synovial sheath of its own it descends in a canal in the medial collateral ligament of the hock to join the large tendon in the proximal half of the metatarsus.

Inflammation of the tarsal sheath, usually unilateral and caused by trauma, is known as tarsal synovitis or *thoroughpin.* An excess of synovial fluid within the sheath bulges the sheath at its proximal extent, about level with the calcanean tuber. Thoroughpin must be differentiated from an excess of synovial fluid in an inflamed tarsocrural joint *(bog spavin)* whose plantar pouches bulge in about the same region.

Retract the tendon of the medial digital flexor and deep flexor tendon strongly and demonstrate their convergence. About the middle of the metatarsus the combined deep flexor tendon is joined by a thin distal continuation of the fibrous layer of the tarsal joint capsule. This is the **accessory (check) ligament;** it plays an insignificant role in the passive stay-apparatus—it may in fact be absent.

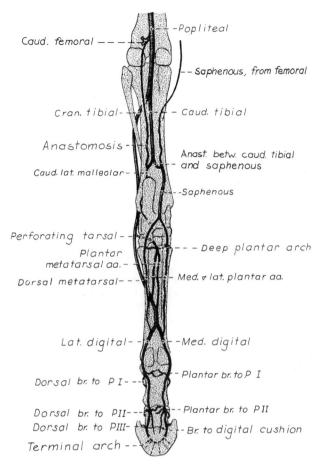

FIGURE 5-23: Arteries of the left hindlimb, caudal view. Schematic.

The **main arterial supply to the digit**, the **dorsal metatarsal artery**, should now be traced with the lateral surface of the limb up. The artery crosses obliquely laterodistally from the dorsal surface of the hock to reach the groove between the large and lateral small metatarsal bones (Fig. 5-22/8), where the pulse may be taken. At the distal third of the metatarsus the artery passes medially between the two bones and lies deep to the interosseus. At the bifurcation of the latter just above the fetlock, the artery (discontinue tracing it) is joined by the small plantar and plantar metatarsal arteries, emerges between the two branches of the interosseus, and bifurcates to form the **medial and lateral digital arteries** (Fig. 5-23). The digital arteries will be traced on the forelimb.

Pick up the **deep peroneal nerve** where it divided at the hock and trace the medial branch, the *medial dorsal metatarsal nerve*. This cannot be done if the fascia on the metatarsal bones has been allowed to dry. The nerve lies at first under the medial edge of the long extensor tendon, but soon leaves the tendon and obliquely crosses the space between the tendon and the medial splint bone. It is a fairly wide, flat nerve accompanied by tiny veins, and lies directly on the large metatarsal bone (Fig. 5-24). It passes the fetlock on the medial surface (discontinue tracing) and ramifies on the medial and dorsal surfaces of the pastern as far distally as the laminar dermis. The smaller *lateral dorsal metatarsal nerve* accompanies the dorsal metatarsal artery. It is distributed to the digit in the same manner as the medial nerve (Fig. 5-25).

The digit, the part of the limb distal to the fetlock joint, is virtually the same on the forelimb and will be studied in detail when the forelimb is studied. There are however some important differences in the innervation of the hind digit which should be mentioned. The differences exist because there are dorsal metatarsal nerves in the hindlimb, and no corresponding metacarpal nerves in the forelimb.

1. The joint capsules of the pastern and coffin joints are largely innervated by the plantar digital nerves. The dorsal parts of the capsules, however,

While retracting the combined deep flexor tendon palpate and expose the **interosseus*** which is largely tendinous in the horse, but is homologous to the fleshy third interosseus muscle of the dog. The interosseus arises from the distal row of tarsal bones and the proximal end of the large metatarsal bone and runs distally between the splint bones. Above the fetlock it splits into two thick branches which attach to the proximal sesamoid bones (Fig. 5-26/2). Thin extensor branches pass obliquely over the fetlock to join the extensor tendon on the front of the digit. Palpate the bifurcation of the interosseus but do not trace the branches. They are arranged similarly on the forelimb where they will be traced to their destinations. (Equine practitioners refer to the interosseus as the suspensory ligament.)

---

*Note this spelling, distinct from interosse*ous*, the adjective we use for interosseous space, artery, membrane, and so forth. Interosseus (without the o) is an adopted noun for naming muscles, similar to deltoide*us*, omohyoide*us* and sternothyroide*us*. The same applies to the cutaneous muscles of the trunk and neck, cutane*us* trunci and cutane*us* colli, respectively.

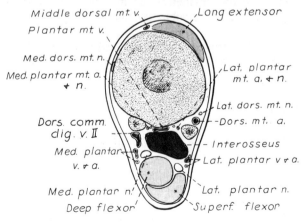

FIGURE 5-24. Transverse section through the middle of the right metatarsus, proximal surface.

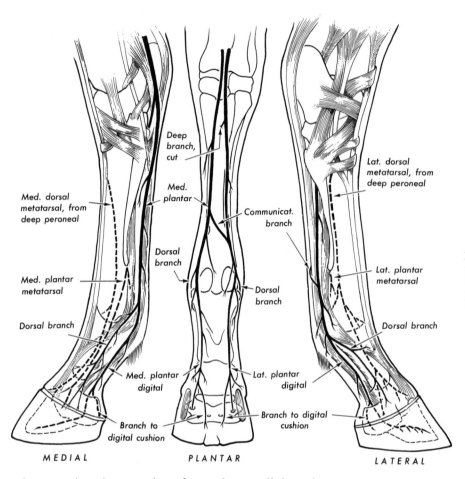

FIGURE 5-25. Nerves on the right tarsus, metatarsus, and digit, semischematic. (Modified with permission from Pohlmeyer and Redecker, 1974.)

also receive innervation from the medial and lateral *dorsal* metatarsal nerves.

2. The medial and lateral dorsal metatarsal nerves (branches of the deep peroneal) innervate the dorsal part of the coronary and laminar dermis.

It is evident from this description that the deep peroneal as well as the tibial nerve must be blocked in order to obtain complete desensitization of the hind digit. A supf. plantar block would fail to anesthetize the branches of the deep peroneal and the plantar metatarsal nerves.

(For an overview of the innervation of the hindlimb muscles and their primary joint action see Appendix B.)

Hock Joint

The two parts of the hindlimb still to be studied are the important hock and stifle joints. Unfortunately, their dissection requires that several structures passing over these joints will have to be displaced or cut. Tagging the stumps of the structures to be reflected will help you when you review the limb.

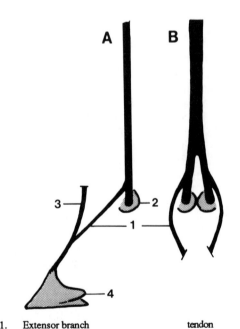

1. Extensor branch	tendon
2. Proximal sesamoid bone	4. Distal phalanx
3. Long or common extensor	

FIGURE 5-26. Isolated interosseus, lateral view *(A)*, plantar view *(B)*.

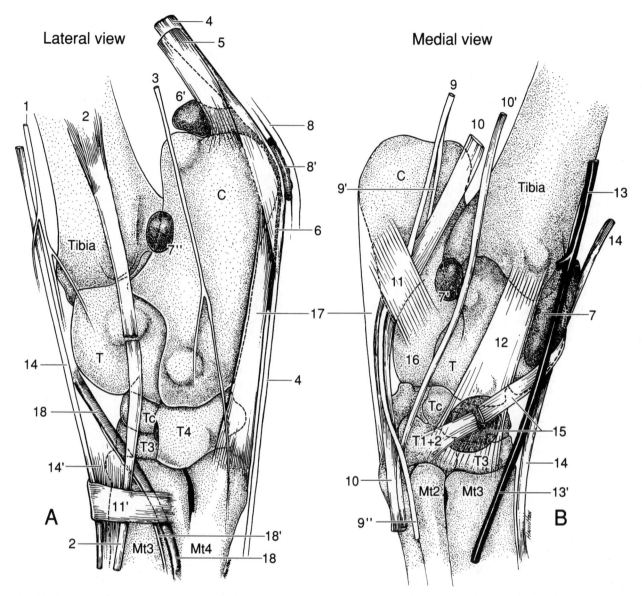

Lateral view

Medial view

1. Supf. peroneal nerve
2. Lat. digital extensor
3. Caudal cutaneous sural n.
4. Supf. digital flexor
5. Gastrocnemius
6. Subtendinous calcanean bursa, extension under gastrocnemius tendon at 6'
7. Dorsal pouch of tarsocrural joint, medioplantar and latero-plantar pouches at 7' and 7"
8. Skin, inconstant subcutaneous calcanean bursa at 8'
9. Tibial n., lat. and med. plantar nn. at 9' and 9"
10. Large deep flexor tendon, tendon of medial digital flexor at 10'
11. Flexor retinaculum, distal extensor retinaculum at 11'
12. Medial collateral ligament
13. Cranial branch of medial saphenous v., dorsal common dig.vein II at 13'
14. Long digital extensor, short extensor at 14'
15. Cunean tendon and bursa
16. Sustentaculum tali
17. Long plantar ligament
18. Dorsal metatarsal a.,

lat. dorsal metatarsal nerve at 18'
C Calcaneus
T Talus
Tc Central tarsal bone
T1+2, T3, T4 Tarsal bones with like number
Mt2, Mt3, Mt4 Metatarsal bones with like number

FIGURE 5-27. Selected structures in schematic lateral (A) and medial (B) views of the dissected hock joint.

In the study of the hock joint particular attention should be paid to the bony, tendinous, and ligamentous structures as they relate to the various joint capsules. An articulated specimen next to your dissection will greatly assist you with this.

The outer fibrous membrane of the **joint capsule** of a composite joint like the hock is common to the component joints—four for the hock. It is attached proximally around the

margins of the tibial articular surface and distally around the margins of the metatarsal articular surfaces and blends, of course, with the collateral ligaments. The synovial membrane on the other hand, is attached around the articular surfaces of each component joint. Its inner surface carries many irregular projections (light brown in preserved specimens) that greatly increase the surface area. A **joint pouch** is a part of a joint capsule that is free to bulge when distended by synovia; it can be palpated as a soft area in the live animal.

The four component joints of the hock are:

1. The **tarsocrural joint** is the largest. Its capsule surrounds the articulation of the tibia with the trochlea of the talus. It communicates with—
2. the **proximal intertarsal joint** between the talus and calcaneus proximally and the central and fourth tarsal bones distally.
3. The **distal intertarsal joint** includes the articulation of the central tarsal with T1+2 and T3 distally and communicates in about 38% of cases with—
4. the **tarsometatarsal joint** which includes the articulation between T1+2, T3, and T4 proximally and Mt2, Mt3, and Mt4 distally. It also includes the articulations between the three metatarsal bones, between T1+2 and T3, and between T3 and T4.

Clean the loose fascia off the hock. On the dorsomedial surface between the tendinous peroneus tertius and the medial malleolus of the tibia palpate and open the **dorsal pouch of the tarsocrural joint** with a *longitudinal* cut. The fibrous membrane of the joint capsule is thin here and is not covered by a collateral ligament or tendon. An excess of fluid in the joint cavity (bog spavin), therefore, can cause the pouch to bulge. Verify that the pouch is a proximodistally oriented oval by cutting it fully open and reflecting the flaps medially and laterally (Fig. 5-27/B,7). With the help of your articulated bone specimen, determine which features of which bones are exposed. Mark the boundaries of the exposure with pencil on your articulated specimen. Would you see more, or less, if the joint was flexed? Would you know in which part of this large joint you are, if you saw the exposed features through an arthroscope?

The cranial branch of the medial saphenous vein and a large anastomosis to the cranial tibial lie on the dorsal pouch (Fig. 5-3). The veins may appear swollen when the pouch is distended (blood spavin). Transect the cranial tibial artery and vein and the deep peroneal nerve and reflect them out of the way. Probe the joint and open it again lateral to the peroneus tertius. The fibrous membrane is thicker here and supported by the long extensor tendon; put the distal stump of the long extensor back in its place and verify that.

On the dorsal surface of the hock probe for the distal extent of the tarsocrural joint. Your probe should stop at the distal end of the trochlear ridges. If it goes beyond this, the probe has passed through the rather wide communication between this and the proximal intertarsal joint.

The proximal and distal intertarsal and tarsometatarsal joints are best viewed on the articulated bone specimen. Virtually no movement occurs in them. Their joint spaces of course, are very narrow in the standing animal. Nevertheless, experienced veterinarians are able to place thin hypodermic needles into the distal two joints taking advantage of the vertical gap between T1+2 and T3 on the medial aspect.

The **medial collateral ligament of the hock joint** is composed of a long supf. and a short deep part; both parts originate from the medial malleolus. The supf. part spreads distally, covering the tendon of the medial digital flexor and merging with the flexor retinaculum. Clean the surface of the ligament and cut its dorsal edge free from the fibrous layer of the tarsocrural joint capsule with which it blends. Transect the ligament at its origin on the medial malleolus. Carefully reflect the supf. part distally cutting it off its attachment to the distal tubercle of the talus. It also attaches to the surface of the distal row of tarsal bones and the proximal ends of Mt2 and Mt3. The Y-shaped deep part of the ligament is now exposed. It arises cranial and deep to the supf. part on the medial malleolus and passes plantarodistally to attach on the proximal tubercle of the talus and on the sustentaculum tali. The deep part is truly Y-shaped only when the hock is flexed. On the basis of fiber analysis the deep part can again be divided into supf., middle, and deep parts (Updike, 1984). Do not attempt the division. The short (deep) medial collateral ligaments are said to be responsible for a snapping motion occurring during the excursion of the tarsocrural joint (see further on).

The **flexor retinaculum** has already been seen and partially removed (p. 99) when the medial and lateral plantar nerves were traced through the flexor canal which the retinaculum forms with the calcaneus. Note that it blends with the medial collateral ligament. See the stumps of the retinaculum where it was cut away from the body of the calcaneus above the sustentaculum tali, from the sustentaculum tali, and from the medial surfaces to Tc, T1+2, and Mt2. Laterally it is continuous with a mass of tendinous tissue on the plantar surface of the calcaneus. Push the point of your scalpel into this tissue and convince yourself that it is tendinous and not, as you might expect, the plantar surface of the calcaneus.

This tendinous tissue is the **long plantar ligament,** a strong flat band attached to the plantar surface of the calcaneus and covering the lateral part of the plantar surface of the hock joint (Fig. 5-27/17). It passes distally to the plantar surface of T4 and Mt4 and steadies the calcaneus against the pull of the common calcanean tendon.

Palpate and open the small **medioplantar pouch of the tarsocrural joint** proximal to the sustentaculum tali and between the tibia and the sheath of the large deep flexor tendon (Fig. 5-27/B/7'). Explore the extent of this pouch with a flexible probe and determine its continuity with

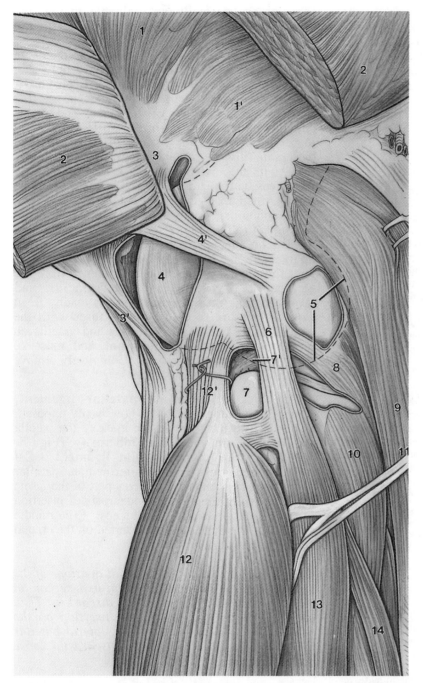

1,1' Rectus femoris and vastus intermedius
2. Vastus lateralis, reflected
3. Patella, patellar ligaments at 3'
4. Lat. ridge of femoral trochlea, lat. femoro-patellar ligament at 4'
5. Lat. femoral condyle exposed through fenestrated femorotibial joint capsule, also outline of condyle
6. Lat. collateral ligament
7. Lat. tibial condyle exposed through fenestrated femorotibial joint capsule, lat. meniscus at 7'
8. Popliteus
9. Lat. head of gastrocnemius
10. Tibialis caudalis (deep dig. flexor)
11. Common peroneal nerve
12. Long. dig. extensor, its tendon combined with that of the peroneus tertius at 12'
13. Lat. digital extensor
14. Soleus

FIGURE 5-28. Lateral view of left stifle. The femoropatellar and femorotibial capsules have been fenestrated. Broken line: distal end of femur.

the dorsal pouch. It is also continuous, deep to the sheath of the deep flexor tendon, with the **latero-plantar pouch of the tarsocrural joint.** Open the latter pouch between the lateral malleolus of the tibia and the calcaneus (Fig. 5-27A/7"). It is freely continuous with the dorsal pouch.

The **lateral collateral ligament of the hock joint** is also composed of long supf. and short deep parts; both originate on the lateral malleolus. The supf. part ends on the lateral surfaces of the calcaneus, T4, Mt3, and Mt4. It forms a groove for the passage of the lateral extensor tendon. Incise the ligamentous tissue over the tendon, cut the tendon free from its mesotendon, and draw it to one side. (What was

the significance of a mesotendon again?) Clean the supf. part of the lateral collateral ligament and transect it just below the malleolar origin. Reflect it carefully distally. The deep part can now be seen passing from the cranial part of the lateral malleolus to the fossa on the lateral surface of the talus and to the adjacent part of the calcaneus. On the basis of fiber analysis the deep part can again be divided into supf., middle, and deep parts (Updike, 1984). Do not attempt the division.

Before attempting to flex and extend the hock joint, the tarsal tendons of biceps and semiten-dinosus, and certainly the large deep flexor tendon opposite the point of the hock (calcanean tuber), must be cut. Also remove all capsular and tendinous structures from the dorsal surface of the joint. The movement in the hock takes place in the tarsocrural joint; the two intertarsal and the tarsometatarsal joints are capable only of limited sliding movements. Can you detect the snapping motion produced by the short deep medial collateral ligaments at about one-third of the distance from the point of full extension to full flexion?

The *hock joint* of the horse is subject to a variety of ills that give rise to lameness. A common one is an osteoarthritis (bone spavin) usually starting on the medial aspect where it involves the adjacent parts of T1+2, T3, and Tc (seat of spavin). ("Spavin" is a nondescript lay term for almost any disorder in the horse's hock.) Tarsal hydrarthrosis (bog spavin) is a chronic distention of the tarsocrural joint capsule by excess synovia that causes the joint pouches to bulge. Blood spavin is an unfortunate choice of a term given to a non-existing condition: it is the apparent swelling of the cranial branch of the medial saphenous vein as it passes over the bulging dorsal pouch of a bog spavin.

The medial tibialis cranialis tendon (cunean tendon) passes over the seat of spavin and is sometimes resected as palliative therapy for bone spavin. The tendon is underlain by a subtendinous bursa which may be inflamed (cunean bursitis) as a separate entity in Standardbred horses. (Most clinicians prefer the term "cunean" for the bursa or tendon to the longer official terms, which for the former is subtendinous bursa of the medial tibialis cranialis tendon.)

The thick long plantar ligament on the plantar aspect of the hock provides an important connection between the calcaneus, T4, and the proximal ends of the metatarsal bones. During the propulsive phase of the limb when the stifle is extended by the powerful thigh muscles, the common calcanean tendon exerts a tremendous pull on the calcanean tuber. The long plantar ligament transfers the pull to the metatarsal bones and assures that the hock is extended with the distal end of the limb moving caudally and the hoof pushing into the ground to move the animal forward. Injury to the ligament, whether from a kick of another horse or during overexertion (partial rupture), causes it to swell. The condition is known as curb (French, *courbe*, curve) because the swelling puts a curve into the otherwise straight supf. flexor tendon that overlies the ligament.

When neighboring component joints communicate as is the case between the tarsocrural and proximal intertarsal capsules, an inflammatory process in one easily enters the other since synovia can flow back and forth between the two joints. Similarly, an injection of material in one joint serves both.

Stifle Joint

Time Saver: During the dissection of the stifle one student of each group should obtain the stored forelimb and remove the skin as directed on page 114.

The stifle should be studied with particular emphasis on the bony and ligamentous structures palpable on the live animal. The bursae and joint capsules are normally not palpable in the live animal but can be located by reference to the bones and ligaments.

There are three **patellar ligaments** in the horse and cow; we and the dog and cat have only one. In order to expose the three patellar ligaments, it will be necessary to remove the aponeurosis that passes from the surface of the biceps and vastus lateralis across the front of the stifle. It is only loosely attached to the surface of the vastus and the cranial division of the biceps, but it is closely fused with the insertion of the middle division of the biceps on the lateral patellar ligament and must be separated from the latter by sharp dissection. The aponeurosis must also be cut off its close attachment to the cranial surface of the patella, but there is no attachment to the intermediate patellar ligament. The lateral aponeurosis is continuous with the medial aponeurosis that comes from the surface of the vastus medialis, gracilis, and sartorius. The medial aponeurosis is readily freed from the vastus medialis, but is fused with the common insertion of the sartorius and gracilis on the **medial patellar ligament** and must be separated by sharp dissection. Completely remove the medial and lateral aponeuroses.

The thick **intermediate patellar ligament,** although embedded in fat, is now easily exposed. It attaches on the front of the apex of the patella and distally on the tibial tuberosity (Fig. 5-30/B,11"). The **lateral patellar ligament** is flat and attached close to the intermediate patellar ligament at both ends. It receives part of the fascia lata and part of the strong aponeurosis of insertion of the middle division of the biceps. (The middle division of the biceps is also inserted on the cranial border of the tibia.)

Separate the middle and cranial divisions of the biceps. Cut the middle division off its insertion on the lateral patellar ligament and discard it. Then cut the cranial division off its insertion on the patella and proximal part of the lateral patellar ligament and discard it also. Discard the loose caudal division of the biceps also.

The thin but distinct **lateral femoropatellar ligament** is now exposed extending from the lateral epicondyle of the femur to the lateral border of the patella. It is fused with the fibrous membrane of the femoropatellar joint capsule (Fig.5-28/4').

The **lateral collateral ligament** arises from the lateral epicondyle, just distal to the femoropatellar ligament, and ends on the head of the fibula where it is continued by the lateral digital extensor.

Demonstrate the common tendon of origin of the long digital extensor and peroneus tertius by tensing the muscles and palpating between the lateral patellar and lateral collateral ligaments, The common tendon arises from the extensor fossa of the femur just cranial to the lateral femoral condyle (Fig. 5-28/12'). Open the **lateral femorotibial joint capsule** between the common tendon and lateral collateral ligament. The lateral joint is accessible clinically at this point. Demonstrate, by probing, the large distal extension of the lateral femorotibial capsule deep to the common tendon; it may already have been opened when the peroneus tertius was separated previously from the tibialis cranialis.

Transect the vastus lateralis and then the vastus medialis close to the patella. Although the **quadriceps** ends on the patella, functionally speaking it is inserted on the tibia to extend the stifle. The **patella** is regarded as a sesamoid bone (embedded in the quadriceps tendon) that articulates with the femur and allows the tendon to slide over the bone with minimal friction during the excursions of the joint.

There are **bursae** between the patella on the one hand and the lateral vastus and cranial biceps division on the other, and subcutaneous ones on the collateral ligaments. The rectus femoris is underlain by a proximal extension of the femoropatellar joint capsule.

The proximal attachments of the medial and intermediate patellar ligaments are rather widely separated on the patella. The ligaments insert close together, however, on the tibial tuberosity. The medial patellar ligament is joined by the aponeurosis of sartorius and gracilis, and its proximal part furnishes insertion for fibers of the vastus medialis. Sever now also the insertions of sartorius and gracilis.

The medial femoropatellar ligament is very thin and not distinct from the underlying joint capsule. It arises above the medial femoral epicondyle and attaches near the medial patellar ligament on the patellar fibrocartilage (Fig. 5-29/3).

Cut the adductor from its insertion on the proximal end of the **medial collateral ligament**. The ligament arises on the medial femoral epicondyle, just cranial to the insertion of the semimembranosus, and passes to the medial condyle of the tibia.

Open the **medial femorotibial joint capsule** between the medial patellar and medial collateral ligaments close to the medial condyle of the tibia. This is the usual point of clinical access.

Isolate as best you can the medial femoropatellar ligament, and with scissors remove the medial wall of the **femoropatellar joint capsule** proximal and distal to the ligament. This exposes the large medial ridge of the femoral trochlea (see skeleton). Find and explore with your finger the large proximal extension of the joint capsule lying on the femur proximal to the trochlea. Turn the specimen over and repeat the removal of the

femoropatellar joint capsule on the lateral side (Fig. 5-28). The lateral ridge of the trochlea is considerably smaller. Open the femoropatellar joint capsule also between the intermediate and medial patellar ligaments close to the apex of the patella by removing the thick cushion of fat between the capsule and the patellar ligaments.

Probe the femoropatellar joint cavity. A narrow communication usually exists between the femoropatellar and the *medial* femorotibial cavities at the distal end of the medial ridge of the trochlea (do not look for it). A similar communication occurs in about 25% of cases between the femoropatellar and the lateral femorotibial cavities. Communication between the lateral and medial femorotibial joint cavities is rare in the horse. Note that the femoropatellar joint cavity extends also under the femoropatellar ligaments. The usual point for clinical injection is between the patellar ligaments close to the patellar apex.

Remove remaining tags of the femoropatellar joint capsule from between the patellar ligaments so that the cranial surface of the trochlea is exposed and its relationship to the patellar ligaments can be observed.

Cut the insertion of the semimembranosus on the medial femoral epicondyle and remove the muscle. Isolate the medial head of the gastrocnemius, cut it close to its origin on the caudal surface of the femur, and reflect the distal stump without injury to the tibial nerve.

Probe the **medial femorotibial joint cavity**. Remove any muscle tags remaining and (with scissors) cut away as much of the capsules as you can especially that enclosing the medial femoral condyle. Note that the joint is incompletely divided into an upper and lower compartment by the **medial meniscus**.

Cut the insertion of the rectus femoris as close to the patella as possible so that the latter remains attached only by the patellar and femoropatellar ligaments. Shorten the proximal stumps of the quadriceps so some of the shaft of the femur is exposed.

Turn the specimen so that the caudal surface is up. Cut and reflect the lateral head of the gastrocnemius (including the supf. flexor) in the same way you did the medial head, fully exposing the popliteal artery.

The **popliteal artery** disappears deep to the popliteus muscle where it gives rise to the cranial and caudal tibial arteries that were seen in the leg. The cranial tibial artery passes forward between tibia and fibula, as in the dog (Fig. 5-23).

Transect the **popliteus** at the level of the popliteal artery and reflect the stumps off the caudal surface of the joint. The strong tendon of origin is attached to the distal depression (not the extensor fossa) on the lateral femoral epicondyle and passes around the lateral meniscus deep to the lateral collateral ligament. Deep to the tendon is an extension of the lateral femorotibial joint capsule that facilitates the movement of the tendon against the meniscus and the tibial condyle below it.

Remove the lateral femorotibial joint capsule and the segment of the popliteal vessels caudal to the stifle, making sure the distal stumps of the vessels are short.

The caudal end of the **lateral meniscus** is now seen to be attached to the tibia, and to the femur by means of the meniscofemoral ligament. The latter crosses obliquely through the intercondylar fossa to the proximal end of the medial femoral condyle. Transect it and remove the synovial structures and small vessels from the intercondylar fossa. This exposes the caudal and cranial **cruciate ligaments,** named according to their attachment on the tibia. The caudal cruciate ligament runs from the popliteal notch of the tibia to the axial surface of the medial femoral condyle. The cranial cruciate ligament runs from the depression in the intercondylar eminence of the tibia to the axial surface of the lateral femoral condyle. Twist the tibia and flex and extend the stifle to demonstrate the action of the cruciate ligaments. They seem to be most effective in limiting extension and, together with the collateral ligaments, pronation—turning the limb distal to the stifle inward.

It is necessary for the demonstration of the **PATELLAR LOCKING MECHANISM** to work together with the group that has the other hindlimb of your horse.

On o n e of the limbs cut the medial and lateral femoropatellar ligaments and reflect the patella distally off the trochlea. Remove the remaining tags of the femoropatellar joint capsule and from between the patellar ligaments so that the articulating surfaces of the trochlea and patella are fully visible.

The **trochlea** consists of medial and lateral ridges separated by a groove. Note that the medial ridge is much larger than the lateral and that it is thickened by a smooth **tubercle** on the proximal end of the medial surface. The articular surface of the trochlea presents an abrupt change of direction at the proximal end, so that the upper portion, a transverse zone about 1.5 cm wide, faces dorsocranially in the standing animal. It may be termed the **resting surface** of the trochlea, and the remaining much larger surface may be called the **gliding surface** (Fig. 5-29).

The articular surface of the **patella** is also divided into resting and gliding surfaces. The **resting surface** is a zone about 1.5 cm wide along the distal border. Between the apex and the medial angle of the patella it forms an angle of about 130 degrees with the medial part of the gliding surface. The resting surface also extends about 2 cm lateral to the apex. The **gliding surface** conforms to the corresponding surface of the trochlea.

Now take the other limb and on it, without reflecting the patella, remove what remained of the femoropatellar joint capsule and fat from the patellar ligaments, patella, and trochlea so the trochlea can be seen through the patellar ligaments.

The **tubercle** on the proximal end of the medial ridge, although not articulating with the patella, is covered with cartilage because it provides a friction catch for the **patellar fibrocartilage** (palpate) and the medial patellar ligament. Strongly flex the stifle and identify the resting and gliding surfaces of the trochlea and patella.

When the horse is standing squarely on both hindlimbs (extend the stifle of your specimen) the patella is at the proximal end of the trochlea, the resting surfaces are in contact, and the cranial border of the medial patellar ligament is about one finger-breadth caudal to the cranial edge of the medial ridge of the trochlea. When the patella is on the resting surface of the trochlea little force is required to prevent the patella from slipping onto the gliding surface (try this by flexing the stifle). Palpation of the quadriceps femoris in the live animal will show that the muscle is relaxed when the horse is standing. However, the biceps femoris and tensor fasciae latae are attached to the lateral patellar ligament and the sartorius and gracilis to the medial patellar ligament and may help to hold the patella in the resting position. The patella reaches the resting position also in the weight-bearing phase of the walk. It is not known whether this occurs also in faster gaits.

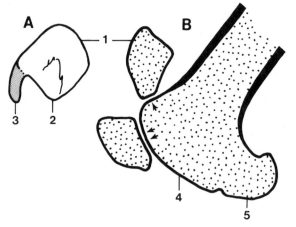

1. Patella
2. Apex
3. Patellar fibrocartilage
4. Femoral trochlea
5. Femoral condyle

Single arrow: resting surfaces of femur and patella engaged.
Double arrows: gliding surfaces of femur and patella engaged.

FIGURE 5-29. Cranial view of left patella *(A)* and sagittal section of distal femur with patella in resting and gliding positions *(B)*.

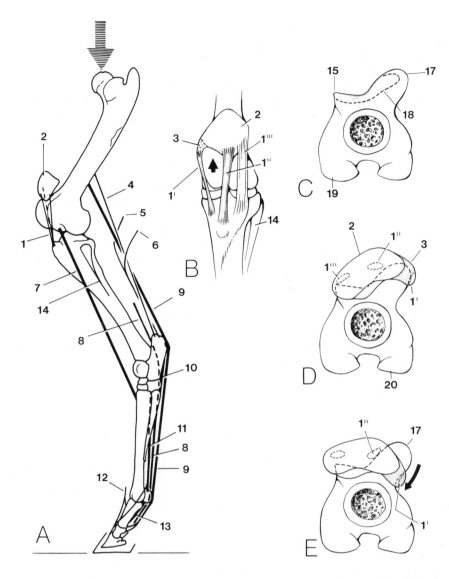

1',1",1'" Medial, intermediate, and lateral
  patellar ligaments
2. Patella
3. Patellar fibrocartilage
4. Fascial band associated with lat. head
   of gastrocnemius
5. Tarsal tendon of semitendinosus
6. Tarsal tendon of biceps
7. Peroneus tertius (theoretically not
   required in the standing horse)
8. Deep flexor tendon
9. Supf. digital flexor
10. Long plantar ligament
11. Interosseus
12. Long digital extensor tendon
13. Sesamoidean ligaments
14. Fibula
15. Lat. trochlear ridge
17. Tubercle on proximal end of medial
    trochlear ridge
18. Resting surface on proximal end of
    trochlea
19, 20 Lat. and med. femoral condyles

FIGURE 5-30. A, The passive stay-apparatus of the left hindlimb, lateral view. (After Schmaltz, 1911.) B, Left stifle joint, cranial view. C-E, distal end of femur, looking distally; in D, position of patella in horse standing squarely; in E, stifle locked.

When the horse rests one hindlimb on the toe of the hoof, the supporting limb undergoes slight flexion with the added weight and the hindquarters sink about 4 cm. The pelvis is tilted with the supporting side higher. In the supporting limb the patella in the resting position rotates medially (about 15 degrees; simulate on your specimen) and the fibrocartilage and medial patellar ligament slide farther caudally on the tubercle. Observe the loop formed by the intermediate and medial patellar ligaments and the patella over the top of the medial trochlear ridge. This mechanism prevents flexion of the stifle and enables the horse to stand with little muscular effort. Some effort must be required, however, because the horse soon tires and shifts his weight to the other hindlimb.

The patellar locking mechanism features a loop of structures that hooks over the tubercle on the proximal end of the medial trochlear ridge (Fig. 5-30/B). The loop, from medial to lateral, comprises the medial patellar ligament, patellar fibrocartilage, patella, and the intermediate patellar ligament.

In *upward fixation of the patella*, the horse (often a young animal) can slip the loop over the tubercle, but cannot pull it off again when it wants to flex the stifle, and thus it swings the extended limb forward in a lateral arc when it is made to walk. The upward fixation of the patella is often intermittent and usually bilateral, with one hindlimb often more affected than the other. Treatment will vary depending on the severity and persistence of the condition. Surgical treatment consists of cutting the loop at the distal end of the medial patellar ligament (medial patellar desmotomy) through a small skin incision under local anesthesia. This releases the lock.

Passive Stay-Apparatus

(When reading this section, re-identify on your specimen the structures set in bold type, and with the help of Figure 5-30 determine or recall their attachments on the bony column of the limb.)

The **patellar locking mechanism** is part of the so-called stay-apparatus of the hindlimb which enables the horse to support the hindquarters with a minimum of muscular effort by preventing flexion in the stifle and hock joints and over-extension in the fetlock and phalangeal joints. The tendinous **peroneus tertius** and **supf. digital flexor** link stifle and hock in such a way that the two joints can move only in unison (Fig. 5-30/A/7,9). Consequently, when the stifle is locked by its patellar mechanism, the hock joint is locked also and will not flex under weight.

The fetlock and phalangeal joints are supported principally by the interosseus and the supf. and deep flexor tendons with the fetlock joint slightly overextended in the standing animal. (Can you explain the difference between extension and overextension of a joint?) The tendinous **interosseus** (/11) arises proximal to the fetlock, attaches on the proximal sesamoid bones, and is functionally continued by **distal sesamoidean ligaments** (/13) that attach on the plantar surface of the proximal two phalanges. (You will see all this in detail when we study the forelimb—hind and fore digits are practically identical.) The **supf. and deep flexor tendons** (/9,8) also attach proximal and distal to the fetlock and lend further support. The tendinous structures are under tension when weight is on the overextended fetlock joint and support the joint by preventing it from overextending further.

6
2
4

L

Exercises on the Live Animal

1---Begin at the stifle by finding the tibial tuberosity which is more distal than is often imagined. Palpate the two dimples between the (distal) attachments of the three patellar ligaments on the tibial tuberosity. The dimples are good starting points for stifle palpation; they are at the level of the femorotibial joint space. Follow the patellar ligaments from the dimples to the patella (easiest on the medial, hardest on the lateral ligament) and palpate (through fat) the smooth medial trochlear ridge between the medial and intermediate ligaments. (The ridge protrudes more cranially when the horse holds the stifle in the locked position.)

2---Still on the stifle, palpate caudolaterally from the dimples and feel the common tendon of origin of the peroneus tertius and long extensor in the extensor groove of the tibia. More caudally you can feel the head of the fibula, the common peroneal nerve passing over it (in which direction?), and proximal to this the lateral collateral ligament. The lateral femorotibial joint can be punctured between the common tendon of peroneus tertius and long extensor and the lateral collateral ligament. On the medial surface, palpate the area between the medial patellar and medial

collateral ligaments at the level of the femorotibial joint space (level with the dimples). The medial femorotibial joint can be punctured here.

3---Systematically examine the leg (crus), preferably on a limb the horse is resting on the toe of the hoof (more relaxed). Working from cranial to caudal on the lateral surface, palpate the long extensor, the lateral extensor, and the separation between these two muscles. This is the site for the deep peroneal nerve block; in the distal half of the separation you can palpate the superficial peroneal nerve. Caudal to the lateral extensor is the tibialis caudalis (one of the three deep flexors). Palpate the gastrocnemius tendon as it spirals around the lateral surface of the supf. flexor tendon from the supf. to the deep position. Working from cranial to caudal on the medial surface, palpate the tibialis cranialis, the cranial branch of the medial saphenous vein (follow it over the hock), the tibia, the medial digital flexor (another one of the deep flexors), and the tibial nerve in the groove cranial to the common calcanean tendon.

4---Outline the extent of the hock by finding the medial and lateral malleoli of the tibia and the proximal end of Mt3. From the malleoli, follow the course of the collateral ligaments, and then find the peroneus tertius tendon in the center of the dorsal surface. Attempt to palpate the medial branch of the tibialis cranialis (cunean) tendon—less difficult when the limb relaxed.

5---Still on the hock, pick up the cranial branch of the medial saphenous vein and follow it over the *soft* dorsal pouch of the tarsocrural joint (the pouch is bounded by the peroneus tertius tendon, medial branch of the tibialis cranialis tendon, medial malleolus, and medial collateral ligament). Find the very much smaller medioplantar pouch between the medial collateral ligament and deep flexor tendon at the level of the medial malleolus. And finally, palpate the lateroplantar pouch between the lateral malleolus and calcaneus.

6---In the metatarsus, palpate the shallow grooves between the large and small metatarsal bones and the rounded distal ends of the latter bones; in the lateral groove take the pulse (with several finger tips) from the dorsal metatarsal artery. Palpate the long and lateral extensor tendons and note where they join. On the plantar aspect, palpate the supf. and deep flexor tendons and the interosseus, which you should follow to the proximal sesamoid bones. The communicating branch between the medial and lateral plantar nerves that crosses the supf. flexor tendon is more easily palpated on the forelimb.

7---Find chestnut and ergot.

8---To palpate the **locking of the stifle** a little more time is required. On a horse standing squarely on both hindlimbs, palpate the medial and intermediate patellar ligaments and the rounded medial ridge of the femoral trochlea between them. Note that the medial ligament is about one finger-breadth caudal to the cranial edge of the ridge. Also note that the quadriceps is relaxed.

Wait until the horse rests one hindlimb on the toe of the hoof and supports the weight with the other. When palpating the supporting stifle you will find that the medial patellar ligament is now about two finger-breadths caudal to the cranial edge of the ridge and that the apex of the patella (deep to the proximal end of the intermediate patellar ligament) is in close contact with the trochlea. Now push the horse off the supporting limb with your shoulder and, as the stifle begins to flex, feel the distinct snap with which the patella is released from the top of the medial ridge. The patella rotates laterally about 15 degrees as the gliding surfaces engage and a notch becomes palpable between the apex of the patella and the trochlea.

6

FORELIMB

A considerable number of pages are devoted to the study of the forelimb, so its features can be seen and explored in detail. Considering that the relatively slender forelimbs have to support such a large weight—often at racing speeds—it is no wonder that injuries abound, particularly in the carpus, metacarpus, and digit. To diagnose and treat these successfully, veterinarians need a thorough knowledge of forelimb anatomy. The following facts illustrate how severe competition and stress in horses can be: among Thoroughbreds in the U.S., only 10 percent of horses that start the training process are still competing after one year of racing. Only 50 percent of horses being trained reach the racetrack. (From Cunha, 1980).

Purpose and Plan of the Dissection

1---To see the vessels and nerves (brachial plexus) supplying the limb, the axillary lymph nodes, and the pectoral muscles on the medial aspect where the limb was removed from the trunk. To see the supplying structures again, and the cubital lymph nodes, on the medial surface of the arm after the pectoral muscles have been removed.

2---To explore the shoulder joint and adjacent structures from both lateral and medial aspects.

3---To follow the radial nerve to the lateral aspect and see it enter the carpal and digital extensor muscles at the level of the elbow joint.

4---To become familiar with the bones of the forearm, carpus, and metacarpus, and to follow the principal arteries and the median and ulnar nerves through the forearm into the metacarpus.

5---To see the internal tendon of the biceps, and its lacertus fibrosus continuation, and to study systematically the muscles (and their tendon sheaths) that surround the radius.

6---To study the passage of the digital flexors

through the carpal canal and the accessory (check) ligaments by which their tendons connect to the bony column distal to their bellies.

7---To study the capsules of the three component joints of the carpus and the interior of the proximal two joints that open during flexion. To become familiar with the major ligaments of the carpus and with the retinacula that guide the tendons of the digital extensors and flexors over this joint.

8---The purpose of the detailed dissection of the digit is to see virtually all features of the phalanges, the digital joints and ligaments, to follow the tendons, vessels, and nerves to their destinations, and to explore the remarkable organization of the hoof in this clinically very important part of the horse's body.

Plan. After the cut surface of the limb has been examined, the pectoral muscles are removed to expose the medial surface of the arm. The muscles connecting scapula and humerus are transected and reflected for the study of the shoulder joint. Then the heads of the triceps are transected to view the course of the radial nerve around the humerus to the cranial surface of the elbow joint.

The subcutaneous veins, principal arteries, and the median and ulnar nerves are traced through forearm and carpus into the metacarpus. After removing the muscle tissue of the biceps to expose the internal tendon and its connections to the radius and (via lacertus and extensor carpi radialis) to the large metacarpal bone, the muscles of the forearm are transected and reflected, their tendon sheaths opened (and probed; optional) and the carpal retinacula cut to expose the tendons at this level. The bellies of the digital flexors are transected several times to see the large amounts of internal fibrous tissue sheets that seem to play a role in preventing the elbow joint from collapsing in the standing animal. The capsules of the radiocarpal and midcarpal joints are removed and the tendons crossing the carpus reflected to expose the articular surfaces of the bones forming these two joints.

After studying its external features, the hoof is removed to expose the hoof dermis, cartilages, and digital cushion for study. The digital vessels and nerves are traced to their terminations, as are the extensor tendons on the dorsal aspect. This necessitates opening the dorsal pouches of the fetlock and digital joints. On the palmar aspect of the digit the annular ligaments associated with the flexor tendons are cut so that the tendons can be reflected to their attachments on the phalanges. This exposes the three bearing surfaces over which the flexor tendons change direction. Then we study the interosseus, the sesamoidean ligaments, the palmar ligaments of the pastern joint, and the collateral ligaments of the joints and of the navicular bone. To conclude, the fetlock and digital joints are disarticulated.

Shoulder Joint and Arm

(A fresh forelimb from the post mortem room can be used for this dissection. Make allowance for added skin reflections and smaller stumps of the pectoral muscles and of the branches of the brachial plexus. The limb should definitely be kept refrigerated.)

To horse owners the "shoulder" of the horse is the region between the dorsal edge of the scapular cartilage and the shoulder joint. Anatomically speaking this is the scapular region (Fig. 6-1/1). The cranial part of the greater tubercle of the humerus on the live animal is known as the **point of the shoulder;** the prominent olecranon is the **point of the elbow.** The **carpus** is also known popularly as the "knee" but it does of course not correspond to our knee. The **fetlock joint** (metacarpophalangeal joint) is often called the "ankle", a false analogy because the human ankle is the talocrural articulation of the pelvic limb. The part of the limb distal to the fetlock is the **digit,** and the part of the digit from the fetlock to the hoof is the **pastern.** The junction between the skin and hoof is known popularly as the coronet. Chestnut and ergot have been described with the hindlimb (p. 82). With help of Fig. 6-1 identify the labeled parts on our specimen.

During the dissection of the forelimb constant reference to the skeleton should be made whenever bony structures are mentioned. Use the

articulated forelimb specimen from your course locker for the distal part of the limb.

On the medial surface of the arm find the cut ends of the axillary artery and vein (Fig. 6-2/21). Clean the axillary vein until the **axillary lymph nodes** are exposed; they drain most of the limb (/28). The supf. lymphatics of the scapular region and arm drain into the supf. cervical lymph nodes.

Note that the supraspinatus extends beyond the cranial border of the scapula and is therefore visible on the medial surface. At the level of the scapular notch (Fig. 6-1/2) about 12 cm dorsal to the axillary vessels, the large **suprascapular nerve** dips between the subscapularis and supraspinatus. Tag the nerve; it will be traced later. The **musculocutaneous nerve** (Fig. 6-2/7) may be identified and tagged as it passes distally lateral to the axillary artery. It forms a loop distal to the artery with the large **median nerve** (/6). The median nerve lies medial to the artery. *You will see this*

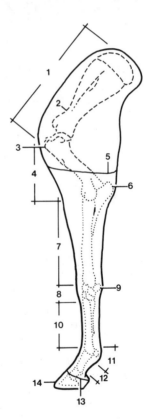

1.	"Shoulder" or scapular region	8.	Carpus
2.	Scapular notch	9.	Accessory carpal bone
3.	Point of shoulder, cranial part of greater tubercle	10.	Metacarpus
		11.	Fetlock
4.	Arm	12.	Pastern
5.	Skin previously reflected to here	13.	Coronet, junction of skin and hoof
6.	Point of elbow, olecranon	14.	Hoof, with contents also known as the foot of the horse
7.	Forearm		

FIGURE 6-1. The forelimb and its parts at the beginning of its dissection.

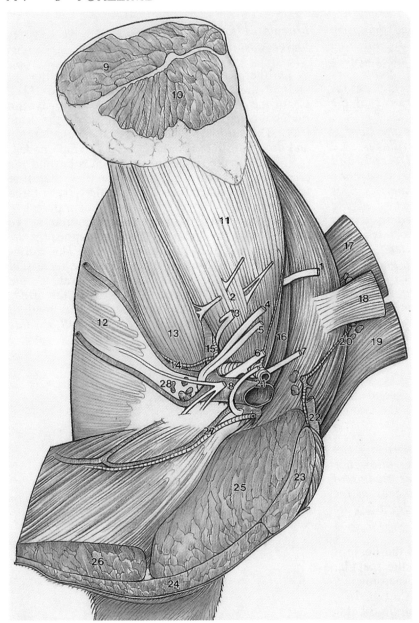

Nerves:
1. Suprascapular
2. Subscapulars
3. Axillary
4. Radial
5. Ulnar
6. Median
7. Musculocutaneous
8. Cranial and caudal pectorals

9. Rhomboideus thoracis
10. Serratus ventralis
11. Subscapularis
12. Latissimus dorsi
13. Teres major
14. Thoracodorsal vessels
15. Subscapular vessels
16. Supraspinatus
17. Omotransversarius
18. Omohyoideus
19. Cleidomastoideus
20. Prescapular br. of supf. cervical artery, and supf. cervical lymph nodes
21. Axillary vessels
22. Deltoid br. of supf. cervical artery, and cephalic vein
23. Pectoralis descendens
24. Pectoralis transversus
25. Subclavius
26. Pectoralis profundus
27. External thoracic vessels
28. Axillary lymph nodes

FIGURE 6-2. Left shoulder and arm with pectoral muscles, medial view.

relationship only if you did cut the axillary vessels and brachial plexus close to the first rib (as directed when the forelimb was removed).

Make a skin incision along the caudal border of the limb, over the point of the elbow, to the beginning of the metacarpus. Reflect the skin carefully off the arm, forearm, and carpus, and then cut it off. Wrap the limb well with plastic at the end of each laboratory period; a skinned specimen dries very quickly and becomes useless if it is left exposed to the air. In addition: because of their clinical importance the digit and hoof will be dissected in detail and must not be allowed to dry. Therefore, keep metacarpus and digit wrapped in cloth soaked with mold-inhibiting solution and plastic while the proximal parts of the limb are studied.

There are four **PECTORAL MUSCLES** in the horse; all originate from the sternum:

Supf. pectoral muscles
  Pectoralis descendens
  Pectoralis transversus
Deep pectoral muscle (Pectoralis profundus)
Subclavius (not present in the dog)

With the help of Fig. 6-2 identify the stumps of the four muscles on your specimen; this should not be difficult if you transected them close to the sternum when the limb was removed. Carefully separate the ventral end of the large **subclavius** (/25) from the pectoralis descendens on its ventral surface and the pectoralis profundus on its deep (lateral) surface. This separation is readily accomplished by close attention to the direction of the muscle fibers. Reflect the subclavius cranially and dorsally noting its loose insertion on the scapular fascia and the proximal part of the supraspinatus (Fig. 6-3/1,9).

Isolate the **pectoralis profundus**. It has medial and lateral insertions on the humerus. The medial insertion is fleshy and attached to the cranial part of the lesser tubercle of the humerus (palpate) just below the fleshy medial insertion of the supraspinatus. The lateral insertion becomes aponeurotic as it crosses over the intertubercular groove to attach to the cranial part of the greater tubercle (palpate). Transect the pectoralis profundus *close* to the medial insertion and *remove* the large caudal stump.

A thin tendinous slip of the **cutaneus trunci** (/15) may now be seen passing cranially to the lesser tubercle, remove it.

Identify the stumps of the supf. pectoral muscles and of the cleidomastoideus and omotransversarius. The **pectoralis transversus** is wide craniocaudally and thin dorsoventrally; it inserts on the medial deep fascia of the forearm below the elbow (Fig. 6-3/16). The **pectoralis descendens** is narrow and thick and closely applied to the cranial part of the preceding muscle.

Turn the limb so the cranial surface is up and see once more the groove between the pectoralis descendens and brachiocephalicus; in the groove is the **cephalic vein** (/12).

Preserving a cutaneous nerve deep to the caudal border of the pectoralis transversus, free this border from the deep fascia of the arm and forearm and reflect this muscle and the pectoralis descendens craniodistally off the medial surface of the arm and discard them.

On the caudal surface of the forearm just below the elbow locate the **caudal cutaneous antebrachial nerve** (from the ulnar). It ramifies on the caudal surface and both sides of the forearm (Figs. 6-7/10 and 6-6).

The brachial vein can now be seen passing distally beneath the deep fascia. Incise the deep fascia over the vein from the shoulder joint to the elbow. Reflect the flaps: cranially off the coracobrachialis to the edge of the fusiform biceps brachii; caudally off the surface of the tensor fasciae antebrachii.

Beginning at the stumps of the axillary vessels, clean the **axillary artery** and trace it into the arm where it is known as the brachial artery and lies cranial to its large satellite vein. Locate the **subscapular artery** which arises from the axillary and passes proximally between the subscapularis and the teres major (Fig. 6-2/15). The **axillary nerve** (/3) passes laterally between the sub-

scapularis and the subscapular artery. It is accompanied by a branch of the subscapular artery, the caudal circumflex humeral artery. The nerve and artery will be seen later on the lateral side. The **radial and ulnar nerves** (/4,5) lie close together and pass distally caudal to the junction of the subscapular and axillary veins.

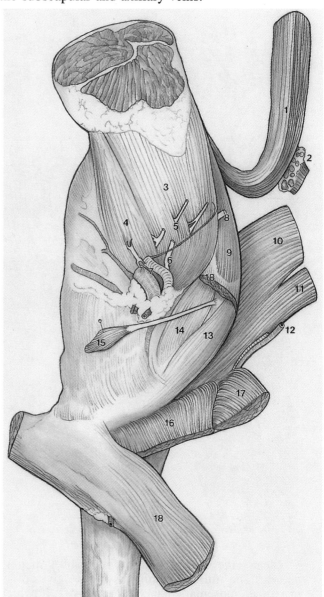

1.	Subclavius	10.	Omotransversarius
2.	Supf. cervical lymph nodes on omohyoideus	11.	Cleidomastoideus
		12.	Cephalic vein
3.	Subscapularis	13.	Biceps, covered by fascia
4.	Teres major	14.	Coracobrachialis, covered by fascia
5.	Subscapular nerves		
6.	Axillary nerve	15.	Cutaneus trunci
7.	Axillary vessels (and associated nerves), reflected dorsally	16.	Pectoralis transversus
		17.	Pectoralis descendens
		18.	Pectoralis profundus, reflected
8.	Suprascapular nerve		
9.	Supraspinatus		

FIGURE 6-3. Left shoulder and arm, medial view. Subclavius, pectoral muscles, and the axillary vessels have been reflected.

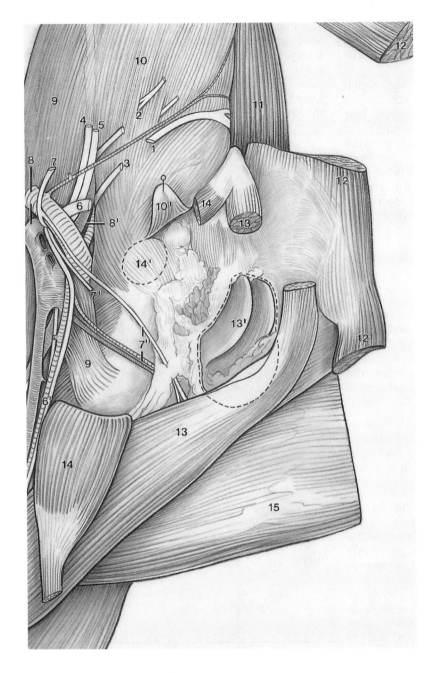

1. Suprascapular
2. Subscapulars
3. Axillary
4. Radial
5. Ulnar
6. Median, covering the brachial artery at 6'
7. Musculocutaneous, branch to coraco-brachialis at 7', with cran. circumflex humeral vessels at 7" (prox. muscular br.)

8. Axillary vessels, reflectred dorsally; sub-scapular vessels at 8'
9. Teres major
10. Subscapularis, part of attachment to lesser tubercle of humerus elevated at 10'
11. Infraspinatus
12. Supraspinatus, transected; stump of pectoralis profundus at 12'
13. Biceps, transected; intermediate tubercle exposed by opening intertubercular bursa at 13'
14. Coracobrachialis, reflected; its subten-dinous bursa at 14'
15. Brachiocephalicus

FIGURE 6-4. Area of left shoulder joint, craniomedial view. The intertubercular bursa has been opened by transection of the biceps tendon.

Clean the musculocutaneous and median nerves. The **musculocutaneous nerve** gives off a proximal muscular branch (Fig. 6-4/7',7")which supplies the coracobrachialis and biceps. The musculocutaneous then joins the **median nerve** below the axillary artery, and the two nerves pass distally cranial to the brachial vein; they are closely adherent but may be pulled apart. Near the middle of the arm the musculocutaneous separates from the median and dips beneath the belly of the biceps where it ends as the distal muscular branch for the brachialis and a cutaneous branch for the medial surface of the limb.

The **cubital lymph nodes** cover the brachial vessels and the median nerve in the distal part of the arm. They receive afferents from the limb below and send efferents to the axillary and supf. cervical nodes.

Reflect the stumps of the axillary vessels and the median and musculocutaneous nerves caudally to expose the deeply lying **brachial artery** more fully. The cranial circumflex humeral artery arises from the proximal part of the brachial and enters the belly of the coracobrachialis close to the proximal muscular branch of the musculo-cutaneous nerve. The deep brachial artery arises from the caudal surface of the brachial near the middle of the arm; do not trace. The **collateral ulnar artery** arises from the caudal surface of the

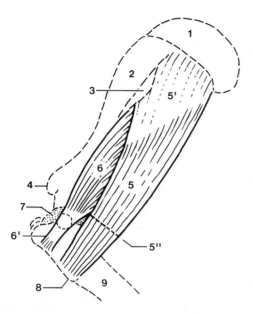

FIGURE 6-5. Attachments of the deltoideus (5) to deltoid tuberosity (8), scapular spine (3), surface of infraspinatus (6), and to the caudal angle of the scapula.

1.	Scapular cartilage	6.	Infraspinatus
2.	Supraspinous fossa	6'.	Infraspinatus tendon
3.	Scapular spine		and bursa (circle)
4.	Supraglenoid tubercle	7.	Head of humerus (stippled)
5,5'	Muscular and aponeurotic	8.	Deltoid tuberosity
	parts of deltoideus	9.	Shaft of humerus
5"	Level of transection of		
	deltoideus		

between the supraspinatus and infraspinatus by palpating distal to the scapular spine. Using the deep fascial septum between the two muscles as a guide, isolate the supraspinatus and transect it just distal to the level of the suprascapular nerve that was seen and tagged on the medial surface. Reflect the proximal stump freeing it from the supraspinous fossa of the scapula.

The **suprascapular nerve** is now fully exposed as it crosses the cranial border of the scapula. It innervates the supra- and infraspinatus muscles (Fig. 6-9).

Damage to the suprascapular nerve results in *sweeny*, a neurogenic atrophy (shrinkage) of the supra- and infraspinatus muscles; it causes the scapular spine to stand out between the two muscles. Damage is from direct trauma as when a horse runs with the shoulder against a door jamb for example.

Reflect the distal stump of the supraspinatus to its insertions. Cut the medial insertion of the supraspinatus and the medial insertion of the pectoralis profundus from their points of attachment on the humerus. The tendon of origin of the **biceps brachii** is now exposed as it passes from the supraglenoid tubercle through the intertubercular groove. Transect the biceps tendon close to the supraglenoid tubercle and reflect it distally off the intertubercular groove.

brachial artery about 5 cm distal to the deep brachial. The **transverse cubital artery** arises from the cranial surface opposite the cubital lymph nodes and disappears under the biceps (Fig. 6-15).

Free the brachial vein sufficiently to expose the course of the ulnar and radial nerves. The **radial nerve** detaches branches to the tensor fasciae antebrachii and the long head of the triceps and passes laterally caudal to the humerus; it will be traced later on the lateral surface of the arm. The **ulnar nerve** accompanies the radial for a short distance and then inclines obliquely to the caudal border of the brachial vein. Near the middle of the arm the ulnar detaches a cutaneous branch to the caudal surface of the forearm.

Separate the thin, flat tensor fasciae antebrachii from the long head of the triceps, working from the caudal border. The tensor may be divided into distinct cranial and caudal portions of which the latter overlaps the caudal edge of the triceps. Transect the tensor at its middle and reflect the distal stump. The ulnar nerve and the collateral ulnar vessels are now exposed as they pass caudodistally toward the point of the elbow; they will be traced in the forearm later.

Cut the already loosened subclavius off the surface of the supraspinatus and discard it. Now turn the limb over so the lateral surface is up. Remove the supf. fascia and locate the groove

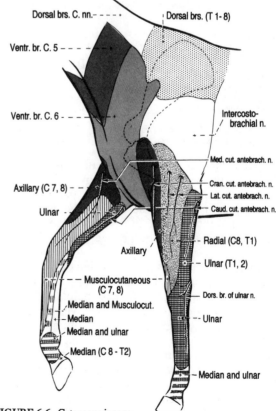

FIGURE 6-6. Cutaneous innervation and named cutaneous nerves of the forelimb, craniolateral view. (Modified from Ellenberger and Baum 1943.)

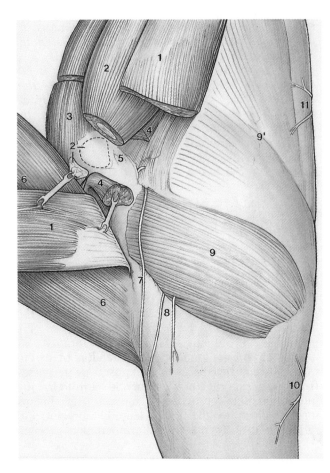

1. Deltoideus
2. Infraspinatus, its supf. tendon and infraspinatus bursa at 2'
3. Supraspinatus
4. Teres minor, transected
5. Shoulder joint capsule
6. Brachiocephalicus
7. Cran. cutaneous antebrachial nerve
8. Lat. cutaneous antebrachial nerve
9. Lat. head of triceps, long head under fascia at 9'
10. Caud. cutaneous antebrachial nerve
11. Intercostobrachial nerve

FIGURE 6-7. Area of left arm, lateral view. Deltoideus, infraspinatus, and teres minor have been transected and reflected.

This opens the large **intertubercular bursa** that lies between the tendon and the groove. The bursa usually does not communicate with the shoulder joint cavity as it does in the dog. The tendon is partly cartilaginous and closely molded to the intermediate tubercle in the groove (Fig. 6-4/13').

For the transection of the **deltoideus** it is best to find first its cranial border (Fig. 6-5/5,5"): Identify the infraspinatus (/6) and palpate distally on it until its tendon is felt passing over a distinct rounded tuberosity. Caudal to the tendon of the infraspinatus is the cranial border of the deltoideus. Push your fingers under the border and the entire muscle and vigorously undermine it until you are stopped by the heavy aponeurosis (/5') with which the deltoideus is attached to the lateral surface of the infraspinatus and the spine of the scapula. Transect the deltoideus level with the previous supraspinatus transection and reflect the

distal stump to its insertion, with part of the cleidobrachialis, on the deltoid tuberosity. (The deltoideus of the horse is not clearly divided into two parts as in the dog and domestic ruminants.)

Branches of the **axillary nerve** and of the caudal circumflex humeral artery are now exposed between the long and lateral heads of the triceps. The nerve supplies the muscles in the vicinity: teres major and minor, deltoideus, and cleidobrachialis (do not trace).

The axillary nerve also furnishes the **cranial cutaneous antebrachial nerve** which emerges from the caudal border of the deltoideus near its insertion. The cutaneous nerve runs craniodistally to the flexion surface of the elbow joint and ramifies on the cranial surface of the forearm (Fig. 6-6). The nerve should be traced with a minimum of dissection but the cutaneus omobrachialis muscle will have to be reflected.

The wide **supf. tendon** of the **infraspinatus**, bound down by a fibrous sheet, is now exposed. Transect the muscle at the musculotendinous

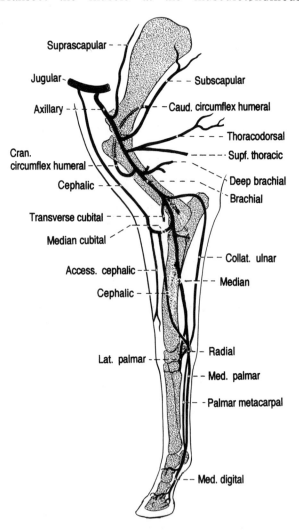

FIGURE 6-8. Veins of the right forelimb, medial view. Variations will be encountered, especially at the level of the carpus.

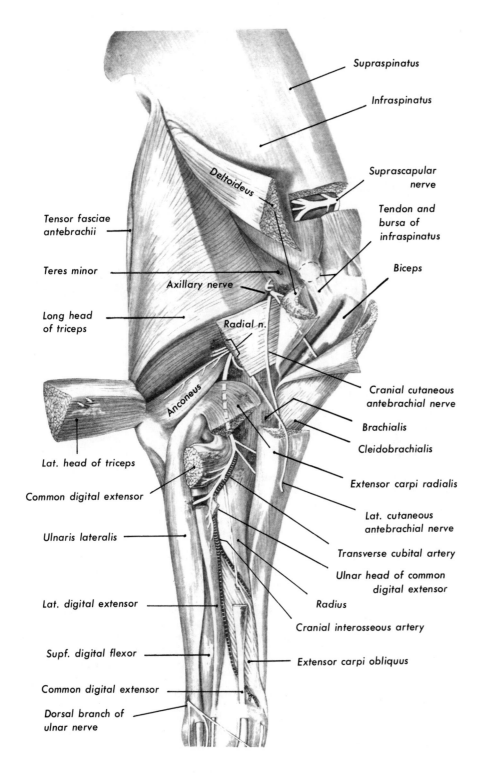

Supraspinatus

Infraspinatus

Suprascapular nerve

Tendon and bursa of infraspinatus

Biceps

Deltoideus

Tensor fasciae antebrachii

Teres minor

Axillary nerve

Long head of triceps

Radial n.

Anconeus

Lat. head of triceps

Common digital extensor

Ulnaris lateralis

Lat. digital extensor

Supf. digital flexor

Common digital extensor

Dorsal branch of ulnar nerve

Cranial cutaneous antebrachial nerve

Brachialis

Cleidobrachialis

Extensor carpi radialis

Lat. cutaneous antebrachial nerve

Transverse cubital artery

Ulnar head of common digital extensor

Radius

Cranial interosseous artery

Extensor carpi obliquus

FIGURE 6-9. Deep dissection of right arm and forearm, lateral view, to show the distribution of the suprascapular, axillary, and radial nerves. (Modified from Hopkins 1937.)

junction and reflect the *tendinous* distal stump to its insertion on the greater tubercle (Fig. 6-7/2,2'). There is a bursa, the **infraspinatus bursa**, between the tendon and the rounded caudal part of the tubercle. Reflection of the infraspinatus tendon reveals a second, deep, *fleshy* insertion of the muscle on the proximal border of the greater

tubercle. The teres minor passes caudal to this to reach its insertion on and above the deltoid tuberosity. Transect the fleshy insertion (of the infraspinatus) and the teres minor close to their attachments and reflect them proximally to expose the lateral surface of the **shoulder joint capsule.** Open the capsule. The articular head of the

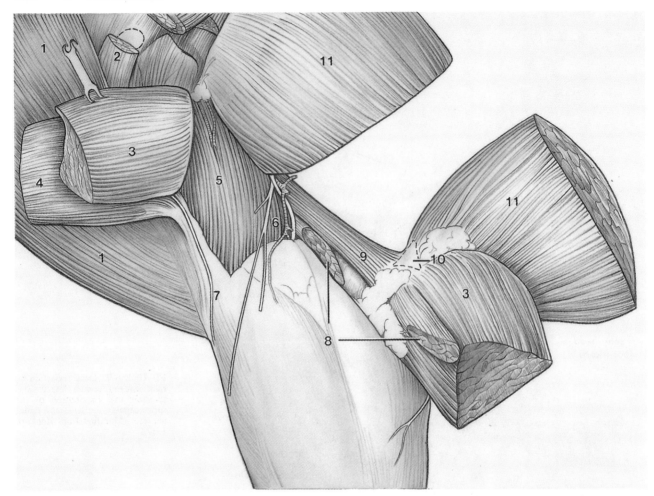

1.	Brachiocephalicus	6.	Radial nerve and br. of deep brachial artery	10.	Subtendinous bursa of triceps
2.	Infraspinatus tendon and bursa	7.	Cran. cutaneous ante-brachial nerve	11.	Long head of triceps
3.	Lat. head of triceps	8.	Anconeus		
4.	Deltoideus	9.	Med. head of triceps		
5.	Brachialis				

FIGURE 6-10. Deep dissection of left arm, lateral view. The lateral and long heads of the triceps and the anconeus have been transected to expose the brachialis and radial nerve.

humerus is much larger than the glenoid cavity of the scapula.

Turn the limb so that the medial surface is up. Find the tendon of the coracobrachialis that arises from the coracoid process of the scapula, transect it near the process, and reflect the muscle distally (Fig. 6-4/14). A bursa lies between the tendon and the broad tendon of insertion of the **subscapularis** (/10,10'). Transect the latter tendon close to its attachment on the caudal part of the lesser tubercle of the humerus. Deep to the tendon is the shoulder joint capsule.

Continue reflecting the coracobrachialis distally, exposing and preserving the proximal muscular branch of the musculocutaneous nerve and the cranial circumflex humeral vessels (/7"). The nerve branch supplies the coracobrachialis and enters the proximal end of the biceps. The combined tendons of the teres major (/9) and latissimus dorsi are inserted on the teres tuberosity distal to the cranial circumflex humeral artery.

There are no collateral ligaments on the **shoulder joint**. The tendons, notably of the subscapularis and infraspinatus take their place.

Dislocations of the shoulder joint are rare in the horse because of the large articular head of the humerus and the width of the infraspinatus and subscapularis tendons acting as collateral ligaments of the joint. The infraspinatus bursa under the former tendon is subject to inflammation. Anesthetic injection for the diagnosis of shoulder lameness may be performed at the cranial border of the infraspinatus tendon dorsal to the greater tubercle. Simulate the injection on your specimen and note the depth and direction the needle will have to be given to locate its tip just cranial to the glenoid cavity of the scapula.

It will be necessary to examine the supf. veins of the forearm before proceeding to deeper structures. Locate again the **cephalic vein** in the groove between the brachiocephalicus and pectoralis descendens on the cranial surface of the arm. The vein has been seen earlier to originate from the external jugular. Trace the cephalic vein to the distal end of the biceps and note its confluence with the **median cubital vein** that connects it to the brachial vein deep to

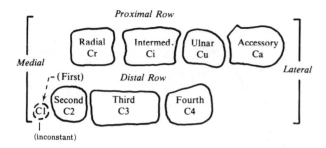

FIGURE 6-11. Schematic dorsal view of the left carpal bones.

the pectoralis transversus (Fig. 6-8). Follow the cephalic vein distally over the medial surface of the radius. At the carpus it usually (variations do occur) becomes the radial vein and this continues into the metacarpus as the medial palmar vein to be seen later (Fig. 1-10). Return to the proximal end of the forearm and find the **accessory cephalic vein** running distally from the cephalic along the medial border of the extensor carpi radialis. It passes to the dorsal surface of the carpus. (The nerves you may have seen accompanying the cephalic and accessory cephalic veins are cutaneous branches of the musculocutaneous nerve.)

Turn the limb so that the lateral surface is up. Remove the remaining supf. fascia from the lateral surface of the arm. By reflecting the distal stump of the deltoideus, locate the origin of the lateral head of the **triceps**. This arises from the deltoid tuberosity and the curved line between the tuberosity and the neck of the humerus. Incise and reflect the deep fascia, exposing the lateral head of the triceps (Fig. 6-7/9).

The **lateral cutaneous antebrachial nerve**, a branch of the radial, emerges from the distal border of the lateral head of the triceps. It ramifies on the lateral surface of the forearm as far distally as the carpus (Figs. 6-6 and 6-7/8). The nerve is often double.

Transect the lateral head of the triceps midway and reflect the stumps. This exposes the **brachialis** winding around the humerus from caudal to lateral to cranial. The **radial nerve**, accompanied by a branch of the deep brachial artery, winds around the humerus on the caudal border of the brachialis. Tense the nerve on the medial side of the arm and demonstrate its continuity. Find the muscular branches to the triceps, and the continuation of the nerve deep to the cranial border of the origin of the extensor carpi radialis. The continuation supplies the extensors of the carpus and digit in the forearm and will be traced when these muscles are exposed.

Transect the long head of the triceps at its middle. Reflect the distal stumps of the lateral and long heads to their insertions on the olecranon (Fig. 6-10/11,3). The small medial head of the triceps (/9) arises from the humerus just distal to the insertion of the teres major and latissimus dorsi. It may be followed to its insertion on the olecranon without transection.

Identify again the insertions of the pectoralis descendens and brachiocephalicus on the deltoid tuberosity and vicinity. Now turn the limb so that the medial surface is up. On the flexion surface of the elbow, distal to the insertion of these muscles, the **medial cutaneous antebrachial nerve** (from the musculocutaneous) emerges between the palpable distal ends of the biceps and brachialis. Trace the nerve distally. It splits to form several branches that accompany the cephalic and accessory cephalic veins. It supplies cutaneous innervation to the medial surface of the forearm and the dorsomedial surface of the carpus and metacarpus as far distally as the fetlock (Fig. 6-6), but it cannot be traced that far grossly. Cut the pectoralis descendens and brachiocephalicus close to their insertions and remove them. Trace the medial cutaneous antebrachial nerve proximally between the biceps and brachialis. It arises deep to the biceps as one of the terminal branches of the musculocutaneous nerve. Free the lateral and medial borders of the biceps and retract the muscle to expose this origin. The other termination of the musculocutaneous enters the brachialis.

Identify the stumps of brachiocephalicus and pectoralis descendens, reflect them to their insertion on the deltoid tuberosity and vicinity, and remove them.

Forearm and Metacarpus

On the articulated specimen from your course locker, study the bony structures of the distal end of the radius, carpus, and metacarpus. The distal end of the **radius** presents three cranial grooves. The lateral groove is for the tendon of the common digital extensor. The middle groove is for the tendon of the extensor carpi radialis. The medial groove is small and shallow and guides the tendon of the extensor carpi obliquus. The lateral styloid process provides attachment for the lateral collateral ligament of the carpus and bears a groove for the tendon of the lateral digital extensor. The medial styloid process provides attachment for the medial collateral ligament.

The **carpus** is composed of seven or eight bones arranged in two transverse rows (Fig. 6-11).

The **accessory carpal** (Ca) presents a groove on its lateral surface for the passage of the long tendon of the ulnaris lateralis. The flexor carpi ulnaris and ulnaris lateralis insert on Ca; no other carpal bone receives tendon insertions. The palmar surface of the carpal bones, in the fresh state, is made smooth by the **palmar carpal ligament** that forms the **carpal canal** with the flexor retinaculum. The latter connects the Ca with the carpal bones (Cr, C2) on the medial aspect. The carpal canal channels the flexor tendons into the metacarpus.

The **large metacarpal bone** (Mc3) is a few cm shorter than the corresponding metatarsal bone and is one of the strongest bones in the skeleton. The dorsomedial surface of the proximal end is enlarged to form the metacarpal tuberosity for the insertion of the extensor carpi radialis tendon. The palmar surface is roughened proximally for the attachment of the interosseus. The distal extremity presents small medial and lateral depressions and tubercles for the attachment of the collateral ligaments of the fetlock joint. The **small metacarpal bones** (Mc2 and Mc4) are practically identical with Mt2 and Mt4.

Turn your specimen so the medial surface is up. Palpate the large metacarpal bone and cut the skin longitudinally over the bone from the carpus to the fetlock joint. Circle the fetlock (shallow cut, skin only) and remove the metacarpal skin. Be sure to keep the digit and hoof moist and well wrapped.

Remove the supf. fascia from the medial surface of the forearm. The supf. fascia blends at the carpus with the deep fascia. Cut the insertion of the distal stump of the tensor fasciae antebrachii on the **deep fascia of the forearm** and remove the muscle. The deep fascia is continued over the carpus, forming two retinacula:

1. The **extensor retinaculum** (Fig. 6-13) which binds down the extensor tendons on the dorsal surface of the carpus, and
2. the **flexor retinaculum** which binds down the flexor tendons in the carpal canal (Figs. 6-13 and 6-18).

These retinacula should be preserved and isolated as was done on the hindlimb.
Pick up the collateral ulnar vessels and the ulnar nerve where they were last seen in the arm. At the

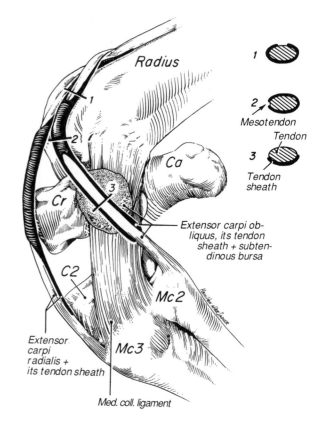

FIGURE 6-12. Medial view of flexed right carpus to show how the radio- and midcarpal joints open dorsally and that the tendon sheaths do not surround their tendon fully at all levels.

elbow the **ulnar nerve** gives off muscular branches to the flexor carpi ulnaris, the supf. digital flexor, and part of the deep digital flexor; do not trace these branches now. Incise the deep fascia along the caudal surface of the forearm and trace the nerve and the collateral ulnar vessels

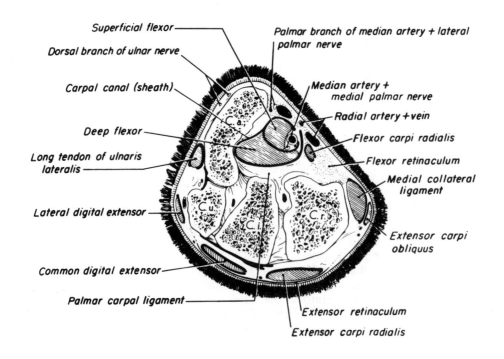

FIGURE 6-13. Transverse section of the right carpus, proximal surface.

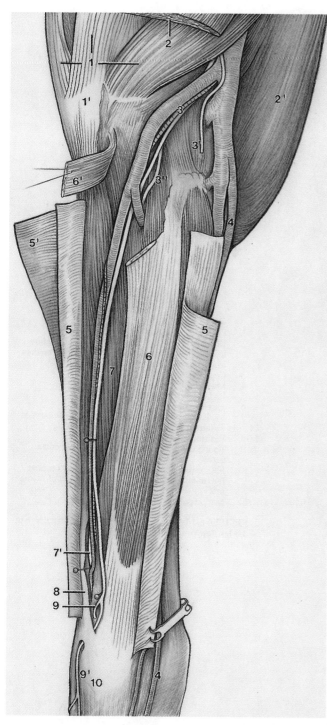

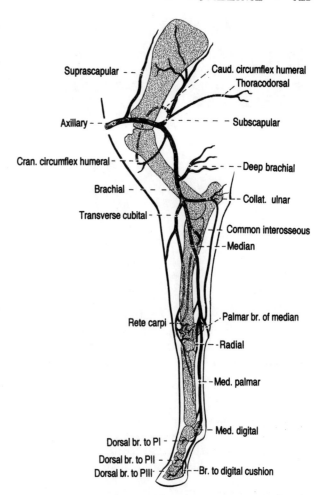

FIGURE 6-15. Arteries of the right forelimb, medial view.

1. Triceps, point of elbow at 1'
2. Prox. stump of tensor fasciae antebrachii, biceps at 2'
3. Ulnar nerve and collateral ulnar vessels
3'. Caud. cutaneous antebrachial nerve
3''. Muscular br. of ulnar nerve
4. Cephalic vein
5. Deep fascia, supf. fascia at 5'
6. Flexor carpi ulnaris, its ulnar head at 6'
7. Deep digital flexor, the tendon of its ulnar head at 7'
8. Tendon of ulnaris lateralis
9,9'. Palmar and dorsal branches of ulnar nerve
10. Position of accessory carpal bone

FIGURE 6-14. The distribution of the ulnar nerve in the caudal part of the left forearm, caudal and slightly medial view.

distally. This will necessitate severing the small ulnar head of the flexor carpi ulnaris (Fig. 6-14/6'). In the distal third of the forearm the nerve and vessels lie between the flexor carpi ulnaris medially and the ulnaris lateralis laterally. At this level the ulnar nerve bifurcates to form a dorsal branch and a palmar branch. The **dorsal branch** perforates the deep fascia between the tendons of the flexor carpi ulnaris and ulnaris lateralis and ramifies subcutaneously over the dorsolateral surface of the carpus and metacarpus (Figs. 6-6 and 6-9); it need not be traced this far. The **palmar branch,** accompanied by the collateral ulnar vessels, dips under the caudal edge of the flexor carpi ulnaris; we will see it again later.

Palpate the medial epicondyle of the humerus and the medial collateral ligament of the elbow joint. Remove the heavy, shiny deep fascia and expose the **median nerve** and the **brachial artery** (and the two brachial veins) lying cranial to the ligament. Note the muscular branches arising from the caudal edge of the median nerve; they supply the flexor carpi radialis and part of the deep digital flexor (Fig. 6-16/4).

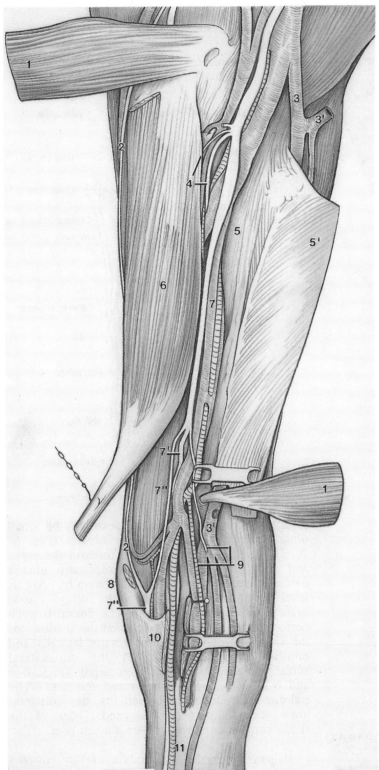

1. Flexor carpi radialis, reflected
2. Ulnar nerve; at the carpus, with its palmar br., joining the lateral palmar nerve from the median
3. Median cubital vein
3' Cephalic vein
4. Muscular branches of median nerve
5. Radius, reflected deep fascia at 5'
6. Flexor carpi ulnaris
7. Median nerve and vessels, medial palmar nerve at 7', lateral palmar nerve at 7''
8. Position of accessory carpal bone
9. Radial artery and cutaneous br. of the median nerve
10. Flexor retinaculum cut and retracted to expose the medial palmar artery (continuation of median artery)
11. Medial palmar nerve, artery, and vein

FIGURE 6-16. The distribution of the median nerve in the left forearm, medial view.

One of the terminal branches of the median artery, the **radial artery,** is supf. just above and at the carpus (Fig. 6-17). Identify and preserve this artery in the following dissection. Reflect the deep fascia cranially off the surface of the flexor carpi ulnaris and the flexor carpi radialis to where the fascia attaches on the radius. Transect the flexor carpi radialis at its middle and reflect the stumps.

The median nerve and vessels may now be traced through the forearm (Fig. 6-16/7).

The **median nerve** crosses the artery obliquely, and proximal to the carpus divides into two terminal branches. One, the **medial palmar nerve,** crosses under the artery to reach its cranial surface. Open the flexor retinaculum at the carpus and the deep metacarpal fascia and trace the nerve

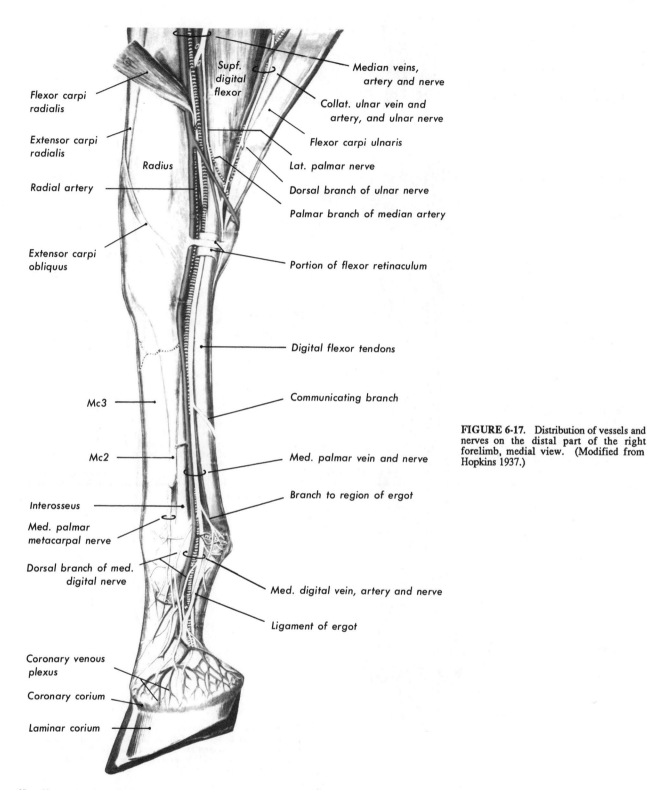

Flexor carpi radialis

Extensor carpi radialis

Radius

Radial artery

Extensor carpi obliquus

Mc3

Mc2

Interosseus

Med. palmar metacarpal nerve

Dorsal branch of med. digital nerve

Coronary venous plexus

Coronary corium

Laminar corium

Supf. digital flexor

Median veins, artery and nerve

Collat. ulnar vein and artery, and ulnar nerve

Flexor carpi ulnaris

Lat. palmar nerve

Dorsal branch of ulnar nerve

Palmar branch of median artery

Portion of flexor retinaculum

Digital flexor tendons

Communicating branch

Med. palmar vein and nerve

Branch to region of ergot

Med. digital vein, artery and nerve

Ligament of ergot

FIGURE 6-17. Distribution of vessels and nerves on the distal part of the right forelimb, medial view. (Modified from Hopkins 1937.)

distally to the fetlock, carefully preserving the accompanying vessels. Note that the metacarpal fascia is thick proximally where it blends with the flexor retinaculum; it becomes progressively thinner toward the fetlock. Near the middle of the metacarpus the medial palmar nerve gives off a large **communicating branch** (Fig. 6-17) that winds obliquely distally over the palmar surface of

the flexor tendons to join the lateral palmar nerve.

The other, smaller, terminal branch of the median nerve, the **lateral palmar nerve,** passes obliquely caudally deep to the tendon of the flexor carpi ulnaris. It communicates with the palmar branch of the ulnar nerve at the level of the accessory carpal bone. Transect the flexor carpi ulnaris tendon close to its insertion on the acces-

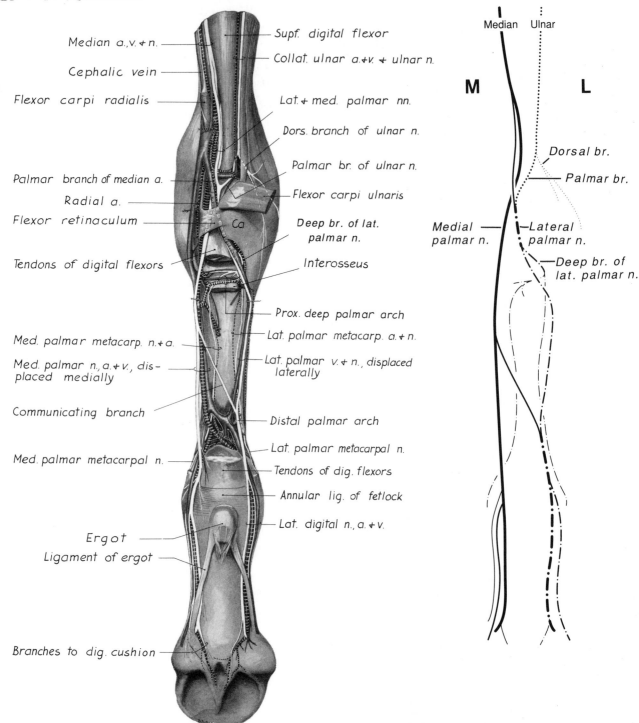

Median a.,v. + n.

Cephalic vein

Flexor carpi radialis

Palmar branch of median a.

Radial a.

Flexor retinaculum

Tendons of digital flexors

Med. palmar metacarp. n. + a.

Med. palmar n., a. + v., displaced medially

Communicating branch

Med. palmar metacarpal n.

Ergot

Ligament of ergot

Branches to dig. cushion

Supf. digital flexor

Collat. ulnar a. + v. + ulnar n.

Lat. + med. palmar nn.

Dors. branch of ulnar n.

Palmar br. of ulnar n.

Flexor carpi ulnaris

Deep br. of lat. palmar n.

Interosseus

Prox. deep palmar arch

Lat. palmar metacarp. a. + n.

Lat. palmar v. + n., displaced laterally

Distal palmar arch

Lat. palmar metacarpal n.

Tendons of dig. flexors

Annular lig. of fetlock

Lat. digital n., a. + v.

Ca

Median   Ulnar

M   L

Dorsal br.

Palmar br.

Medial palmar n.

Lateral palmar n.

Deep br. of lat. palmar n.

FIGURE 6-18. Distribution of median and ulnar nerves and blood vessels in a deep dissection of the distal part of the right forelimb; the nerves have been duplicated schematically on the right to show the mixing of median and ulnar components; caudal view. (Modified from Hopkins 1937.)

sory carpal and demonstrate the communication between the nerves (Fig. 6-16/7", 2).

On the lateral side of the metacarpus locate the lateral palmar nerve in the groove between the interosseus and the flexor tendons (palpate). It is

accompanied by a small artery and a larger vein (Fig. 6-19). Tense the nerve and demonstrate its continuity with the nerve proximal to the carpus.

The brachial artery gives off the **common interosseous artery** in the proximal part of the forearm and becomes the **median artery** (Fig. 6-15). The latter continues distally with nerve and

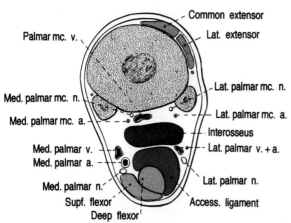

FIGURE 6-19. Transverse section through the middle of the right metacarpus, proximal surface.

veins of like name and gives rise to two branches above the carpus whose hookup with lesser arteries distal to the carpus is shown schematically in Fig. 6-32. The median artery itself accompanies the medial palmar nerve through the carpal canal and in the metacarpus becomes the **medial palmar artery**. Trace the latter to the distal fourth of the metacarpus where it dips in between the flexor tendons and the interosseus.

The following facts are of clinical and surgical importance:

1. The medial palmar artery is the main blood supply to the digit. It lies on the medial surface of the flexor tendons. (Where was the principal artery to the hoof in the metatarsus?)
2. In the proximal two thirds of the metacarpus the medial palmar nerve lies behind (palmar to) the medial palmar artery in the groove between the interosseus and the flexor tendons. The medial palmar vein lies dorsal to the artery. In the distal third of the metacarpus the artery is more deeply placed and the nerve lies behind the vein (Fig. 6-17).
3. The lateral palmar nerve maintains the same relationship except that the accompanying lateral palmar artery is small.
4. There is a constant communicating branch between the medial and lateral palmar nerves (Fig. 6-18). Palmar nerve block is best performed distal to the communication on both sides of the metacarpus. (Why would such a nerve block at the level of the communication not work?)

Muscles of the Forearm

The **flexor carpi radialis**, already transected, arises from the medial epicondyle of the humerus. Its tendon passes through a canal formed within the substance of the flexor retinaculum of the carpus to be inserted on Mc2. Incise the heavy fascia that covers the tendon and open its synovial

sheath. The sheath extends from a few cm above the carpus, almost to the metacarpal insertion.

Pull the brachial vessels and median nerve caudally out of the way and clean the long part of the **medial collateral ligament of the elbow**. Transect the long part of the ligament opposite the distal end of the biceps and reflect the stumps. The short tendon of insertion of the biceps is now exposed as it attaches on the radial tuberosity. The thin, fleshy insertion of the brachialis can be seen distal to the biceps insertion (Fig. 6-20/5,6). The short deep part of the medial collateral ligament attaches to the medial epicondyle of the humerus and the medial side of the radius. Transect it and open the joint capsule. Note the position of the ligament caudal to the axis of elbow joint rotation (/3). In order to flex the extended joint the ligament must be stretched: in other words, the ligament impedes initial flexion of the elbow joint.

Remove the fleshy part of the **biceps** and locate the heavy tendinous band (internal tendon) that runs through the length of muscle. The tendinous band is continuous proximally with the tendon of origin. Distally it ends on the radius but splits off the **lacertus fribrosus** (Fig. 6-20/5',5").The lacertus fibrosus blends with the deep fascia of the forearm and joins the tendon of the extensor carpi radialis. The internal tendon of the biceps, together with the pressure and friction of the molded tendon of

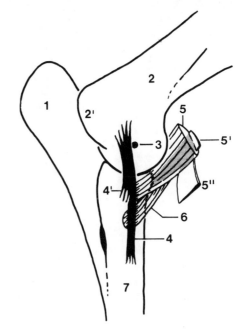

1.	Olecranon	5.	Biceps near its insertion
2.	Humerus, medial epicondyle		on radius
	at 2'	5'	Internal tendon of biceps
3.	Axis of rotation	5"	Lacertus fibrosus
4.	Long supf. part of medial	6.	Brachialis
	collateral ligament, short deep	7.	Radius
	part at 4'		

FIGURE 6-20. Medial view of left elbow joint to show the eccentrically placed collateral ligament and the insertions of biceps and brachialis. The internal tendon (gray) of the biceps splits off the lacertus fibrosus from the lateral surface of the muscle.

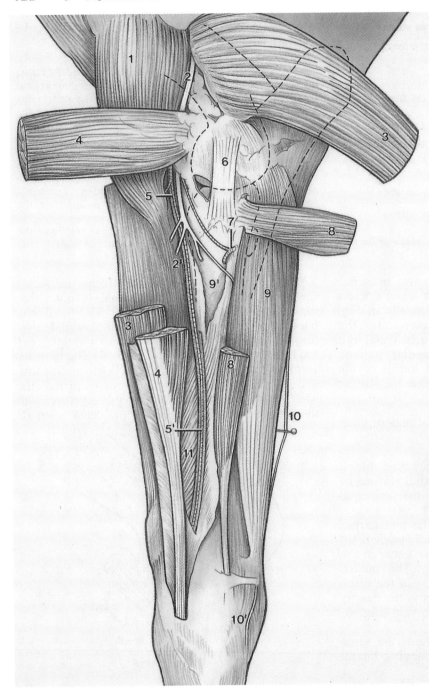

1. Brachialis
2. Radial nerve, its muscular branches at 2'
3. Extensor carpi radialis
4. Common digital extensor
5. Transverse cubital artery, its continuation to the rete carpi dorsale at 5'
6. Lat. collateral ligament of elbow joint
7. Cranial interosseous artery emerging from the interosseous space (broken line) and anastomosing with the transverse cubital artery
8. Lat. digital extensor
9. Ulnaris lateralis
9' Radius
10. Ulnar nerve, its dorsal branch at 10'
11. Extensor carpi obliquus

FIGURE 6-21. Distribution of the radial nerve in the left forearm, lateral view. The broken lines give the position of the bones forming the elbow joint.

origin in the intertubercular groove forms an efficient mechanical system (Fig. 6-42/A,2,6,10): without muscular effort it prevents flexion of the shoulder joint in the normal standing position.

Turn the limb over so the lateral surface is up. Remove the supf. fascia from the lateral surface of the forearm. Palpate the extensor carpi radialis. Incise and reflect the deep fascia ensheathing the muscle. Proximal to the carpus the tendon of the **extensor carpi obliquus** climbs over the tendon of the extensor carpi radialis to reach the oblique groove on the distal end of the radius (Fig. 6-12). Trace the obliquus tendon to its insertion on Mc2,

preserving the wide extensor retinaculum of the carpus. A synovial sheath envelops the tendon as it crosses the radius and carpus; and between the sheath and the medial collateral ligament of the carpus is a bursa.

Palpate the course of the tendon of the **extensor carpi radialis**. It passes over the dorsal surface of the carpus bound down by the extensor retinaculum to insert on the metacarpal tuberosity. Its synovial sheath begins several cm above the carpus and extends almost to the metacarpal tuberosity. Transect the extensor carpi radialis at its middle and reflect the proximal stump. It originates from the craniolateral aspect of the distal end of the humerus and from the deep fascia of the area. Sever the origins from the deep fascia and reflect the muscle to the humeral origin. The deep face of the origin adheres to the elbow joint capsule; open it. The radial nerve detaches muscular branches to the extensor carpi and disappears under the common extensor (Fig. 6-9).

Incise and reflect the deep fascia covering the **common digital extensor** (Fig. 6-21/4). Its synovial sheath begins several cm above the carpus and extends to the proximal end of the metacarpus. Clean the tendon, preserving the retinaculum, and trace it to the fetlock. Transect the common extensor proximal to the carpus and

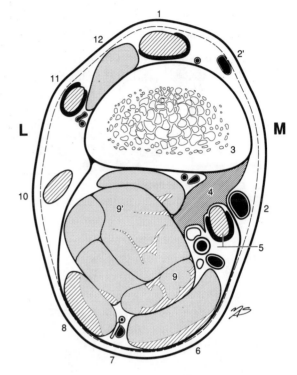

1.	Extensor carpi radialis	6.	Flexor carpi ulnaris
2,2'	Cephalic and accessory cephalic veins	7.	Ulnar nerve and collat. ulnar vessels
3.	Radius	8.	Ulnaris lateralis
4.	Accessory (check) lig. of supf. digital flexor	9,9'	Supf. and deep digital flexors
5.	Flexor carpi radialis, median artery, and med. & lat. palmar nerves	10.	Lat. digital extensor
		11.	Common digital extensor
		12.	Oblique digital extensor

FIGURE 6-23. Transverse section of left forearm 5.5 cm proximal to the proximal border of Ca, to demonstrate the topography of the accessory (check) ligament (4) of the supf. digital flexor; proximal surface. The hatched areas are tendons or tendinous tissue, the gray areas are muscle tissue.

reflect the proximal stump. Sever its fleshy origins from the radius and ulna and from the lateral collateral ligament of the elbow. Reflect the strong wide tendon of origin from the humerus, exposing and opening the elbow joint capsule. Note the muscular branches of the radial nerve entering the deep face of the muscle (/2').

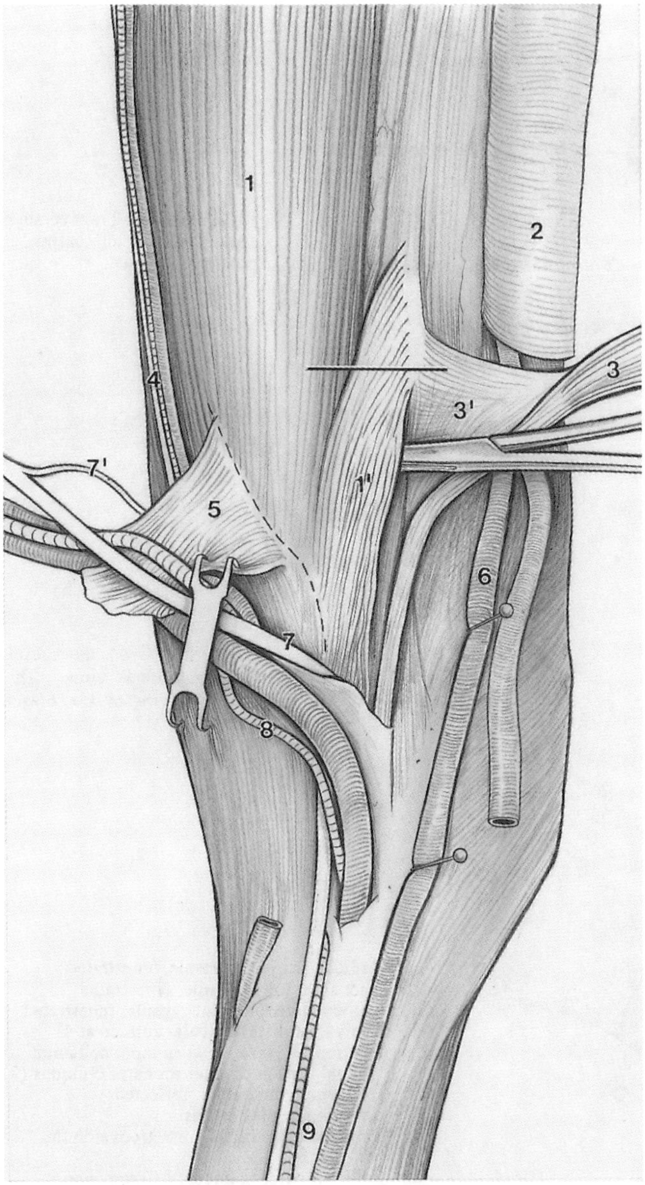

The **lateral collateral ligament of the elbow** is short and thick. It attaches to the lateral epicondyle of the humerus and the lateral surface of the head of the radius. Its position and function relative to the axis of rotation and flexion of the elbow joint is the same as for the medial ligament.

1.	Supf. digital flexor, its accessory ligament at 1'; the line crossing the ligament is the level of section shown in Fig. 6-23B.		ulnar vessels
2.	Deep fascia, reflected	5.	Wall of carpal sheath, reflected
3.	Flexor carpi radialis, its mesotendon at 3'	6.	Cephalic vein
4.	Ulnar nerve and collateral	7,7'	Medial and lateral palmar nerves
		8.	Radial artery
		9.	Medial palmar n., a. & v.

FIGURE 6-22. Deep dissection proximal to the left carpus to show the accessory (check) ligament of the supf. digital flexor, caudomedial view. The hemostat indicates the proximal extent of the opened carpal sheath.

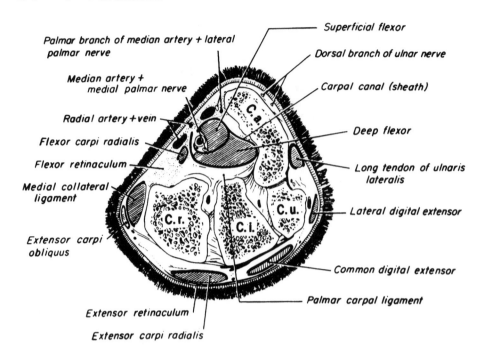

Palmar branch of median artery + lateral palmar nerve

Median artery + medial palmar nerve

Radial artery + vein

Flexor carpi radialis

Flexor retinaculum

Medial collateral ligament

Extensor carpi obliquus

Superficial flexor

Dorsal branch of ulnar nerve

Carpal canal (sheath)

Deep flexor

Long tendon of ulnaris lateralis

Lateral digital extensor

Common digital extensor

Palmar carpal ligament

Extensor retinaculum

Extensor carpi radialis

FIGURE 6-24. Transverse section of the left carpus, proximal surface.

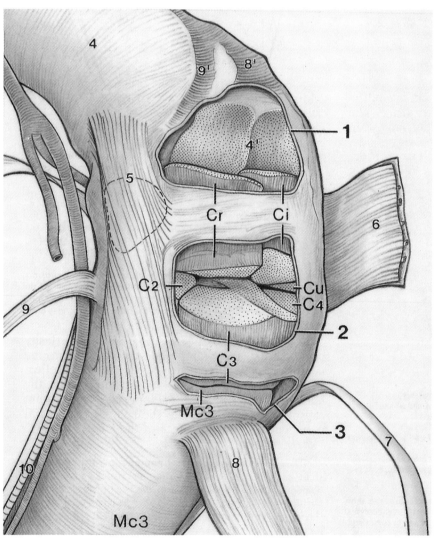

1. Radiocarpal joint capsule, fenestrated
2. Midcarpal joint capsule, fenestrated
3. Carpometacarpal joint capsule, fenestrated
4. Radius, its distal articular surface at 4'
5. Position of bursa between med. collateral lig. and tendon of extensor carpi obliquus (9)
6. Extensor retinaculum, reflected
7. Common digital extensor
8. Extensor carpi radialis, its groove on the radius at 8'
9. Extensor carpi obliquus, its groove on the radius at 9'
10. Medial palmar nerve, artery, and vein.

FIGURE 6-25. Flexed left carpus, dorsomedial view. The articular surfaces are stippled.

Remove the deep fascia from the narrow **lateral digital extensor.** Its tendon passes through the groove on the lateral styloid process on the distal end of the radius and over the carpus in a canal formed by the lateral collateral ligament. Below the carpus the tendon receives a slip from the common extensor and passes to the fetlock. The synovial sheath of the lateral extensor begins a few cm above the carpus and extends to the proximal end of the metacarpus. Transect the lateral extensor and reflect the proximal stump to its origin on the lateral surface of the head of the radius (Fig. 6-21/8). Preserve the vessels and nerves on its deep surface. The radial nerve is now seen sending terminal branches into the lateral extensor, the extensor carpi obliquus, and the ulnaris lateralis (Fig. 6-9).

Locate the origin of the **common interosseous artery** from the brachial artery on the medial surface of the proximal part of the forearm and follow it to the interosseous space between radius and ulna (Fig. 6-15). Probe the artery and find its continuation, the cranial interosseous artery, on the lateral side of the interosseous space, where several small branches and usually an anastomosis to the transverse cubital are given off. The cranial interosseous passes distally on the caudal edge of the extensor obliquus and forms the **rete carpi dorsale** with the transverse cubital which also descends to the carpus. The cranial interosseous may be absent and replaced by the transverse cubital.

Remove the rest of the deep fascia from the forearm and isolate the **ulnaris lateralis.** The ulnar head of the deep flexor and its long thin tendon lie on the caudal border of the ulnaris lateralis and should be preserved. Transect the muscle and reflect the proximal stump to its origin from the lateral epicondyle of the humerus caudal to the lateral collateral ligament. The elbow joint capsule adheres to the deep surface of the muscle at its origin. The wide tendon of the ulnaris lateralis bifurcates just proximal to the accessory carpal bone (Ca). The short tendon is inserted on Ca; it has no synovial sheath. The long tendon passes in the groove on Ca, enveloped by a synovial sheath, and ends on Mc4.

Reflect the proximal stump of the previously transected **flexor carpi ulnaris** off the surface of the **supf. digital flexor.** Both muscles originate from the prominent medial epicondyle of the humerus and receive muscular branches from the ulnar nerve. Expose these branches. The ulnar nerve also concurs with the median nerve in the innervation of the deep digital flexor.

A short distance above the carpus the **accessory ligament of the supf. flexor** (proximal check ligament) arises from the caudal surface of the radius and fuses with the supf. flexor tendon. The ligament may be exposed by reflecting the flexor carpi ulnaris and flexor carpi radialis and by pushing the median vessels and associated nerves

between the supf. flexor tendon and the radius aside (Figs. 6-22/1' and 6-23/4).

The thin tendon of the ulnar head of the deep flexor joins the main tendon of the **deep digital flexor** (humeral head) just above the carpus. The bellies of the supf. and deep flexors are usually fused; do not separate them. The tendons of the supf. and deep digital flexor pass through the carpal canal enveloped in a common **carpal synovial sheath.** This sheath is longer than the others, beginning several cm proximal to the carpus and extending to the middle of the metacarpus.

The flexor tendons and interosseus in the metacarpus are under great and repeated strain during the fast gaits. This unfortunately results in partial, often internal, tearing of tendon fibers, especially in immature horses or others who are worked too hard. Inflammation with hemorrhage inside the tendon sets in where the tears have occurred (*acute tendinitis*). Scar tissue laid down during healing causes the affected tendon to thicken and to bow caudally in the metacarpal region (*bowed tendon*). Ultrasonography is commonly used to localize the acute lesion and to determine its severity.

Transect the bellies of the ulnaris lateralis, flexor carpi ulnaris, and supf. digital flexor several times and note that they contain large quantities of tendinous tissue. The origins of these muscles lie caudal to the axis of rotation of the elbow joint. Therefore, in the standing animal the tendinous portions of these muscles are tense and mechanically prevent flexion of the elbow joint. The collateral ligaments of the elbow also assist in preventing flexion as noted earlier (Fig. 6-42/A). If the limb is not to collapse, the elbow has to remain extended. This will become clearer when the entire passive stay-apparatus is studied at the end of this chapter. The stay-apparatus enables the horse to support its weight with a minimum of muscular effort.

Carpus

(The articulated specimen from your course locker should lie next to your dissection whenever you are working on it.)

The carpus is a composite joint consisting of three distinct articulations. The fibrous membrane of the joint capsule is common to all three articulations, while the synovial membranes enclose the individual articulations.

1. The **radiocarpal joint capsule** surrounds the articulation of the radius and the proximal row of carpal bones.
2. The **midcarpal joint capsule** surrounds the

articulation between the proximal and distal rows of carpal bones. It communicates with:

3. the **carpometacarpal joint capsule** which surrounds the articulation between the distal row of carpal bones and the metacarpal bones.

Palpate the medial and lateral styloid processes of the radius and the proximal end of the large metacarpal bone (Mc3). Remove the remaining supf. fascia from the carpus. Transect (with a longitudinal i.e., proximodistal cut) the **extensor retinaculum** and reflect the stumps off the surfaces of the extensor carpi radialis and common digital extensor tendons (Fig. 6-24). The retinaculum is thickened deep fascia without distinguishable proximal and distal borders.

Free the common extensor tendon from its mesotendon and reflect it distally off the carpus. Transect the extensor carpi obliquus where it crosses the extensor carpi radialis. Now free the latter muscle from its mesotendon (proximal half of carpus) and the fibrous layer of the joint capsule (distal half of carpus) and reflect it distally to its insertion (Fig. 6-12).

Strongly flex the carpus to form an angle of about 80 degrees and palpate the radiocarpal joint. Open the fibrous and synovial membranes of the **radiocarpal capsule.** Palpate the midcarpal joint and open the **midcarpal capsule.** The **carpometacarpal capsule** is tight and need not be opened. Flex and extend the carpus and note the movements of the three joints: the articular surfaces of the radiocarpal and midcarpal joints are widely separated during flexion, the carpometacarpal joint is relatively fixed.

Now with thumb forceps and scalpel remove all the tags of the radio- and midcarpal joint capsules so that the interior of the two joints can be fully seen when the carpus is maximally flexed (Fig. 6-25).

At the radiocarpal level: The distal (articular) surface of the radius is divided by a central crest. The surface lateral to the crest is larger than the other and may present a notch and a line proceeding from it, indicating where the distal end of the ulna was incorporated into the radius. Note that the intermediate carpal bone rises in relation to the radial carpal as the joint opens. This is clearly shown on lateral radiographs of the flexed carpus.

At the midcarpal level: The distal surface of the intermediate carpal bone bears a crest that occupies the junction between third and fourth carpal bones when the joint is closed in extension. The proximal surface of the large third carpal is also divided by a crest that occupies the junction between radial and intermediate bones.

Flex the joint maximally and observe that the axes around which both joints rotate lie in the palmar portion of radius and carpal bones, causing the joints to open in the front (dorsally) during flexion (Fig. 6-12). Conversely, when the carpus is extended—forcefully during the fast gaits—the dorsal portions of the articular surfaces are driven together to prevent overextension.

Do not dissect but visualize the **medial collateral ligament** on your dissection and articulated specimen. The ligament extends from the radius to Mc2 and Mc3. It blends with the fibrous membrane of the joint capsule and with the extensor and flexor retinacula. With the latter it forms a canal for the tendon of the flexor carpi radialis as this passes distally to end on Mc2 (Fig. 6-24). The short deep parts of the collateral ligament connect the individual bones on the medial side.

The **flexor retinaculum** (Fig. 6-24) has already been opened when we traced the medial and lateral palmar nerves into the metacarpus. It fans from Ca to Cr and C2, and blends with the medial collateral ligament. Its proximal and distal borders are ill-defined.

Transect the supf. and deep flexor tendons at the level of the accessory (check) ligament of the supf. flexor and reflect them distally out of the **carpal canal.** The **palmar carpal ligament** is the thickened palmar part of the common fibrous joint capsule and forms, with the flexor retinaculum, the carpal canal (Fig. 6-24). The palmar carpal ligament is continued distally as the accessory ligament of the deep flexor tendon (distal check ligament) which blends with the tendon of the deep flexor near the middle of the metacarpus. There are, therefore, two accessory ligaments in the forelimb (Fig. 6-42/C, close to labels 9 and 11). The accessory ligament of the deep flexor is much stronger than that of the hindlimb.

On the lateral side: Between the styloid process of the radius and the long tendon of the ulnaris lateralis there is a palmarolateral pouch of the radiocarpal joint capsule (Fig. 6-26/6). Distention of the radiocarpal capsule may manifest itself here as well as on the dorsal surface.

Open the canals lodging the long tendon of the ulnaris lateralis and the tendon of the lateral extensor. Reflect the tendons off the carpus. Palpate the **accessory carpal bone** (Ca) and note that its distal border is continued by a strong ligament (/9') that anchors the bone to C4 and Mc4 and transfers the pull of the muscles attaching on its proximal border to the metacarpus (Fig. 42/A).

The **ligaments of the accessory carpal bone** can be divided into three units: The proximal ligament of Ca is a short band that extends from Ca, dorsal to the groove for the ulnaris lateralis tendon, to the lateral styloid process of the radius, palmar to the groove for the lateral extensor tendon. A middle ligament connects Ca and Cu. The two strong bands of the distal ligament arise from the distal border of Ca and attach to C4 and the proximal end of Mc4. The proximal and middle ligaments of Ca blend dorsally with the lateral collateral ligament.

Do not dissect but visualize on your specimen and on the skeleton: The **lateral collateral ligament** extends from the radius to Mc3 and Mc4. It forms a canal for the lateral extensor tendon and blends with the extensor retinaculum and the fibrous membrane of the joint capsule. The short deep parts of the ligament connect the individual bones on the lateral side.

We have mentioned that the dorsal portions of the carpal bones are driven together hard during the fast gaits. This unfortunately causes so-called chip or slab fractures predominantly in the radial and third carpal bones. Surgical removal of the fragment is the only effective treatment.

Distensions of the radiocarpal and/or midcarpal capsules appear clinically as puffs between the tendons on the dorsal surface but also on the lateral side between the styloid process of the radius and the long tendon of the ulnaris lateralis (palmarolateral pouch).

The synovial sheaths and the radiocarpal and midcarpal joint cavities may be involved in traumatic injury to the dorsal surface of the carpus, often by kicks from other horses.

(For an overview of the innervation of the forelimb muscles and their primary action see Appendix D.)

Digit and Hoof

Before considering the **SUPF. STRUCTURES OF THE DIGIT** it is well to remember that the digit of the horse is the homologue of the middle (3rd) finger of your hand. It contains proximal, middle, and distal phalanges which for the sake of brevity may be referred to as PI, PII, and PIII, respectively. The knuckle at the root of your finger is the metacarpophalangeal articulation known in the horse as the **fetlock joint.** (The fetlock is the tuft of hair that grows distally from the metacarpophalangeal joint caudal to the digit.) The joint between PI and PII is the **pastern joint,** because the narrow part between the enlargement of the fetlock joint and the hoof is the pastern. (The shackle by which horses were hobbled [fettered] at pasture was attached to the narrow part and was known as a pastern (Fig. 6-27). Hence the narrow part of the digit became the pastern.) The joint between PII and PIII is known as the **coffin joint** in the horse, because PIII, the coffin bone, is entirely enclosed in the hoof as in a "coffin". Note that both the hoof and your fingernail are associated with PIII. What is loosely known as the horse's "foot" is the hoof and its contents. That is why the front and rear of the hoof are called "toe" and "heels", as you will learn

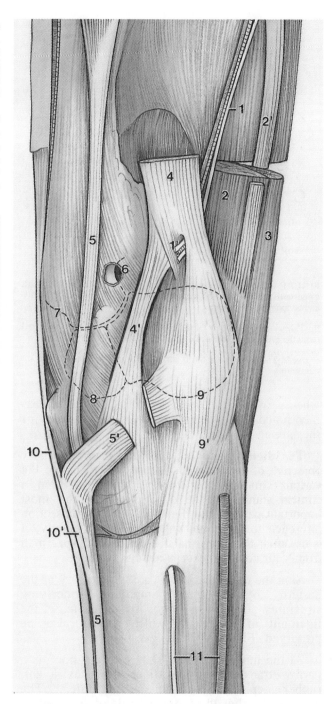

1.	Ulnar nerve, its dorsal branch at 1'	7,8,9	Outlines of distal end of radius, ulnar carpal, and accessory carpal, respectively
2	Deep digital flexor, tendon of its ulnar head at 2'		
3.	Supf. digital flexor	9'	Distal ligament of accessory carpal connecting Ca with Mc4
4	Ulnaris lateralis attaching on accessory carpal, its long tendon at 4'		
5.	Lat. digital extensor, band from accessory carpal joining it at 5'	10.	Common dig. extensor, tendon of its radial head at 10'
6	Palmarolateral pouch of the radiocarpal joint	11.	Lat. palmar nerve and vein

FIGURE 6-26. Structures passing the left carpus, lateral and slightly palmar view. Broken lines give the position of the distal end of the radius and the ulnar and accessory carpal bones.

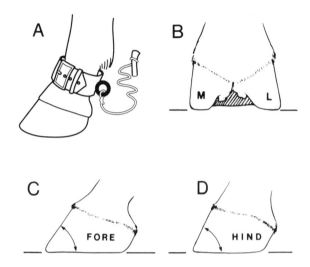

FIGURE 6-27. *A*, In former days, horses at pasture were hobbled with a "pastern"; this is why the narrow part of the limb above the hoof is known today as the pastern.

B, Palmar (plantar) view of the foot; the lateral angle of the wall (with the ground) is more acute than the medial.

C and D, The angle at the toe is more acute in the fore- than in the hindlimb.

when we study the hoof. None of the three last-mentioned terms designates the same structure on the human foot.

The digit should be studied with the primary objective of learning to palpate and visualize the various structures on the live animal. From a clinical standpoint the digit is one of the most important parts of the horse. During its dissection reference to the bones will be made constantly; it is essential therefore that the articulated specimen from your course locker is always available.

Skin the digit; particular care is necessary at the pastern not to destroy important underlying structures. Raise the ergot so as to tense the **ligament of the ergot** which should also be preserved (Fig. 6-28/7).

At the junction of the skin with the hoof is a narrow transitional zone which produces a soft rubbery epidermis known as **periople.** The periople overlies the proximal part of the wall of the hoof where it forms a band 1-2 cm in width. The band becomes wider on the palmar aspect where it covers the bulbs of the heels and blends with the frog. As the periople is carried distally with the growth of the hoof it gradually dries and forms a glossy layer on the surface of the hoof. In embalmed specimens the periople is dryer and more flaky than in the natural state.

Examine the external surface of the wall of the **HOOF** either on the limb or on the dried hoof from your course locker. The surface of the **wall** has a smooth, glossy appearance below the

periople. Note the fine parallel lines, the **horn tubules,** which extend from the coronary border to the sole border. Smooth ridges parallel to the coronary border indicate variations in the growth activity of the hoof. The wall is divided into three topographical regions: the **toe** or dorsal part and the two (medial and lateral) **quarters.** The quarters end at the **heels,** the most caudal parts of the hoof (Fig. 6-29/B). Note that the horny wall is thickest at the toe and gradually thins toward the heels. This is of importance to farriers when rasping or driving nails into the wall. The curve of the wall is wider on the lateral side and the angle of the wall with the ground therefore is steeper on the medial side. The angle of the toe is about 50 degrees on the forelimb and 55 degrees on the hindlimb (Fig. 6-27/C,D). The toe angle is carefully adjusted on gaited and racing animals.

The wall reflects upon itself at the heels to form the **bars** which are visible on the ground surface. The bars are continuous with the sole but are separated from the frog by the **paracuneal grooves.** The **frog** (cuneus) presents a central

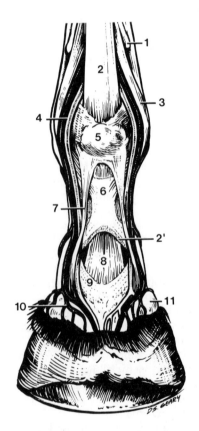

1.	Distal end of splint bone	7.	Ligament of ergot
2.	Supf. digital flexor, its bifurcation at 2'	8.	Deep digital flexor emerging from the bifurcation of the supf. flexor
3.	Interosseus		
4.	Digital vein and artery	9.	Distal digital annular lig.
5.	Ergot	10.	Coronary part of venous plexus
6.	Proximal digital annular lig. covering supf. digital flexor	11.	Hoof cartilage

FIGURE 6-28. Digit, palmar view. (From Ellenberger-Dittrich-Baum by Horowitz/Geary.)

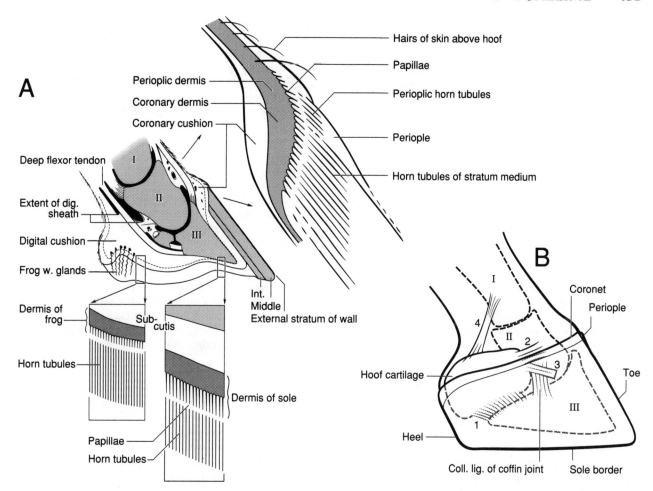

FIGURE 6-29. *A:* Axial section of foot, and enlargements to show the structure of the dermis and overlying epidermis. *B:* Foot with hoof cartilages and some of their ligaments.

I-III, Proximal, middle, and distal phalanges; 1, Lig. chondroungulare; 2, Lig. chondrocoronale; 3, Lig. chondrotendineum, cut; 4, Lig. chondrocompedale.

groove, an apex, and two crura. The crura form the axial walls and the bars the abaxial walls of the paracuneal grooves. The frog is expanded on the palmar surface and covered by periople to form the **bulbs of the heels.** The **sole** fills in the ground surface between the sole border of the wall and the frog. Note that it is slightly concave in all directions. The angles of the sole fill the space where wall and bars meet at the heels.

Now you need the dried hoof and the sagittal sections from your course locker. The inner surface of the hoof is excavated at the proximal border to form the **coronary groove.** The groove is perforated by innumerable small openings which contain the papillae of the coronary dermis in the intact state.

Distal to the coronary groove the wall bears about six hundred **horny** or **epidermal laminae** which extend to the sole border. The laminar wall reflects upon itself to form the laminar part of the

bars. The horny laminae seen here interlock with the dermal laminae of the laminar dermis. The significance of this interlocking will be discussed when we examine the dermis.

Examine sections of the **wall.** The outermost layer, **stratum externum,** is composed of the periople proximally and a very thin layer of glossy horn derived from the periople and carried distally with the growth of the wall. The middle layer, **stratum medium,** forms the bulk of the wall; it is pigmented in dark hooves except in its deepest part. The laminar layer, **stratum internum,** consists of the horny laminae and is non-pigmented (Fig. 6-29).

The inner surface of the **sole** is perforated by numerous small holes which contain the papillae of the dermis of the sole. The **frog** presents a central spine ("frog-stay") bounded by two deep depressions corresponding to the crura on the external surface. The two rounded ridges correspond to the paracuneal grooves on the external surface.

To remove the hoof capsule:
(Your course leader may have you study the dermis of the hoof on stock specimens. If so, skip

the following three paragraphs set in italics.)

If there is evidence of dried blood at the coronet, the digit of your limb did not receive sufficient preservative during embalming. This has the advantage that the hoof capsule will come off easily—in fact you may be able to just pull it off after loosening it at the coronary border; consult an instructor. The underlying dermis will largely be undisturbed for study; wash the blood off with a sponge.

If the digit is well preserved, you will need more time and considerable effort to remove the hoof. Test the periople: if it is still moist and pliable, the hoof may be removed without further preparation. If the periople is dry and hard, the hoof will have to be soaked for 10 minutes in water at 60 degrees Celsius before removal and may have to be taken off piece-meal.

Pare off the periople and, with a cartilage knife or a <u>stiff-bladed</u> scalpel, loosen the horny wall and bulbs from the dermis, <u>all around the coronary border</u> to a depth of about 2 cm. (These are deep cuts; detachable blades often break; the fragment left in the tissue presents a hazard.) Make two parallel saw cuts 5 cm apart and also about 2 cm deep through the wall of the hoof as shown at A and B in Figure 6-30. With a chisel free this small section of the wall sufficiently to grasp it with heavy pincers. Exerting traction with the pincers, free the section of the wall from the dermis, working from the sole toward the coronary border, and remove it. Now grasp the cut edge of the wall at B with the pincers and, by drawing outward and downward, free it from the dermis. Repeat on the opposite side and continue loosening the hoof from the dermis until the hoof can be removed in one piece. Carefully wrap the digit with cloth soaked in mold-inhibiting solution and plastic to prevent drying until it is examined.

Study the five areas of the **DERMIS OF THE HOOF.** The dermis (corium) is the modified and highly vascular continuation of the connective tissue layer (dermis) of the skin. It provides

attachment for, and supplies nutrition to the hoof. The microscopic living layers of epidermis (stratum basale and spinosum) cover the dermis and by their growth and keratinization form the horny components of the hoof. The relationship here is the same as that of the dermis and epidermis of the skin. The perioplic dermis and coronary dermis have probably been destroyed on your specimen. Study these and the underlying subcutis on demonstration specimens and on the sections in your course locker.

Embedded in dermis and subcutis is an extensive **venous plexus** that forms a continuous network of veins all around the part of the digit that is covered by the hoof capsule (Figs. 6-17 and 6-28/10). Do not dissect.

1. The **perioplic dermis** is a narrow band of thin papillae which is continuous proximally with the dermis of the skin. It is separated distally from the coronary dermis by a shallow groove. At the heels it widens and blends with the dermis of the frog.

2. The **coronary dermis** is the thick raised band (coronary band) distal to the perioplic dermis (Fig. 6-29/A). It bears long papillae in the natural state; most of these are pulled off when the hoof is removed. The epidermis covering the papillae and nourished by the coronary dermis produces the stratum medium, the bulk of the hoof wall. The wall grows by the production of new horn at the coronary dermis which pushes the older horn toward the ground where it is worn away. When a defect occurs in the wall, the laminar epidermis deep to it forms scar horn directly and fills the wound. This scar horn has to be replaced by the growth of new horn from above. The coronary dermis is attached to the extensor tendon and the cartilages of the hoof by the subcutis, which because of its thickness is known here as the **coronary cushion.**

3. The **laminar dermis** is composed of about 600 **dermal laminae** which extend distally from the coronary dermis and end in small terminal papillae. They of course interdigitate with the horny, or epidermal, laminae seen on the hoof capsule. Since the dermal laminae contain nerve endings and the epidermal do not, the two sets are also known as the sensitive and insensitive laminae. The dermal laminae bear microscopic secondary laminae on their surfaces. By the interlocking of the two sets of laminae, PIII is suspended from the inside of the horny wall. The laminar dermis folds upon itself at the heels to form the dermis underlying the bars.

The laminar epidermis does not produce any significant amount of horn in the intact hoof because it is prevented from doing so by the

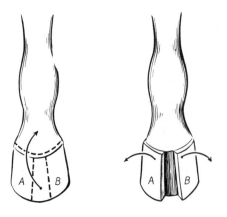

FIGURE 6-30. Removal of the hoof. (After Bourdelle.)

tightly fitting horny wall that covers it. If the wall is separated from the living epidermis by laminitis or in case of a wall defect, this epithelium will produce horn. The epidermis on the terminal papillae, however, continually produces pigmented horn that fills the spaces between the distal ends of the horny laminae.

The deep layer of the laminar dermis is attached to the dorsal surface of PIII and to the lower parts of the hoof cartilages (Fig. 6-29/B). When the distal border of the horny wall strikes the ground, the impact is transmitted through the horny and sensitive laminae to PIII which sinks a little from the weight above and slightly deforms the hoof.

4. The **dermis of the sole** is pigmented and bears long papillae. It is attached to the sole surface of PIII by a modified periosteum.

5. The **dermis of the frog** is pigmented and bears long papillae. The epidermis produces flexuous horn tubules which are relatively soft and not completely keratinized. The frog dermis is attached deeply to the digital cushion.

Return to the hoof and pare the dry horn off the junction of the wall and sole. The ends of the nonpigmented horny laminae are now seen to be united with the pigmented sole by the horn produced by the terminal papillae. The so-called **white line** (zona alba) at the junction of wall and sole gains its whiteness from that of the nonpigmented horny laminae, from the non-pigmented deepest layer of the stratum medium of the wall, and to a significant degree from the thin but very bright line of cap horn that was elaborated by the laminar epidermis and connects the bases of the horny laminae.

And finally, study the cartilages of the hoof and the digital cushion by means of the sections of the entire foot from your course locker and other demonstration material. Develop a mental picture of the relationships of the various components of the horse's foot.

The **cartilages of the hoof** are sagittal plates attached to the palmar processes of PIII and projecting a little above the hoof (Fig. 6-29/B). They facilitate the slight expansion of the hoof at the quarters when weight is placed on the limb. Holes in the cartilages transmit veins of the venous plexus present in the hoof dermis.

Find the **digital cushion** on the sections. It is a wedge-shaped mass of fibrous and adipose tissue that is related to the frog distally, the deep flexor tendon proximally, and the cartilages of the hoof medially and laterally. The caudal portion is partly subcutaneous and divided by a central

depression into the two bulbs of the cushion. The bulbs of the cushion underlie the **bulbs of the heels** which are soft and fatty in texture. The cushion is denser and more fibrous in structure in its central and dorsal parts. Tubular glands occur in the cushion chiefly over the spine of the frog (Fig. 6-29/A). Their ducts pass through the dermis and horn of the frog—the glands and ducts are not visible grossly.

When you reflect on the considerable weight of a horse and its small footing surface, it becomes clear that the hoof is easily injured, though owner's neglect is partly to blame. All hoof injuries make horses lame.

When horses have to stand in urine or feces-soaked bedding, a foul-smelling bacterial infection (*Thrush*) can develop on or about the frog. When barefoot (unshod) horses are worked on hard, rough terrain, *Sole bruises* may result—those in the angles of the sole being known as *Corns:* the horse steps with its sole on a sharp stone, for example, the momentary pressure injures the underlying dermis, and a non-infected hemorrhagic lesion similar to a black eye results. Penetrating wounds, from a nail for instance, carry infection below the sole (*Subsolar abscess*) that, if left untreated, may fester inside the hoof until it breaks through the skin at the coronet (path of least resistance). If the nail punctures the coffin joint or the navicular bursa or enters bone, the infection of course becomes that much more severe and more difficult to treat. Cracks in the hoof wall (*Sand or Quarter cracks*) arise from various causes. They may extend the full length of the hoof, go partway down from the coronary border, or partway up from the sole border. They may be supf., or involve the laminar dermis and then are very painful.

Have an entire hoof capsule handy when reading the following section on the **ACTION OF THE HOOF**. The hoof is remarkably adapted to accommodate the concussion produced by contact with the ground. The wall bears most of the impact and weight. This is especially true in draft horses when they are shod with the frog off the ground.

In the normal unshod hoof the frog strikes the ground first, followed by the heels, bars, quarters, and toe. The frog expands, spreading the bars, and transmits its initial impact to the digital cushion. The major part of the impact is transmitted from the sole border of the quarters and toe to the wall. The impact is converted to tension from the inside of the wall through the laminae and periosteum to PIII, supporting much of the weight of the horse. This tension causes a retraction at the coronary border of the toe, while the heels are spread by the distortion of the wall, frog, and digital cushion. The coffin joint yields under the pressure from PII because the navicular bone gives downward and backward with the stretching of its collateral ligaments and the deep flexor tendon. Depression of the sole by PIII is slight; the sole does not support weight on dry terrain.

This discussion shows that the weight of the horse does not pass from PIII through the sole (as may have been suspected), but is transmitted to the wall, with the result that the sole border of the wall is the principal weight bearing area. The union between PIII and wall by means of the inter-digitating laminae is therefore a very strong one. The union is also very special----and enigmatic---- because it allows the wall to grow distally(!) *against* the weight of the horse.

In essence then, the hoof is a flexible struc-ture that yields under the pressure of the impact with the ground, dissipating the concussion by causing a depression, compression, and lat-eral expansion of the various parts. The slight deformation of the hoof compresses the valveless **venous plexus** that is embedded in the underlying dermis and in the coronary and digital cushions. This forces the blood proximally into the digital veins, which again have valves to prevent the blood from re-entering the hoof when the foot is off the ground. The hoof mechanism thus aids in blood return that in the limbs is largely the responsibility of contracting and relaxing muscle bellies, but these are absent in the horse distal to carpus and hock.

The venous plexus deep to the hoof is of considerable importance in the surgical resection of the hoof cartilages for the relief of quittor. *Quittor* is a purulent infection of the cartilages with necrosis and break-through where the cartilages are palpable above the hoof. *Sidebone*, another disorder of the hoof cartilages, is their gradual ossification that impedes the elastic hoof mechanism; poor conformation and faulty shoeing are said to be causes.

A grave disease of the hoof is *Laminitis* or "founder". It is an inflammation (from several causes) of the dermal laminae that leads to the destruction of the strong union between the hoof wall and PIII. The bone rotates away from the wall and pushes through the thin sole. Many horses are euthanatized when the disease has progressed to this worst-scenario stage. (The separation of the laminae and the descent of PIII in laminitis is proof that, in the sound horse, most of the weight is borne by the wall of the hoof.)

In the dissection of the **DIGIT** *work on the medial side; the lateral side will then be available for a review dissection.* **Note:** *Only the medial digital nerves and vessels are described. The lateral digital nerves and vessels are distributed similarly.*

Locate the small fibrous mass that underlies the ergot on the palmar surface of the fetlock. (The ergot was removed with the skin.) A narrow white band, the **ligament of the ergot,** extends distodorsally to disappear deep to the veins covering the cartilage of the hoof (palpate). Isolate the ligament as far as the proximal border of the cartilage (Figs. 6-17 and 6-28/7).

Pick up the **medial palmar nerve** where it was last seen in the metacarpus. Trace it distally over the fetlock by incising and reflecting the supf. fascia. Clean the nerve and the accompanying digital vessels, but do not displace them and lose important relationships. The medial palmar nerve becomes the **medial digital nerve** which at the fetlock gives off the dorsal branch (Fig. 6-31).

The **dorsal branch** descends at first between the digital vein and artery and then crosses over the vein to ramify on the dorsal surface of the fetlock and form an extensive plexus on the dorsal and medial surfaces of the pastern including the coronet. (The plexus is often reinforced by a second dorsal branch of the digital nerve.) Trace the larger branches of the dorsal branch. The first of these is given off at the fetlock and crosses the digital vein and the medial palmar metacarpal nerve (Fig. 6-17).

The **medial palmar metacarpal nerve** emerges at the distal end of Mc2 (Fig. 6-31). It is small and very difficult to find; don't try to find it.

The **medial palmar metacarpal nerve** is derived from the deep branch of the lateral palmar nerve, which leaves the lateral palmar nerve after the exchange of fibers between the median and ulnar nerves at the carpus; it supplies the interosseus, and also gives off the **lateral palmar metacarpal nerve** (Fig. 6-18). The latter is distributed on the lateral side of the digit in much the same manner as the medial nerve.

The **medial digital nerve** passes distally on the palmar surface of the digital artery. It is larger than its dorsal branch. Note the oblique course of the ligament of the ergot over the nerve and artery. Just before the nerve disappears medial to the cartilage of the hoof it gives off a branch to the digital cushion.

(Appendix C presents a summary of the inner-vation of the fetlock joint and the structures of the digit.)

The digital nerves are sometimes resected *(digital neurectomy)* for the relief of chronic navicular disease. The removal of the segment of nerve is done as close to the palpable cartilages of the hoof as possible. The ligament of the ergot crosses the area; it must not be mistaken for the nerve.

Pick up the **medial palmar artery** where it was last seen in the metacarpus. The artery bifurcates between the flexor tendons and interosseus to form the medial and lateral digital arteries. (The small palmar metacarpal arteries, which have not been studied, and the small lateral palmar artery accompanying the lateral palmar nerve join the lateral digital artery at this level (Fig. 6-32). Do not trace these small arteries.)

Trace the **medial digital artery.** Above the fet-lock it lies deep to the accompanying digital vein

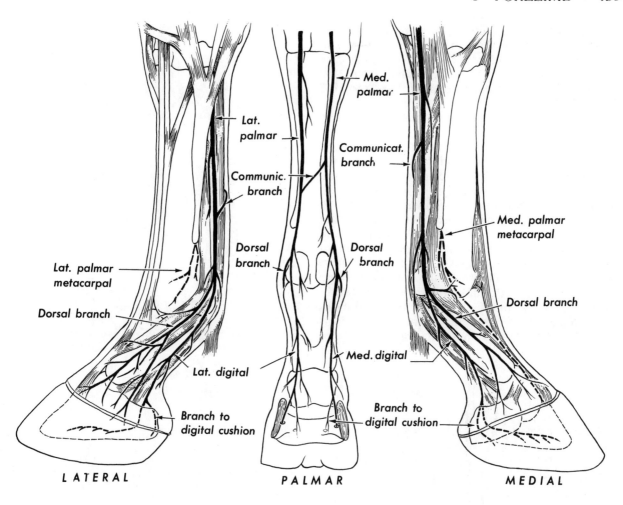

FIGURE 6-31. Nerves on the left metacarpus and digit, semischematic. (Modified with permission from Pohlmeyer and Redecker 1974.)

and the medial palmar nerve. At the fetlock the artery becomes more supf. and lies between the vein and the palmar digital nerve. The main trunk of the medial digital artery continues distally and gives off a **branch to the digital cushion** before disappearing deep to the cartilage of the hoof (Fig. 6-40/B,7) . The branch to the digital cushion accompanies the like-named nerve seen earlier. The termination of the medial digital artery within PIII (Fig. 6-32) will be seen after the digital cushion has been removed.

Near the middle of PI, and again opposite PII, the **medial digital artery** releases small dorsal and palmar branches to these bones; the branches encircle the bones with corresponding branches from the lateral digital artery (Figs. 6-32 and 6-40/B, 6,6',8,8').

Hold the limb on the table so the dorsal surface of metacarpus and digit is up. Incise the supf. fascia along the mid-dorsal line and reflect the flaps to expose the lateral extensor tendon, the common extensor tendon, and the **extensor branches of the interosseus** (Fig. 6-33/2,1,7).

Note how the latter join the common extensor tendon near the distal end of PI. Their origin will be seen shortly.

The **lateral extensor tendon** (/2) passes over the fetlock joint to insert on the proximal mid-dorsal surface of PI. Transect the tendon at the middle of the metacarpus and reflect it distally to its insertion, separating it from the common extensor tendon and cutting it off the fetlock joint capsule.

The **common extensor tendon** passes over the fetlock and widens considerably at the junction with the extensor branches of the interosseus. Weak insertions are detached to the proximal mid-dorsal surfaces of PI and PII. The main insertion is on the extensor process of PIII. (Find these points of insertion on the skeleton of the digit. Why is the tendon ending on the PIII extensor process of the hindlimb called the *long* extensor and not the *common* extensor as in the forelimb?) Transect the tendon at the middle of the metacarpus and reflect it distally off the fetlock joint capsule. Note the bursa that lies between the tendon and the capsule.

Open the **fetlock joint capsule** that lies deep to the tendons. The fibrous membrane is thick and supported by the extensor tendons. Note the **capsular fold** that extends distally from the proximal edge of the articular surface of Mc3 (Fig. 6-34/3).

Transect the two extensor branches of the interosseus at their junction with the common extensor tendon. Continue reflecting the tendon distally, opening the small dorsal pouch of the **pastern joint.** Small capsular folds may be present. (Pathological changes in the digital joints will obscure normal structures. It is therefore useful to examine joints and tendon sheaths also on another specimen.) By palpation on your specimen and reference to the skeleton note the relationship of the distal collateral tubercles of PI to the pastern joint. Palpate dorsally from the tubercles along the articular line to the edge of the extensor tendon. This is how you palpate the landmarks for an injection of the pastern joint; the needle is inserted under the tendon and advanced to enter the dorsal pouch.

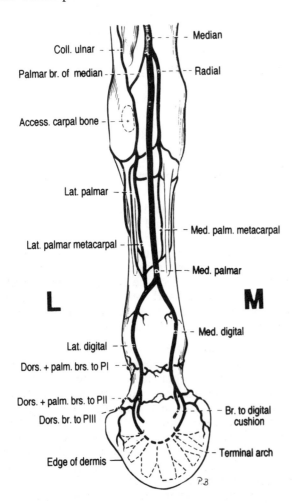

FIGURE 6-32. Arteries of the left carpus, metacarpus, and digit, palmar view. The principal artery to the foot, the medial palmar, continues the median on the medial aspect of the flexor tendons. (See also Fig. 6-40/B)

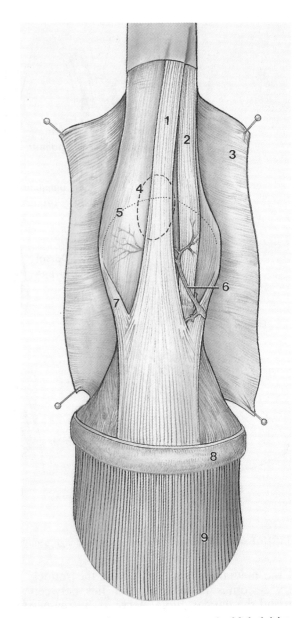

1.	Common digital extensor tendon		pouch of fetlock joint
2.	Lat. digital extensor tendon	6.	Dorsal branch of lateral digital vein
3.	Supf. fascia	7.	Extensor br. of interosseus
4.	Bursa between common extensor tendon and dorsal pouch of fetlock joint		joining common extensor tendon
5.	Proximal extent of dorsal	8.	Coronary dermis
		9.	Laminar dermis

FIGURE 6-33. Termination of common and lateral digital extensor tendons in the left digit, dorsal view.

Reflect the common extensor tendon to its insertion on the extensor process of PIII, opening the dorsal pouch of the **coffin joint.** Note the relationship of the coronary dermis to the coffin joint. On your articulated specimen, find the mark on PII level with the coronary border of the hoof. The coffin joint is within the hoof, only the dorsal pouch protrudes a little above it (Fig. 6-34). The dorsal pouch may be punctured in similar fashion to what was described for the pastern joint. The needle must be placed between the tendon and PII;

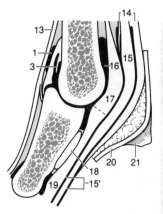

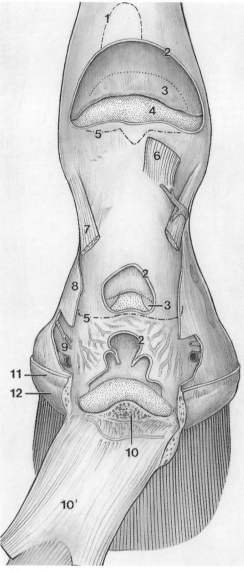

1. Position of bursa deep to the common extensor tendon
2. Cut edge of joint capsule
3. Capsular fold
4. Three stippled areas: distal articular surfaces of Mc3, PI, and PII
5. Position of fetlock and pastern joint spaces
6. Insertion of lat. digital extensor, on PI
7. Extensor branch of interosseus
8. Fascia
9. Dorsal brr. of dig. vessels, to PII
10. Extensor process of PIII, from which the common digital extensor (10') has been detached
11. Perioplic dermis
12. Coronary dermis
13. Common digital extensor
14. Supf. digital flexor forming sleeve around deep digital flexor
15. Deep digital flexor, digital tendon sheath at 15'
16. Prox. palmar pouch of fetlock joint
17. Palmar ligament
18. Oblique sesamoidean ligament
19. Straight sesamoidean ligament
20. Skin
21. Ergot

FIGURE 6-34. The dorsal pouches of the three digital joints exposed by reflection of the common and lateral digital extensor tendons, dorsal view. The visible articular surfaces are stippled. The inset shows the fetlock joint in axial section and the disposition of the capsular fold (3).

the edge of the tendon, unfortunately, is too thin to be palpated in the live horse.

During the fast gaits the fetlock joint is extremely overextended and sinks toward the ground, especially in fatigued horses at the end of a race, for example. Your articulated specimen may allow you to simulate this—try it. Note that the proximodorsal border of PI rides up against the dorsal surface of Mc3 and impinges on the capsular fold. If contact is severe or repetitive, the fold may become inflamed and thicken (*villinodular synovitis*) or the dorsal border of PI may chip, both lesions causing lameness.

Hold the limb on the table so the palmar surface of metacarpus and digit is up. The deep fascia of the fetlock and pastern by and large is thinner than the deep fascia of the limb above. Nevertheless, three annular ligaments represent definite identifiable thickenings of the deep fascia over the palmar surfaces of the flexor tendons. The most proximal is at the fetlock joint, the second at the pastern, and the distalmost just above the digital cushion. We identify only the first, the palmar annular ligament. The other two (known as proximal and distal digital annular ligaments) are optional; see the next paragraphs set in small type.

Incise the supf. fascia over the palmar surface of the metacarpus and fetlock and reflect the flaps. Trace the supf. flexor tendon distally. At the fetlock it is bound down by the **palmar annular ligament** that is attached to the palmar borders of the proximal sesamoid bones (Fig. 6-35/3). Identify the transverse direction of its fibers.

Incise the palmar annular ligament from its proximal edge to the transverse plane of the palpable distal ends of the proximal sesamoid bones, no farther. Make a transverse incision across the distal end of the previous incision and reflect the flaps. This reflection opens the **digital (synovial) sheath.** This important sheath

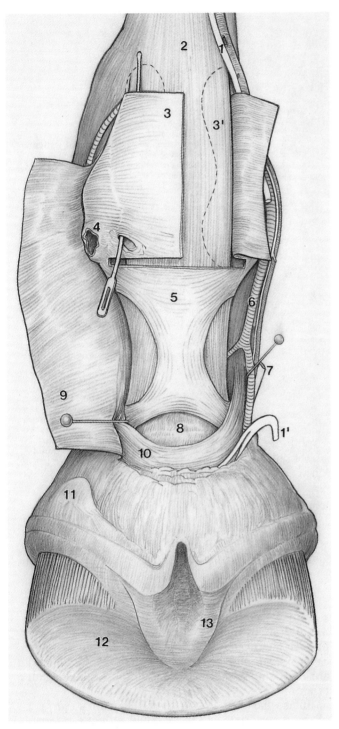

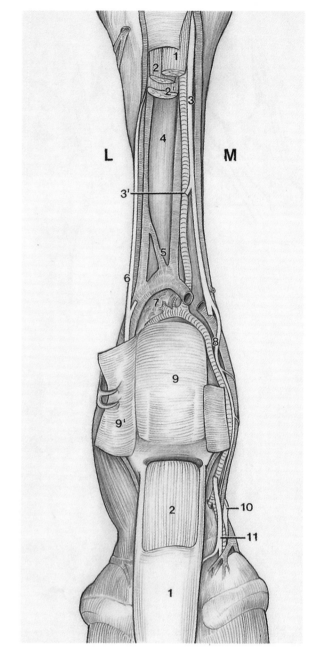

1.	Med. dig. nerve and vein, distal stump of nerve at 1'		dorsal br. of the med. dig. n.
2	Supf. flexor tendon	7.	Distal stump of ligament of the ergot
3.	Palmar annular ligament, med. half reflected	8.	Digital sheath covering deep digital flexor tendon
3'	Extent of digital tendon sheath under palmar annular ligament	9.	Supf. fascia
		10.	Distal digital annular lig.
4	Palpable access to distal palmar pouch of fetlock joint	11.	Hoof cartilage
		12.	Dermis of the sole
5.	Prox. digital annular ligament	13.	Dermis of the frog
6.	Digital artery, dorsal to it is a		

FIGURE 6-35. Palmar view of digit. Removal of skin and superficial fascia reveals three annular ligaments.

1.	Supf. digital flexor tendon	8.	Med. digital vessels and dorsal branch of digital nerve
2	Deep digital flexor tendon, its accessory ligament at 2'		
3.	Med. palmar nerve and vessels, the nerve's communicating branch at 3'	9.	Palmar ligament connecting proximal sesamoid bones (proximal scutum)
4	Interosseus	9'	Palmar annular ligament, reflected
5.	Veins deep to flexor tendons		
6.	Lateral palmar nerve	10.	Stump of ligament of ergot
7.	Lateral palmar and metacarpal arteries joining lat. dig. artery	11.	Med. digital nerve with branch to digital cushion

FIGURE 6-36. Palmar view of left metacarpus after reflection of superficial and (common) deep flexor tendons.

envelops the deep and supf. flexor tendons and is a frequent site of inflammation. Probe its proximal extent, to about the level of the distal ends of the splint bones. The distal extent will be exposed later.

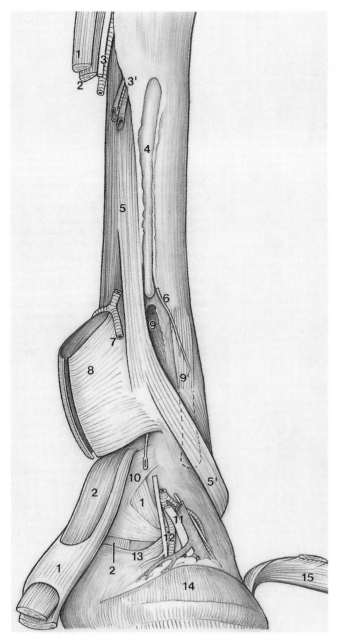

1. Supf. digital flexor tendon
2. Deep digital flexor tendon (its accessory lig. is not shown)
3. Med. palmar nerve and artery, metacarpal vessels at 3'
4. Mc2
5. Interosseus, its extensor branch at 5'
6. Med. palmar metacarpal nerve
7. Med. digital artery
8. Palmar annular ligament
9. Opened palmar pouch of fetlock joint, med. collateral ligament at 9'
10. Prox. digital annular lig.
11. Lig. of ergot and digital vein
12. Digital nerve and artery
13. Distal digital annular lig.
14. Hoof cartilage
15. Common digital extensor tendon

FIGURE 6-37. Medial and slightly palmar view of metacarpus and digit after reflection of supf. and deep flexor tendons. The probe is in the palmar pouch of the fetlock joint.

Locate the proximal and distal bands that attach the four corners of the X-shaped **proximal digital annular ligament** to the proximal and distal collateral tubercles of PI (Fig. 6-35/5). The ligament itself closely adheres to the surface of the supf. flexor. The proximal bands are readily traced to the tubercles, and the proximal part of the ligament is easily separated from the underlying tendon. The distal half of the ligament adheres to the tendon and its borders are indistinct. Furthermore, the (smaller) distal bands are covered by the attachments of the *distal* digital annular ligament, also on PI.

The **distal digital annular ligament** is only partially visible at this stage (Fig. 6-35/10). It forms a crescentic sling over the palmar surface of the deep flexor tendon and arises by two attachments from an oblique crest on the distal half of the medial and lateral borders of PI. Find the crest on the articulated specimen. The deep (dorsal) surface of the ligament fuses with the deep flexor tendon; its supf. surface lies against the digital cushion.

Transect the flexor tendons and the accessory (check) ligament of the deep flexor in the proximal third of the metacarpus. Separate the supf. from the deep flexor tendon and reflect them distally.

Note the sleeve formed by the supf. around the deep tendon at the fetlock. While one student holds the *reflected* flexor tendons, remove the layer of deep fascia that separated the flexor tendons from the interosseus. This exposes several deep veins and the bifurcation of the **medial palmar artery** into medial and lateral digital arteries (Fig. 6-36). The veins are variable and should be transected so as to be able to reflect them laterally.

With the reflection of the veins the **interosseus** is exposed. It arises from the distal row of carpal bones and the proximal end of Mc3, passes distally, applied to the palmar surface of that bone, and divides into two branches proximal to the fetlock. The medial branch of the interosseus (the lateral branch is exactly the same) attaches on the abaxial hollowed surface of the medial sesamoid bone, but sends a thin extensor branch dorsodistally over the fetlock to the common extensor tendon (Fig. 6-42/B,15).

The extensor branch of the interosseus blends with the **medial collateral sesamoid ligament**. This is a triangular plate of fibers that fans out from the palmar border of the proximal sesamoid bone to the tubercle of Mc3 and to the proximal collateral tubercle of PI. (Find the tubercles and their relation to the sesamoid bones on the skeleton.) The ligament is best examined by reflecting (not cutting) the digital vessels and nerves, by palpating and then slicing thin layers off its surface (blade flat against the ligament) until its fibers become visible.

The (proximal) **palmar pouch of the fetlock joint capsule** may be opened distal to the splint bone between the cannon bone and the interosseus (Fig. 6-37/9). Probe the extent of the pouch. Distension of the fetlock joint manifests itself at this point (wind puffs, galls). This is also the usual site for puncturing the joint. (Why does the palmar pouch distend more readily than the dorsal pouch?)

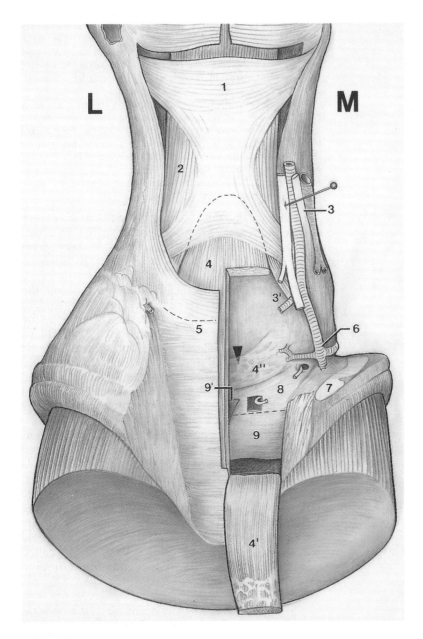

1. Prox. digital annular ligament
2. Supf. digital flexor tendon; its bifurcation is shown by the broken line
3. Lig. of ergot with digital nerve (pin) and vessels, branches to digital cushion at 3'
4. Deep digital flexor tendon, medial half reflected at 4', medial half cut away from the palmar surface of PII at 4"; the arrow head indicates the distalmost extent of the digital sheath on the *dorsal* surface of the deep flexor tendon
5. Lat. half of distal digital annular ligament, the broken line near the 5 is the distalmost extent of the digital sheath on the *palmar* surface of the deep flexor
6. Digital artery with dorsal and palmar branches to PII
7. Cut surface of hoof cartilage
8. Collateral (suspensory) ligament of navicular bone (9); the wire passes through the proximal palmar pouch of the coffin joint
9. Navicular bone; the distal navicular ligament has been removed to permit a view into the distal palmar pouch of the coffin joint (see Fig. 6-38/A)
9' Prox. extent of navicular bursa between deep flexor tendon (4) and navicular bone (9)

FIGURE 6-38. Palmar view of left digit. The digital cushion and the medial half of the deep flexor tendon have been reflected to expose the navicular bursa and the distal extent of the digital sheath.

Remove the deep fascia between the extensor branch of the interosseus and the extensor tendon, and locate the **medial collateral ligament of the fetlock** (Fig. 6-37/9'). Free the previously transected extensor branch and reflect it proximally. Clean the surface of the collateral ligament. It attaches proximally on the tubercle of Mc3 and distally to the rough area in front of the proximal collateral tubercle of PI (palpate and see on articulated specimen).

Examine the fibrocartilaginous **palmar ligament** that unites the proximal sesamoid bones, forming a smooth bearing surface (proximal scutum) for the passage of the flexor tendons (Fig. 6-36/9). The ligament extends proximally beyond the sesamoid bones where its deep surface is grooved to receive the central crest of Mc3 during extreme overextension. (Where would the proximal extension of the ligament contact Mc3 during flexion?)

Cut the digital vessels and nerves a few cm above their disappearance deep to the hoof cartilage and reflect the stumps off the medial surface of the pastern. Remove the supf. fascia from the palmar and medial surfaces of the pastern.

Palpate the bifurcation of the supf. flexor tendon near the distal end of PI. Open the **digital sheath** between and distal to the bifurcation. This is the lowest accessible point for clinical drainage of the sheath (Fig. 6-29/A). (The sheath actually extends 2 cm farther distally on the *deep (dorsal) surface* of the deep flexor tendon, as shown in Fig. 6-38/4.) Opening the sheath exposed the deep flexor tendon passing through the bifurcation of the supf. flexor.

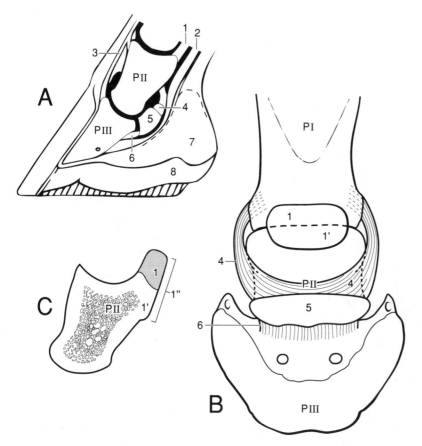

1. Complementary fibrocartilage continued proximally by the straight sesamoidean ligament; the fibrocartilage and the smooth palmar patch of PII (1') form the middle bearing surface (scutum; 1") for the flexor tendons
2. Deep digital flexor tendon surrounded by digital sheath
3. Common digital extensor tendon
4. Collateral (suspensory) ligament of the navicular bone
5. Navicular bone (5 and the central part of 4 form the distal bearing surface (scutum) for the deep flexor tendon)
6. Distal navicular ligament
7. Digital cushion
8. Frog

FIGURE 6-39. A, Axial section of digit and hoof. B, Palmar view of digital skeleton with the collateral and distal navicular ligaments and the middle and distal bearing surfaces for the flexor tendons. C, Axial (sagittal) section of PII; the complementary fibrocartilage (stippled) enlarges the proximal articular surface and takes part in forming the middle scutum (1").

To remove the digital cushion: Make a longitudinal incision as close as possible along the axial surface of the hoof cartilage down to the medial edge of the deep flexor tendon; carry the incision distally along the laminae of the bars to the apex of the frog dermis. Repeat on the lateral side. Reflect the cushion distally, separating it from the distal digital annular ligament on the palmar surface of the tendon.

Examine the **digital cushion,** noting its texture and yielding nature. When, during extreme overextension of the fetlock joint, it is compressed between PII and frog, the cushion presses against the cartilages and promotes the outward movement of the quarters.

Transect the medial half (only) of the flat deep flexor tendon where it passes through the bifurcation of the supf. flexor (Fig. 6-38/4,2). The deep tendon widens considerably below this point and inserts on the flexor surface of PIII. Reflect the medial half of the tendon distally, dividing it sagittally from the lateral half (/4'). Also remove the medial half of the distal digital annular ligament that is fused with the tendon. As half the tendon is reflected it must be cut free from underlying structures; it is important to make these cuts as close to the deep tendon as possible.

The reflection opened the **navicular bursa** and exposed the medial half of the navicular bone (/9).

Probe the extent of the bursa under the lateral half of the tendon that is still in place and relate its proximodistal extent to the navicular bone that appears wider (proximodistally) than it actually is. To determine the width of the navicular bone refer to Fig. 6-38 and walk the point of your scalpel from the distal border of the bone proximally, until the blade sinks into soft tissue. The soft tissue is the central portion of the U-shaped **collateral ligament of the navicular bone.** This arises from PI and with its bottom part attaches to the proximal border of the navicular bone (Fig. 6-39/B,A,4). The proximodistal extent of the navicular bursa, therefore, is greater than the width of the navicular bone and collateral ligament combined. (We will see the navicular bone more fully later.)

Nail wounds penetrating and infecting the *navicular bursa* may be treated surgically by removing part of the frog and digital cushion and resecting the flexor tendon to expose the bursa and navicular bone for drainage.

Time saver: One student of each group should obtain the appropriate half of the split head and skin it according to the instruction on page 154.

Remove the proximal 3 cm of the hoof cartilage by cutting it parallel to the coronary dermis. Note the venous anastomoses that pass through the cartilage and connect the parts of the venous plexus on its axial and abaxial surfaces.

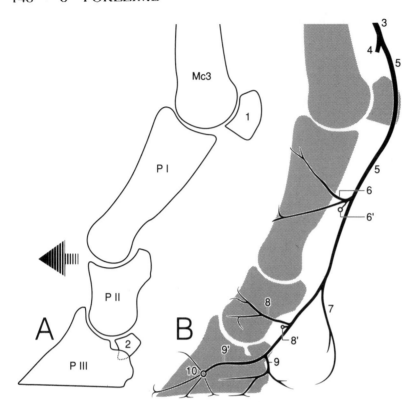

1. Proximal sesamoid bone
2. Distal (navicular) sesamoid bone
3. Medial palmar artery
4. Stump of lateral digital artery
5. Medial digital artery
6,6' Dorsal and palmar branches to PI
7. Branch to digital cushion
8,8' Dorsal and palmar branches to PII
9. Dorsal branch to PIII
9' Continuation of digital a.
10. Terminal arch

FIGURE 6-40. *A*, Position of the phalanges when the pastern joint buckles forward; side view. *B*, Skeleton of digit showing the principal branches of the medial digital artery, side view; drawn from an angiograph.

Pick up the distal stump of the **medial digital artery** and trace it distally. Just proximal to the level of the navicular bone it gives off the dorsal and palmar branches to PII that encircle that bone with corresponding branches of the lateral digital artery (Fig. 6-40/B,8,8'). The medial digital artery continues distally (do not trace) to supply the dorsal (parietal) branch to PIII (/9) and terminates by anastomosing with the lateral artery in the sole canal, forming the **terminal arch** within PIII (/10; and Fig. 6-32).

Study the **termination of the medial digital artery** on the articulated specimen, using the following description: The dorsal branch to PIII passes through the foramen in the palmar process of PIII and runs dorsally in the parietal groove, giving off ascending and descending branches to the laminar dermis. The continuation of the digital artery (i.e., the palmar branch) enters the sole canal through the sole foramen. The terminal arch gives off numerous branches that pass through the bone to ramify in the laminar dermis and the dermis of the sole.

Open the proximal palmar pouch of the coffin joint by cutting the collateral navicular ligament as shown in Figure 6-38/8. Probe the pouch; its continuity, deep to the navicular bone, with the distal pouch will be seen later when the coffin joint is opened. The proximal palmar pouch extends proximally to the middle of PII. The digital sheath ends at this level and is separated from the pouch by a fibrous membrane (Fig. 6-29/A).

At the level of the fetlock joint find and cut open the sleeve of the **supf. flexor tendon** around the deep flexor tendon. Now palpate and then transect the medial insertion (to PI and PII) of the supf. flexor tendon. Transect also the distinct proximal band of the proximal digital annular ligament (Fig. 6-41/4). Separate the two flexor tendons and reflect only the supf. flexor tendon laterally, hooking or holding it to that side of the digit. Palpate the distal stump of the supf. flexor tendon and demonstrate its insertion on both PI and PII.

Now reflect the entire deep flexor tendon distally to expose the navicular bone fully; for this you need to cut down to the lateral border of the tendon as you did when you reflected the medial stump.

With both supf. and deep tendons out of the way the entire channel in which they lay is exposed and the three **bearing surfaces** (scuta, plural of scutum, shield) over which the tendons change direction are clearly visible (Fig. 6-41). The proximal bearing surface is formed by the proximal sesamoid bones and the palmar ligament that connects them; the middle bearing surface is formed by a smooth patch near the proximal border of PII (see articulated specimen) and the **complementary fibrocartilage** of this bone (Fig. 6-39/C); and the distal bearing surface consists of the navicular bone and the central part of the collateral ligament of the navicular bone that attaches to its proximal border.

The **digital sheath** surrounds and protects the two tendons as they slide against each other and over the bearing surfaces. The synovial tissue of

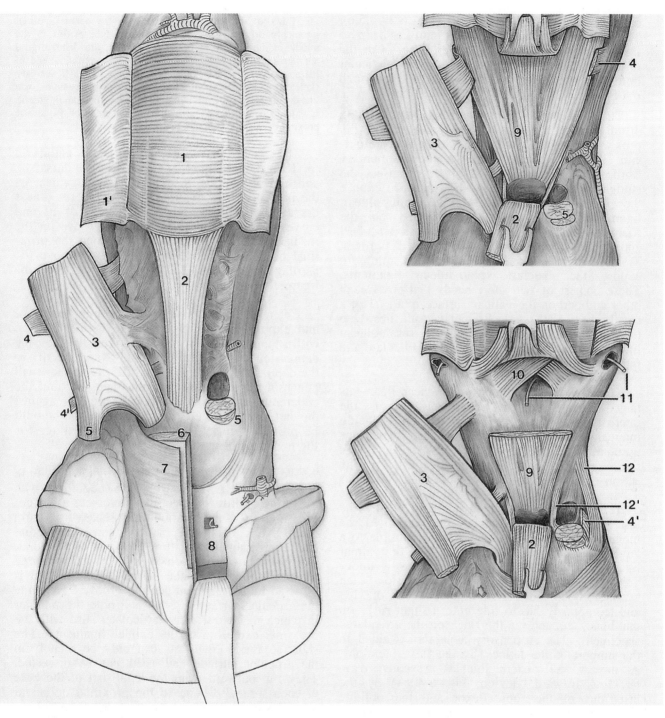

1. Palmar lig. connecting proximal sesamoid bones, palmar annular lig. at 1'
2. Straight sesamoidean lig.
3. Supf. flexor tendon, reflected
4. Stump of proximal attachment of prox. digital annular ligament

4' Stump of distal attachment of prox. digital annular ligament
5. Stump of supf. flexor
6. Stump of deep flexor
7. Distal dig. annular lig.
8. Navicular bone, probe in prox. palmar pouch of coffin joint

9. Oblique sesamoidean lig.
10. Cruciate sesamoidean lig.
11. Probe in distal palmar pouch of fetlock joint
12. Abaxial palmar lig. of pastern joint

12' Axial palmar ligament of pastern joint, the dark area to each side of it is the opened palmar pouch of the joint

FIGURE 6-41. *Left*: Deep dissection of digit, exposing the straight sesamoidean ligament, palmar view. *Right*: Two deeper dissections, exposing the oblique and cruciate sesamoidean ligaments, on the palmar surface of PI.

the sheath is best shown opposite PI in the form of irregular brownish tufts (which should be removed).

Identify again the collateral ligament of the navicular bone. See also the short fibers of the wide **distal navicular ligament** that connects the distal border of the bone to PIII (Fig. 6-39/4,5,6). The **palmar pouch of the coffin joint** lies deep to these ligaments and the navicular bone. Cut the distal navicular ligament close to the navicular bone and open the small distal part of the pouch (/A,6).

There are three sesamoidean ligaments passing distally from the basal (distal) aspect of the proximal sesamoid bones. The **straight sesamoidean ligament** passes to the complementary fibrocartilage of PII (Fig. 6-41/2). Transect the straight ligament and reflect the stumps to expose the medial and lateral **oblique sesamoidean ligaments** (/9). These are inserted on the triangular rough area on the palmar surface of PI and form a triangle with thick rounded borders. Transect them and reflect the proximal stumps to expose the **cruciate sesamoidean ligaments.** These consist of two short bands that cross each other and end on the palmar surface of PI (/10); a small recess of the fetlock joint capsule lies deep to them (/11). (Lesser, short sesamoidean ligaments will be seen when we disarticulate the fetlock joint.)

The straight and oblique sesamoidean ligaments may be regarded as continuations of the interosseus, the proximal sesamoid bones being intercalated in the course of this **suspensory apparatus.** (This is why the interosseus is often referred to as the suspensory ligament.). The action of the suspensory apparatus becomes apparent when the fetlock is visualized in extreme overextension to which it is subjected during the fast gaits or when landing after a jump. At the moment of impact, the thrust of Mc3 is borne to a large extent by the sesamoid bones and the palmar ligament, and the suspensory apparatus is under great tension. In extreme overextension each sesamoid bone slides around the distal end of Mc3 and temporarily has to ride onto a slight ridge on that bone; feel and see the ridge on the articulated specimen. The suspensory apparatus is aided in the support of the fetlock by the flexor tendons. At impact, the pastern joint is prevented from buckling forward (flexion; Fig. 6-40/A) by the insertions of the supf. flexor and the oblique sesamoidean ligaments. The coffin joint is prevented from flexing by the extensor branches of the interosseus to keep the hoof level during footing. The extensor branches counteract the pull of the deep digital flexor tendon (which is also under tension) that wants to flex the joint and dig the toe of the hoof into the ground.

There are three pairs of **ligaments associated with the pastern joint;** see their attachments also on your articulated specimen. The axial palmar ligaments originate from points medial and lateral to the palmar triangular area of PI (Fig. 6-41/12'). They attach distally on the fibrocartilage of PII between the straight sesamoid ligament and the insertions of the supf. flexor tendon. The abaxial palmar ligaments originate on the intermediate tuberosities in the middle of the borders of PI and blend with the distal digital annular ligament. They attach distally on the proximal end of PII abaxial to the insertions of the supf. digital flexor (see skeleton). The medial collateral ligament of the pastern joint lies dorsal to, and blends with, the abaxial palmar ligament. It extends from the distal collateral tubercle of PI to the proximal collateral tubercle of PII.

The medial part of the U-shaped **collateral navicular ligament** (Fig. 6-39/B,4) lies dorsal to, and blends with, the medial collateral ligament of the pastern joint. It originates on the roughness dorsal to the distal collateral tubercle of PI and curves distally through the oblique groove on the medial border of PII. It attaches along the proximal border of the navicular bone. Remove the cartilage of the hoof as necessary to trace the ligament.

Cut away what remains of the hoof cartilage and expose the medial collateral ligament of the **coffin joint.** It attaches proximally to the depression on the distal end of PII and distally to the depression on the side of PIII. Note the small pouch of the joint capsule immediately behind the collateral ligament. This pouch projects against the cartilage, especially during flexion, and should be protected during resection of the cartilage for the treatment of quittor (see p. 138).

We finish the dissection of the digit with a look at the **ARTICULAR SURFACES,** beginning with the **fetlock joint.** Transect the interosseus a few cm proximal to its bifurcation and separate it from Mc3. Cut the joint capsule and the medial collateral ligament and turn Mc3 out of the joint. The joint cavity is formed by PI, the proximal sesamoid bones, and the palmar ligament, and is bisected by a prominent central groove. Examine the articular surface of Mc3 and note the manner in which its central ridge articulates also with the proximal extension of the palmar ligament. The short sesamoid ligaments can only be seen from the articular surface and need not be dissected. They run outward from the axial part of the base of each sesamoid bone to the proximal collateral tubercles of PI. Probe the part of the distal palmar pouch that lies abaxial to the short ligament and note its supf. position. It may be used for access to the joint.

Cut the joint capsule, the medial collateral and medial abaxial palmar ligaments of the **pastern joint,** and turn PI out of the joint. For better exposure cut the axial palmar ligaments also. Note that the **complementary fibrocartilage** is firmly attached to the palmar border of PII and enlarges the joint cavity substantially. It supports the pastern joint at the moment of thrust during the fast gaits. There is no central groove.

Cut the medial collateral ligament of the **coffin joint** and medial part of the U-shaped collateral ligament of the navicular bone and turn PII out of the joint. The joint cavity is formed by PIII, the navicular bone, and by the bottom part of the U-shaped collateral ligament of the navicular bone that is attached to the proximal border of the bone. There is no central groove.

By manipulating the specimen determine the action of the interosseus, palmar ligament, the straight and oblique sesamoidean ligaments, and the fibrocartilage of PII when Mc3 delivers its thrust at the moment of impact of the foot on the ground.

Appendix E lists the bony prominences of the digital skeleton and correlates them with the tendons and ligaments attaching on them. Working through the list with an articulated specimen will enhance your understanding of this concentration of anatomical structures.

Passive Stay-Apparatus

(When reading this section, re-identify on your specimen the structures that are mentioned, and with the help of Figure 6-42 determine or recall their attachments on the bony column of the limb.)

Because of the long cranial extension of the trunk formed by neck and head, the forelimbs support more weight than the hindlimbs. The weight supported by the forelimb is received at the proximal end of the scapula through the attachment of the serratus ventralis. A plumb line from this attachment passes caudal to the shoulder joint, through the elbow joint, through or slightly cranial to the carpal joint, cranial to the fetlock and pastern joints, and then through the hoof. If unsupported, the jointed bony column of the limb would collapse, therefore, by flexion in the shoulder and elbow joints, and by overextension (possibly flexion, buckling forward) in the carpus, and by overextension in the fetlock and pastern joints, those caudal to the vertical. The coffin joint actually flexes when the fetlock sinks under weight and can be disregarded.

The ligamentous structures that prevent this collapse in most of the joints form the stay-apparatus (Fig. 6-42/A) which, like the one of the hindlimb, helps reduce the muscular effort required to support this heavy animal.

The **fetlock joint** is prevented from excessive overextension by the interosseus, the proximal sesamoid bones, and the straight, oblique, and cruciate sesamoidean ligaments. These structures form a functional unit consisting of a ligamentous component proximally, intercalated bones, and a ligamentous component distally. The unit is firmly attached on the palmar surface of the bones proximal and distal to the joint and is placed under tension when the joint is overextended. The proximal attachment is on the carpus and the proximal end of Mc3, and the distal attachment is on PI and PII. The fetlock joint is further supported by the supf. and deep flexor tendons which are also firmly attached on the palmar surface of the bones proximal and distal to the joint. The supf. flexor is attached with its accessory (check) ligament to the radius and extends to PI and PII; the deep flexor is attached with its accessory (check) ligament to the carpus and extends to PIII.

The **pastern joint** is prevented from overextension by its palmar ligaments, the straight sesamoidean ligament, and the deep flexor tendon. The four palmar ligaments are short and just span the joint space, coming under tension when the joint is overextended. So does the straight sesamoidean ligament which arises from the proximal sesamoid bones and is attached on the complementary fibrocartilage on the proximal palmar border of PII. Possible buckling forward (flexion) of the joint (Fig. 6-40/A) is prevented by the attachment of the supf. flexor tendon to the palmar surface of the joint: when weight is on the limb the supf. flexor is under tension and pulls back on the joint.

Overextension of the **carpus** is blocked primarily by the flat dorsal parts of the articular surfaces in the radiocarpal and midcarpal joints, and secondarily by the thick palmar carpal ligament that unites the bones on the palmar surface. The constant upward pull of the extensor carpi radialis tendon through the lacertus fibrosus (see next paragraph) assists in preventing the joint from possibly buckling forward (flexing).

Flexion of the **shoulder joint** is prevented by the tendons of the biceps. The main (internal) tendon connects the supraglenoid tubercle of the scapula directly to the proximal end of the radius, while a supf. branch of the tendon, the lacertus fibrosus, is attached to the proximal end of Mc3 by means of the tendon of the extensor carpi radialis. Flexion of the shoulder joint by the weight of the trunk acting on the proximal end of the scapula tenses the biceps tendons. Since the distal attachments of the tendons are fixed by the weight of the standing animal, the shoulder is prevented from flexing.

The forces tending to flex the **elbow joint** are relatively small since the weight of the horse (with the shoulder joint fixed) presses directly on the upper end of the nearly vertical radius. Flexion is prevented principally by the passive tension within the fibrous components of the carpal and digital flexors in the forearm, and by the eccentrically placed collateral ligaments of the elbow joint. The triceps, the principal extensor of the elbow joint, is flaccid in the standing animal and does not seem to be required.

Exercises on the Live Animal

Students at Cornell should view the two video-tapes on the forelimb to appreciate how many structures can actually be palpated. (The tapes are "Shoulder Region and Arm" and "Distal Forelimb" in the series *Equine Anatomy Reviewed on the Live Animal*.) It is very helpful to be able to refer to a skeleton or your articulated specimen while doing these exercises.

1---Begin on the scapula and proceed distally. Palpate the scapular cartilage, the spine of the scapula, and the supra- and infraspinatus muscles. Locate the supf. tendon of the infraspinatus and palpate the *round* protuberance over which it passes. The protuberance is the caudal part of the greater tubercle of the humerus; a few cm cranial to it is the cranial part of the tubercle, which is the point-of-the-shoulder. The shoulder joint can be punctured by inserting the needle at the cranial border of the supf. infraspinatus tendon and just dorsal to the greater tubercle—find that point.

2---Palpate the deltoid tuberosity; it is a landmark for the injection of the intertubercular bursa that facilitates the biceps tendon's passage over the shoulder joint.

3---Note the flaccid, apparently inactive triceps. Is the triceps not the principal extensor of the elbow joint? What keeps the elbow extended in the standing horse?

4---Find the lacertus fibrosus about 10 cm ventral to the deltoid tuberosity and at the cranial aspect of the elbow joint; it feels as hard as a bone, because it is under tension in the standing animal. Now try to roll the medial cutaneous antebrachial nerve as it crosses the lacertus. The nerve is sometimes blocked—not difficult because (running over a hard surface) it is palpable.

5---Palpate the structures that lie under the skin in midforearm. Begin on the medial surface with the radius, which is flanked by the cephalic and accessory cephalic veins. Trace the (larger) cephalic vein proximally on the caudal border of the bone, over the lacertus, and into the palpable groove between the brachiocephalicus and pectoralis descendens to its origin from the external jugular vein. Return to the radius and proceed around the cranial border of the fore-arm and then all around to the radius again,

palpating the extensor carpi radialis, common digital extensor, lateral digital extensor (small), ulnaris lateralis (which takes you to the caudal border of the limb), flexor carpi ulnaris, and flexor carpi radialis. (See these structures on a transverse section in your textbook; the supf. and deep digital flexors are encased by the last three [flat] muscles you palpated.)

Estimate the extent of the seven synovial sheaths at the carpus. They cannot be palpated in the normal animal. In general, the sheaths extend from 7-8 cm above the carpus to about the proximal end of the metacarpus. The carpal sheath (for the supf. and deep flexors) reaches the middle of the metacarpus.

6---Palpate the medial and lateral styloid processes of the radius, the proximal end of the meta-carpus, and the accessory carpal bone. Run your fingers down the medial and lateral collateral ligaments and the distal ligament of Ca. Lift up the horse's foot and on the dorsal surface of the flexed carpus explore the gaping radiocarpal and midcarpal joints. Feel the tendon of the extensor carpi radialis cross the joint spaces; the joints are punctured medial to the tendon. (Which of the three component joints communicated again?)

7---In the metacarpus locate the large and small metacarpal bones, the interosseus, and the flexor tendons. The point of injection for palmar nerve block is in the palpable groove between the interosseus and the flexor tendons. Palpate the oblique communicating branch from the medial to the lateral palmar nerve as it climbs over the supf. flexor tendon.

Identify by palpation the four landmarks for the palmar pouch of the fetlock joint: distal end of splint bone, caudal border of cannon bone, proximal sesamoid bone, and the interosseus.

---

1. Weight of trunk
2. Biceps
3. Triceps
4. Brachiocephalicus and brachial fascia to elbow joint
5. Axis of elbow rotation
6. Lacertus fibrosus
7. Ulnaris lateralis
8. Flexor carpi ulnaris, its ulnar head at 8'
9. Supf. digital flexor and accessory lig., its sleeve around the deep flexor at 9'
10. Extensor carpi radialis
11. Deep digital flexor and accessory ligament; its radial, humeral, and ulnar heads at 11'
12. Common digital extensor
13. Interosseus
14. Proximal sesamoid bones
15. Extensor br. of interosseus
16,17,18 Cruciate, oblique, and straight sesamoidean ligs.
19. Axial palmar ligaments
20. Distal sesamoid (navicular) bone, its collateral ligament at 20'
21. Stump of flexor carpi radialis
22,22' Medial collat. ligaments of elbow and carpal joints
23. Palmar carpal ligament covering the palmar surface of the carpal bones
24. Distal lig. of accessory carpal bone

FIGURE 6-42 *A,* Passive stay-apparatus of the left forelimb, lateral view. (After Schmaltz 1911.) *B,* Detail of digit, lateral view. *C,* Digital flexors and interosseus of right forelimb, caudomedial view. (Modified after B. and B. Premiani: *El Caballo,* Buenos Aires, Ediciones Centauro, 1957.)

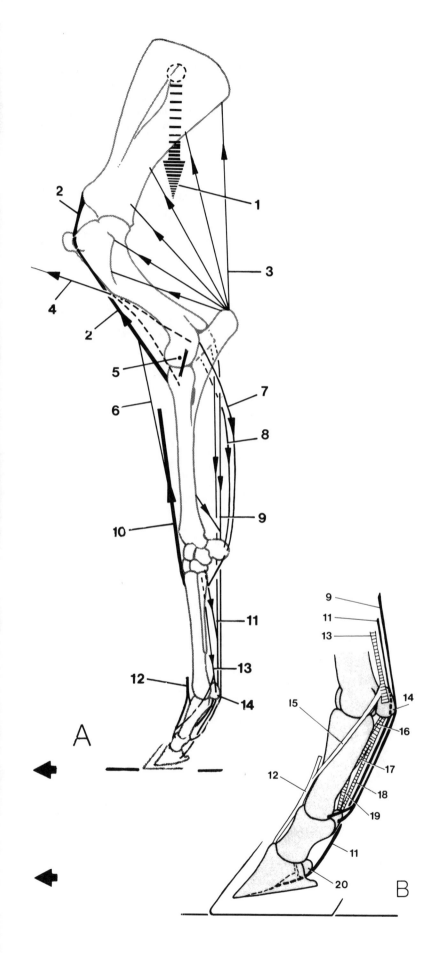

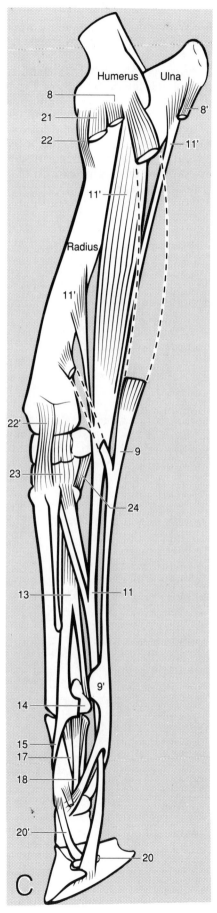

8---With reference to your articulated specimen palpate the following structures:

a) proximal and distal collateral tubercles, and the medial and lateral borders of PI
b) digital artery (i.e., digital pulse) and nerve between the flexor tendons and the border of PI
c) extensor branches of the interosseus
d) insertions of the supf. flexor tendon
e) border of the deep flexor tendon from the insertion of the supf. flexor to the digital cushion
f) hoof cartilages

9---Palpate the landmarks for the injection of the pastern and coffin joints. Palpate dorsally from the distal collateral tubercles of PI, along the articular line of the pastern joint to the (nonpalpable) border of the extensor tendon (2 cm from the dorsal midline of the digit). The needle is directed toward the dorsal midline and pushed under the extensor tendon (Fig. 6-34).

The coffin joint is accessible for injection 1.5 cm proximal to the hoof at the border of the extensor tendon. The needle is directed distally and toward the dorsal midline of the digit and pushed under the tendon.

7

HEAD

Purpose and Plan of the Dissection

1---To see the features of the head that lie directly under the skin and cutaneous muscle, notably the buccal branches of the facial nerve, facial artery where its pulse is commonly taken, parotid duct, mandibular lymph nodes, and the infraorbital foramen and nerve.

2---To note the position of the large veins deep to the masseter, and the masseteric artery and vein, that are at risk in the repulsion of cheek teeth.

3---In the important retromandibular fossa to explore the topography of the parotid and mandibular salivary glands, branches of external jugular vein and common carotid artery, glossopharyngeal and hypoglossal nerves, retropharyngeal lymph nodes, and the guttural pouch.

4---To become familiar with the nasal diverticulum and the orifice of the nasolacrimal duct in the nostril, and the nasal and ethmoidal conchae in the nasal cavity. In the mouth and pharynx, to see the openings of the salivary ducts, tonsils, the soft palate and palatopharyngeal arches, normal appearance of the laryngeal entrance, and the pharyngeal opening of the auditory tube.

5---To see the interior of the paranasal sinuses, how they communicate with each other and with the nasal cavity, and to note their surgical boundaries.

6---To make a full study of the larynx both in situ and after removing it from the head; to understand especially its innervation, the relations of the cartilages to each other and how they are connected, the shape of the laryngeal cavity and the topography of the laryngeal ventricle, and to see the muscles that regulate the width of the glottic cleft.

7---To see the adnexa of the eye, notably the structure of the lids, the conjunctiva, third eyelid, and the lacrimal structures. To understand the orbital fasciae, and to explore the topography of the bulbar muscles and the nerves that accompany them. To see the structures in the interior of the eyeball such as the lens and its suspension by the ciliary body, the iris and retina, and to examine the layers of the wall of the eyeball and the role each of them plays. To become familiar with the innervation and blood supply of the eyeball, eyelids, and conjunctiva.

8---To study the very specialized features of the teeth and to learn the criteria by which horses can be aged by their teeth.

Plan. The heads will have been split in the median plane with a bandsaw. After skinning and removal of the cutaneous muscles to expose supf. structures, the facial artery is traced across the face and the parotid duct is probed. The masseter is reflected to expose the large veins on its deep surface. For the study of the retromandibular fossa the salivary glands are reflected and the maxillary vein and occipitomandibular part of the digastricus (and the digastricus itself) are transected.

If necessary, the nasal septum is removed to expose the conchae. Then the frontal and maxillary sinuses are opened using a chisel and mallet. After larynx and associated esophagus have been detached from the head, the pharyngeal constrictors are transected and reflected, and the thyroid lamina is either fenestrated or reflected ventrally to expose several intrinsic laryngeal muscles.

153

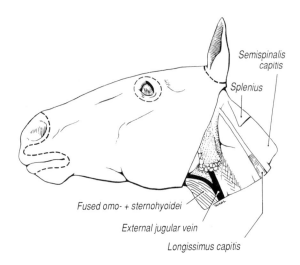

Semispinalis
capitis

Splenius

Fused omo- + sternohyoidei

External jugular vein

Longissimus capitis

FIGURE 7-1. Skin incisions on the head.

On the eye, the lids are skinned and the orbicularis oculi transected and reflected to expose the orbital septum. Then, with a saw, a piece of the zygomatic arch ventral to the eye is removed and the periorbita opened for the study of the retrobulbar structures. The bulbar muscles and optic nerve are transected in succession until the eyeball can be removed. The cornea is removed to expose the iris, and then the eyeball is divided at the equator for the study of the interior during which the lens is taken out. A meridional cut through corneoscleral junction, iris, and ciliary body exposes these structures in profile.

Finally, the ciliary body is pulled away from the sclera to expose the ciliary muscle. No dissection is required for the study of the teeth.

Superficial Structures

Obtain the half-head from your side of the horse. The head will have been split as close to the median plane as possible, but the division will probably be slightly off-center. It is advisable, therefore, to know where the other half-head from your horse is. Keep the half-skull from your course locker always next to your dissection.

Remove the skin, leaving the supf. fascia and the cutaneous muscles on the head. Do not skin the ear. Leave a 2 cm wide rim of skin around the eye, nose, and lips (Fig. 7-1).

Carefully remove the thin cutaneous muscle (cutaneus faciei) from the side of the face; it has a fairly substantial labial part that extends rostrally to the angle of the mouth (Fig. 7-2). The **dorsal and ventral buccal branches of N. VII** crossing the glistening surface of the masseter are now exposed (Fig. 7-3). The buccal branches arise as the direct continuations of the facial nerve emerging from under the parotid gland. They supply motor innervation to the muscles of facial expression. Clean the branches to about the rostral border of the masseter and note their course over the side of the face.

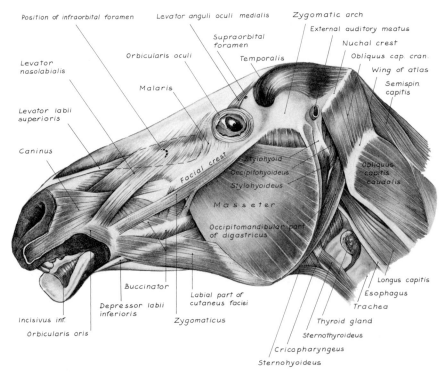

FIGURE 7-2. Muscles of the head. (From Ellenberger-Baum, 1943, by Horowitz/Geary.)

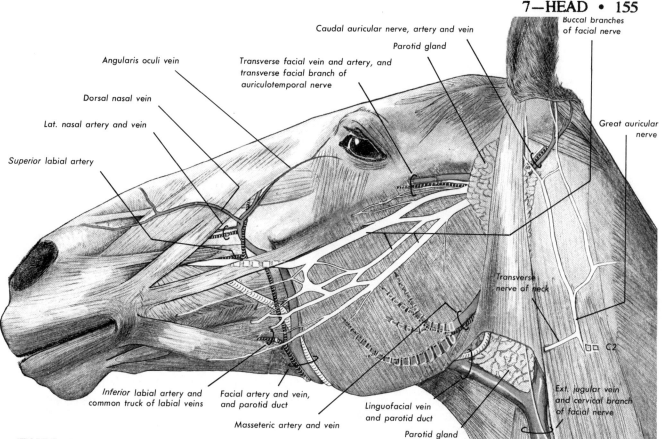

Caudal auricular nerve, artery and vein

Buccal branches of facial nerve

Parotid gland

Transverse facial vein and artery, and transverse facial branch of auriculotemporal nerve

Angularis oculi vein

Great auricular nerve

Dorsal nasal vein

Lat. nasal artery and vein

Superior labial artery

Transverse nerve of neck

C2

Inferior labial artery and common truck of labial veins

Facial artery and vein, and parotid duct

Masseteric artery and vein

Linguofacial vein and parotid duct

Parotid gland

Ext. jugular vein and cervical branch of facial nerve

FIGURE 7-3. Superficial vessels and nerves. (Modified from Hopkins 1937.)

The facial nerve is vulnerable to traumatic, neoplastic, or inflammatory processes, producing facial paralysis. Trauma is common and the signs of paralysis will vary depending on where the facial nerve is affected. The nerve can be damaged by improperly padding the horse's face during anesthesia.

Find and clean the subcutaneous segment of the **masseteric artery** (Fig. 7-7/13); the pulse may be taken here in Thoroughbreds who have thin skin and a short hair coat. Remove the fascia and expose the structures that obliquely cross the ventral border of the mandible and ascend in the palpable groove on the rostral border of the masseter. In rostrocaudal order these are: the facial artery, facial vein, and parotid duct. Clean and trace them caudally on the medial side of the mandible (Fig.7-4/4,5,6,). For this you need temporarily to hold the head so the ventral surface is up. Trace the facial vein caudally to the point near the angle of the mandible where it arises with the lingual vein from the linguofacial, and trace the latter back to its origin with the maxillary vein at the termination of the external jugular. (The linguofacial artery lies much deeper than the vein.)

Find and clean the **mandibular lymph nodes** in the intermandibular space. Right and left nodes are arranged in two elongated groups joined rostrally and diverging caudally in the form of a V. They are related deeply to the palpable body

and lingual process of the hyoid bone and drain the supf. structures of the face, the intermandibular space, the mouth, and the rostral part of the nasal cavity.

The pulse rate is usually taken from the **facial artery** where it turns around the ventral border of the mandible. Trace the artery distally, preserving the parotid duct. On the lateral side of the mandible it gives off the inferior labial artery (/4') which passes beneath the depressor labii inferioris (/1) toward and into the lower lip.

With the aid of Fig. 7-6/18,64' displace the depressor labii inferioris and palpate (press hard) the mental foramen from which the **mental nerve** emerges. The mental nerve arises from the **inferior alveolar nerve,** one of the terminal branches of the mandibular nerve (N. V). Visualize the course of the inferior alveolar nerve on your half-skull; it enters the mandibular foramen and passes rostrally within the mandibular canal, supplying twigs to the cheek teeth and gums. After giving off the mental nerve to the lower lip it continues within the bony canal to supply the canine and incisor teeth and their gums. Identify the mandibular canal on lateral radiographs of the head.

Anesthesia of the lower lip can be obtained by blocking the *mental nerve* at the foramen—an easy block because the nerve can be palpated against the mandible. To desensitize also the canine and incisor teeth, the deposit has to be made 3-5 cm *within* the mental foramen.

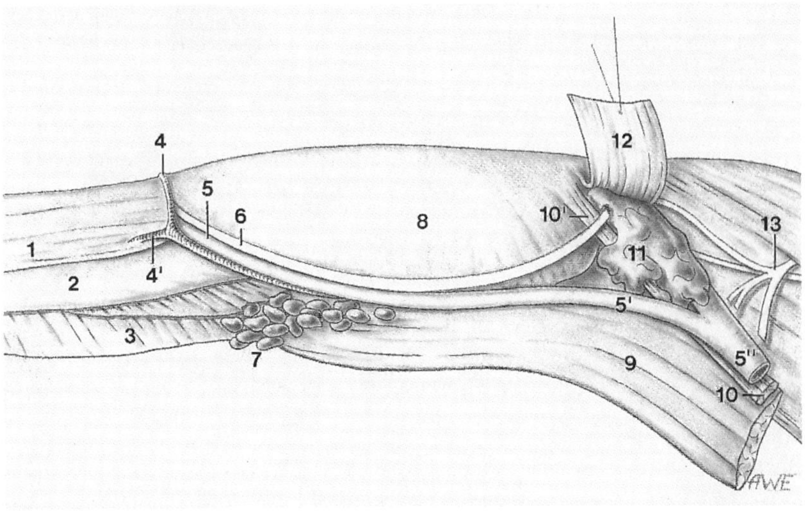

1. Depressor labii inferioris
2. Mandible
3. Mylohyoideus
4. Facial artery, inferior labial artery at 4'
5. Facial vein, linguofacial at 5', external jugular at 5"
6. Parotid duct
7. Mandibular lymph nodes
8. Masseter
9. Fused omo- and sternohyoidei
10. Sternocephalicus, its tendon at 10'
11. Parotid gland
12. Parotidoauricularis
13. C2, crossing accessory nerve

FIGURE 7-4. Ventral view of left half of head to show the facial artery crossing the ventral border of the mandible, and the mandibular lymph nodes.

The **facial artery** continues dorsally across the face and detaches branches as shown in Fig. 7-6.

Tansect the levator nasolabialis to locate and palpate the levator labii superioris (Fig. 7-2). The latter muscle arises rostral to the eye and with a long tendon passes between the nostrils into the upper lip, which it raises. Isolate the muscle belly and push it dorsally so you can find the **infraorbital foramen** and the large infraorbital nerve. Find the foramen on the half-skull and note that it lies a little caudal to the midpoint of a line connecting the rostral end of the **facial crest** with the **nasoincisive notch.** The latter is the prominent angle between the nasal and incisive bones—easily palpated in the live animal.

The **infraorbital nerve** is entirely sensory and is the continuation of the maxillary nerve (N. V). It enters the maxillary foramen and passes rostrally through the infraorbital canal, supplying the upper cheek teeth and gums; a small branch continues within the bone for the upper canine and incisor teeth and their gums. Transect the levator labii superioris and trace the infraorbital nerve for a short distance toward nose and upper lip; its branches mingle with those of the buccal branches of N. VII (Fig. 7-6/67), and its autonomous zone is shown in Fig. 7-5/3.

Anesthesia of the upper lip and nose (to suture lacerations, for example) can be obtained by blocking the *infraorbital nerve* at the infraorbital foramen—also an easy block because the nerve is palpable. Making the deposit 2.5 cm *within* the infraorbital canal desensitizes (in addition) deep structures of the face to the level of the medial eye angle, the first two upper cheek teeth, and the canine and incisor teeth.

Locate the **supraorbital foramen** (Fig. 7-2) on the skull. It pierces the root of the zygomatic process·of the frontal bone. Palpate the borders of the process on your specimen and find the **supraorbital nerve** (usually only a stump)

emerging from the foramen. It innervates the upper eyelid and the skin between the eyes. It may be blocked at the foramen (Figs. 7-5/1 and 7-6/66).

Open the **parotid duct** and (with the flexible probe) probe it forward, deep to the facial vessels, as far as possible. We will see the opening where it penetrates the cheek opposite the 2nd or 3rd upper cheek tooth later. Probe the duct caudally to the mandibular angle of the parotid gland which should be exposed.

Remove the fascia from the surface and borders of the parotid gland. It will be necessary to transect and reflect the thin parotidoauricularis and zygomatico-auricularis muscles that cross the dorsal end of the gland (Fig. 7-7/3,2). The **parotid gland** is roughly rectangular; it lies between the caudal border of the masseter and the wing of the atlas and extends from the base of the ear to the linguofacial vein.

Reflect the rostral border of the parotid gland and trace the buccal branches to their origin from the facial nerve. The **transverse facial artery and vein** emerge a little dorsal to this . The **transverse facial branch** of the **auriculotemporal nerve** (N. V, mandibular) emerges with the artery, having already divided into two branches. Clean these structures. One branch usually accompanies the artery but may join the dorsal buccal branch, and the other branch joins the ventral buccal branch (variations occur; see Figs. 7-3 and 7-8/2). The branches of the auriculotemporal nerve that run in the buccal branches of the facial nerve bring *sensory* innervation to the cheeks.

The purpose of the following dissection is to expose the large vessels that are buried within, and lie deep to, the masseter muscle. Trace the **transverse facial vessels** rostrally, cutting away the masseter in their path. The artery breaks up in the muscle, but the vein reaches the rostral border of the masseter and anastomoses with the **facial vein** ventral to the end of the facial crest (Fig. 7-6/31). Trace the facial vein ventrally, freeing the rostral border of the masseter and reflecting the muscle caudally. About 2 cm ventral to the above anastomosis the facial vein connects with the **deep facial vein** (/30). Trace the latter caudally by reflecting the masseter until the vein can be seen curving medially into the deep part of the orbit. Note the large fusiform dilatation of the vein as it turns into the orbit.

Continue tracing the facial vein ventrally and locate its connection with the **buccal vein** (/29). The latter runs caudally between the masseter and the mandible and along the ventral border of the conjoined depressor labii inferioris and buccinator muscles. Reflect the masseter and note the course of the vein. It also presents a large fusiform dilatation. (What is the function of the dilatations in these veins? Recall that horses at pasture spend about 70% of their waking hours grazing.)

Diseased cheek teeth are generally removed by repelling them into the oral cavity using a punch placed over the root of the involved tooth and a hammer to pound the tooth out in the direction of its growth. The roots of cheek teeth may be either housed in a sinus (caudal maxillary cheek teeth) or within alveolar spaces in the maxilla or mandible. In either case, the root of the tooth to be repulsed is exposed by removing a small disc of bone (trephination) or by creating a bone flap over the sinus. Cheek teeth, as we will see later, are long and packed tightly together and this interferes with loosening a firmly anchored tooth before it can be extracted. Also, horses cannot "open wide" (Why not? Compare with the dog.) This means that dental instruments or the surgeon's hand cannot easily be put into the mouth to perform an oral extraction. Oral extraction of certain cheek teeth has been described and involves incising the cheek (a buccotomy) and the rostral part of the masseter muscle to achieve lateral exposure of the maxilla and tooth. The facial vessels, parotid duct, and large deep veins must be protected during this procedure.

The transverse facial vein may be used for "facial vein venipuncture"; the needle is inserted at 90 degrees to the surface of the masseter one finger-breadth ventral to the facial crest even with the medial canthus of the eye.

Expose the entire lateral surface of the mandibular salivary gland, working from the ventral end of the gland which lies deep to the linguofacial vein on the medial aspect of the mandible. The **mandibular gland** is long and narrow and lies in a curve medial to the angle of the mandible and the parotid gland (Fig. 7-8/8). It is crossed by the **tendon of insertion of the sternocephalicus** (/10) and ends dorsally in the atlantal fossa. To expose the gland fully, the parotid gland has to be reflected dorsally to the base of the ear. This is difficult because the maxillary vein (/9; continuation of external jugular) passes through it. So, either cut the vein as it enters and leaves the parotid gland or

carefully detach the gland tissue from the vein, which takes longer. Now free the dorsal end of the mandibular gland and reflect it ventrally and rostrally.

Trace the transverse facial artery proximally to its origin, with the small rostral auricular artery, from the **supf. temporal artery.** The supf. temporal is not longer than 2 cm and arises as one of the terminal branches of the **external carotid artery** (Fig. 7-9). The other terminal branch, the **maxillary artery,** is much larger and may be located where it passes under the caudal border of the mandible. The external carotid gives off the caudal auricular artery dorsally (do not trace) and the masseteric artery ventrally which was seen already entering the masseter. If the maxillary vein is still crossing the retromandibular space, transect it now and reflect the stumps. Reflect also the sternocephalicus rostrally to its insertion on the mandible.

With the salivary glands and the maxillary vein out of the way and with the help of Figure 7-10, identify and palpate the following structures in this important retromandibular area: caudal border of the mandible, wing of atlas, base of ear, combined

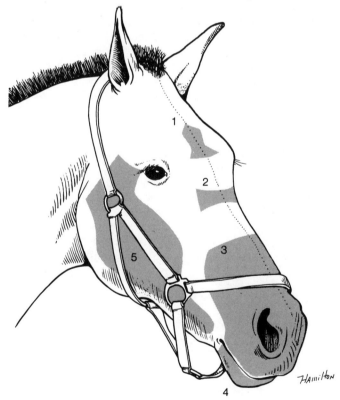

1. Supraorbital
2. Infratrochlear
3. Infraorbital
4. Mental
5. Transverse facial br. of auriculotemporal

FIGURE 7-5. Five autonomous zones of the cutaneous innervation of the head. (Courtesy Drs. H. N. Engel and L. L. Blythe, Oregon State University, Corvallis, Oregon.)

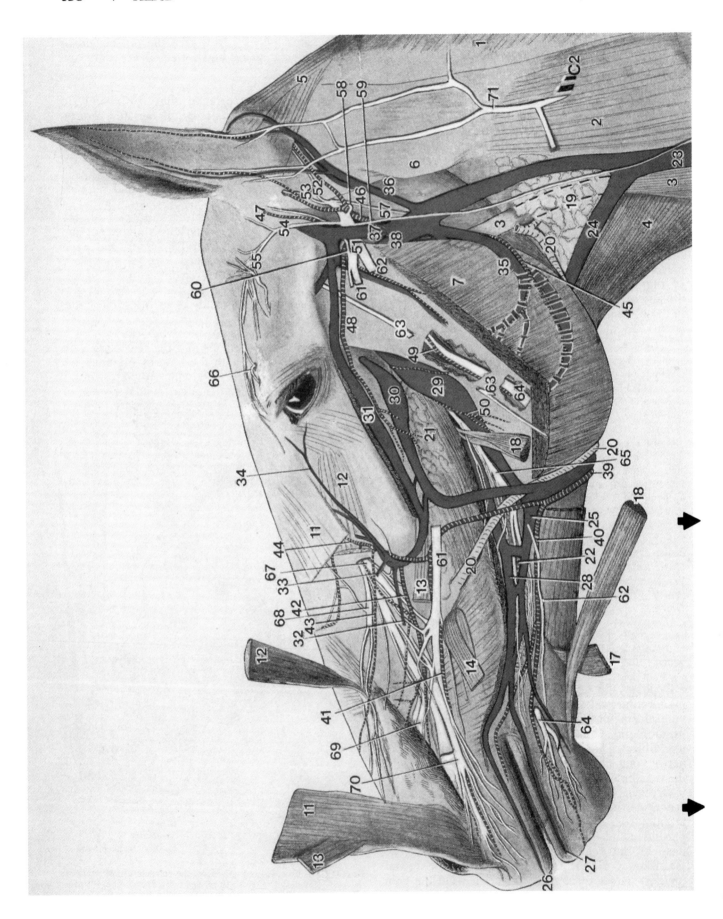

omo- and sternohyoidei, insertion of sternocephalicus, occipitomandibular part of digastricus, cranial deep cervical lymph nodes, thyroid gland, common carotid artery, obliquus capitis cranialis, facial nerve, supf. temporal artery, auriculopalpebral nerve, and auriculotemporal nerve.

The palpebral branch of the *auriculopalpebral nerve* crosses the highest point of the zygomatic arch where it can be palpated and blocked to eliminate blinking—during an examination of the eye, for example. Horses are capable of closing their eyes tightly (blepharospasm) and resist manipulation.

1. Splenius
2. Cleidomastoideus
3. Sternocephalicus
4. Omohyoideus
5. Deep and superficial cervico-auricularis muscles
6. Wing of atlas
7. Masseter, partly removed
11. Levator nasolabialis
12. Levator labii superioris
13. Caninus
14. Zygomaticus
17. Cutaneus faciei, labial part
18. Depressor labii inferioris
19. Parotid gland, mostly removed
20. Parotid duct
21. Dorsal buccal glands
22. Ventral buccal glands
23. External jugular vein
24. Linguofacial vein
25. Common labial vein
26. Dorsal labial vein
27. Ventral labial vein
28. Buccal venous plexus
29. Buccal vein
30. Deep facial vein
31. Transverse facial vein
32. Lateral nasal vein
33. Dorsal nasal vein
34. Angularis oculi vein
35. Masseteric vein
36. Caudal auricular vein
37. Superficial temporal vein
38. Maxillary vein
39. Facial artery
40. Inferior labial artery
41. Superior labial artery
42. Lateral nasal artery
43. Dorsal nasal artery
44. Angularis oculi artery
45. Masseteric artery
46. Caudal auricular artery
47. Rostral auricular artery
48. Transverse facial artery
49. Inferior alveolar artery, exposed
50. Buccal artery
51. Facial nerve
52. Caudal auricular nerve
53. Auricular branch
54. Auriculopalpebral nerve
55. Rostral auricular branches
57. Branch to digastricus
58. Nerve loop around caudal auricular artery
59. Cervical branch of facial nerve
60. Transverse facial branch of auriculotemporal nerve
61,62 Dorsal and ventral buccal branches of facial nerve
63. Masseteric nerve
64. Inferior alveolar nerve
64' Mental nerve
65. Buccal nerve
66. Supraorbital nerve
67. Infraorbital nerve
68. External nasal branches
69. Internal nasal branches
70. Superior labial branches
71. Great auricular nerve

FIGURE 7-6. The distribution of the blood vessels and nerves. The dorsal portion of the masseter has been removed and the mandibular canal fenestrated twice. (From Hopkins 1937.)

The arteries that have been described lie between the caudal border of the mandible and the fusiform **occipitomandibular part of the digastricus** (Fig. 7-10/4). The occipitomandibular part arises from the paracondylar process of the occipital bone and inserts on the angle of the mandible (Fig. 7-11/6). Transect the occipitomandibular part at its middle and reflect the ventral stump to its insertion. Transect and reflect the remainder of the digastricus lying on its medial surface. (You may have to shorten the stumps to see the deeper lying structures better.)

The termination of the **common carotid artery** is now exposed. Find the origin of the internal carotid and occipital arteries from the caudodorsal surface of the common carotid. The **occipital artery** (Fig. 7-9) arises just cranial to, or by a common trunk with, the internal carotid. It passes under the wing of the atlas where it anastomoses with the vertebral artery and sends branches to the brain. The **internal carotid artery** also supplies the brain by passing through the foramen lacerum.

The **occipital artery** may be traced dorsally under the wing of the atlas where it gives rise to the small condylar artery and the larger caudal meningeal artery (both of which pass to the skull) and ends by joining the vertebral artery (Fig. 7-9). The **vertebral artery,** last seen at the thoracic inlet, ascends by passing through the transverse foramina of the cervical vertebrae. It arrives under the wing of the atlas by emerging from the transverse foramen of that bone. After anastomosing with the occipital, the vertebral passes dorsally through the alar foramen and then medially through the lateral vertebral foramen of the atlas into the vertebral canal where it joins the ventral spinal artery to form the basilar.

From the origin of the occipital, the common carotid is continued as the **external carotid** which gives off the linguofacial artery and continues dorsally along the caudal border of the mandible, where it was previously exposed.

Find the large **hypoglossal nerve** (N. XII) as it crosses the lateral surface of the external carotid artery near the origin of the linguofacial. The smaller **glossopharyngeal nerve** (N. IX) lies medial to the artery on the delicate mucous membrane of the **guttural pouch.** Pass your finger into the pouch from the median (cut) surface of the head and verify that. You may have to cut a hole in the thin partition between right and left pouches to get your finger into the pouch on your side. The guttural pouches are ventral diverticula of the auditory tubes and are peculiar to the Equidae among domestic animals. They will be considered in more detail later.

The important retropharyngeal lymph nodes may now be examined with a minimum of dissection. The (larger) and more numerous

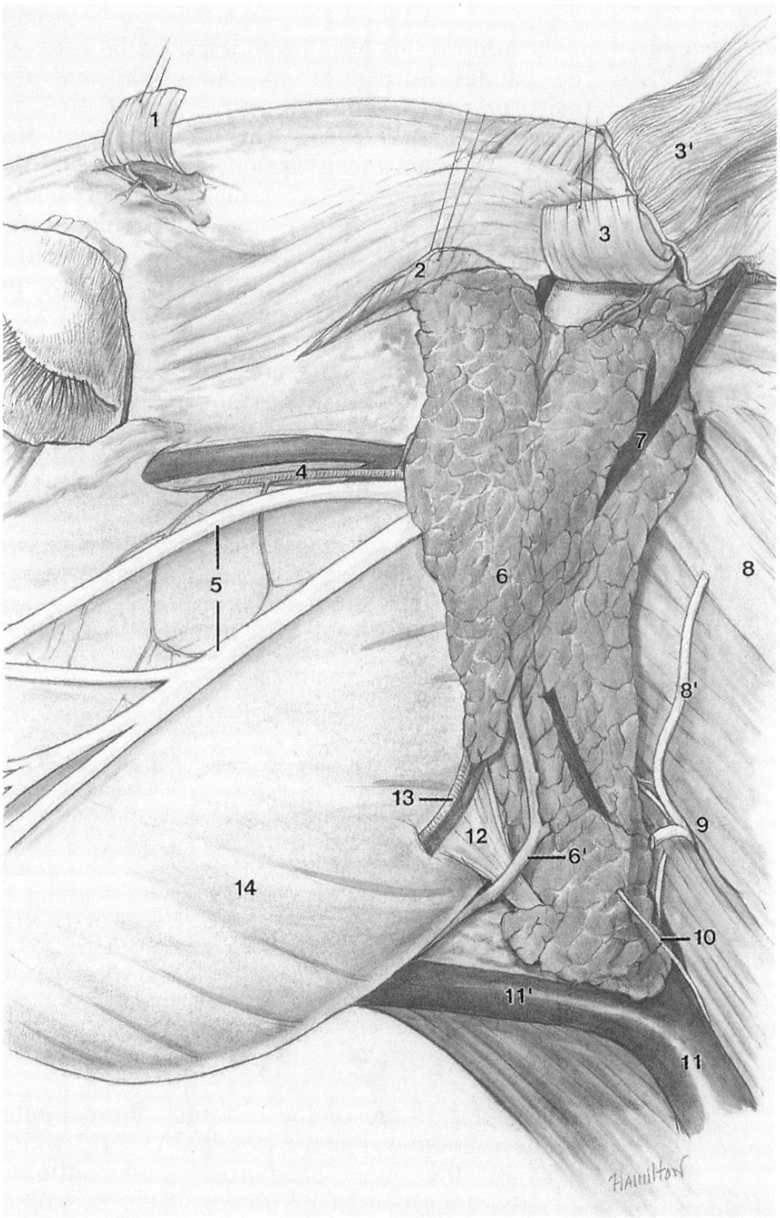

1. Corrugator supercilii, reflected to expose supraorbital foramen, nerve, and artery
2. Zygomaticoauricularis
3. Parotidoauricularis, reflected, exposing auricular cartilage, base of ear at 3'
4. Transverse facial artery and vein
5. Buccal branches of facial nerve
6. Parotid gland, its duct at 6'
7. Caudal auricular vein
8. Tendon of longissimus capitis
8' Great auricular nerve
9. C2
10. Cervical br. of facial nerve
11. External jugular vein, linguofacial vein at 11'
12. Insertion tendon of sternocephalicus
13. Masseteric artery, where the pulse may be taken in thin-skinned horses
14. Masseter

FIGURE 7-7. The left parotid gland and associated structures.

medial retropharyngeal lymph nodes lie in the (lateral) groove between the pharynx and the guttural pouch, medial to the external carotid and linguofacial arteries, the digastricus, and the mandibular gland. The **lateral retropharyngeal lymph nodes** lie on the caudodorsal surface of the guttural pouch near the wing of the atlas. They are close to the internal carotid artery and the vagosympathetic trunk. (In short, the medial nodes are more rostral and ventral, the lateral nodes more caudodorsal.) The retropharyngeal nodes drain nearly all structures of the dorsocaudal part of the head. The lymph from the parotid and mandibular nodes passes through them before reaching the cranial deep cervical lymph nodes.

Replace all structures and study the landmarks that form **Viborg's triangle**, i.e., the linguofacial vein, the tendon of the sternocephalicus, and the caudal border of the mandible (Fig. 1-13/8). Viborg's triangle is used to outline the region where abnormal swelling in the guttural pouch would be observed clinically. The normal guttural pouch is actually quite far from the skin and dorsal to Viborg's triangle. A variety of surgical approaches have been described to access a distended guttural pouch. In the most commonly used approach (modified Whitehouse) the skin is incised ventral and parallel to the linguofacial vein. All surgery in this area is risky because of the many important structures that are vulnerable. With the aid of Figs. 7-7, 7-8, and 7-10 find on your specimen the following structures that must be avoided by the surgeon: parotid duct, linguofacial vein, common and external carotid arteries, and the hypoglossal and glossopharyngeal nerves. (Discuss among yourselves, or with an instructor, why accidentally opening the parotid duct is not a good idea.)

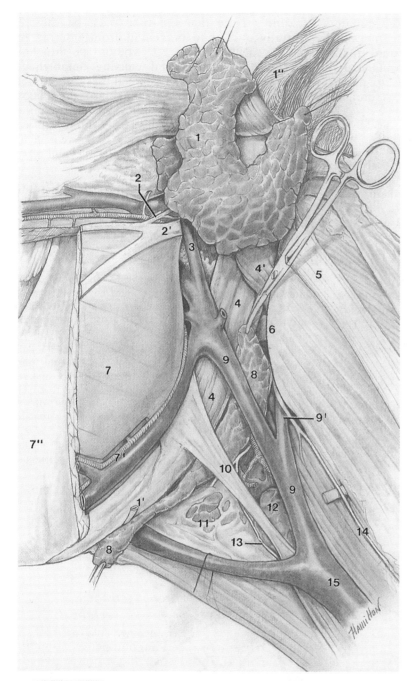

1. Parotid gland reflected dorsally, its duct at 1', base of ear at 1"
2. Transverse facial branch of auriculo-temporal nerve (from N.V.)
2' Facial nerve
3. Supf. temporal vein
4. Occipitomandibular part of digastricus, obliquus capitis cranialis at 4'
5. Tendon of longissimus capitis
6. Wing of atlas
7. Masseter, masseteric vessels at 7', mandible at 7"
8. Mandibular gland held between two hemostats
9. Maxillary vein, occipital vein at 9'
10. Insertion tendon of sternocephalicus
11. Cranial deep cervical lymph nodes
12. Thyroid gland
13. Ventral branch of C1
14. Dorsal branch of accessory nerve, crossing stump of C2
15. External jugular vein

FIGURE 7-8. Retromandibular space with parotid gland reflected and mandibular gland exposed.

The retropharyngeal lymph nodes are commonly abscessed in *strangles,* a streptococcal infection.

The *guttural pouches,* as we will see later, communicate with the nasopharynx and thus may be involved in respiratory infections, or they may be invaded directly from diseased retropharyngeal lymph nodes, which lie against their wall. Accumulation of pus or other exudate causes them to swell. Mycotic infections usually affect the roof of a pouch where substantial blood vessels lie against it. The fungus is capable of eroding both pouch and vessel wall which causes bleeding from the nostril and may in catastrophic cases result in fatal exsanguination.

Nasal Passages, Mouth, and Pharynx

Examine the **nostril.** It is bounded by two wings (alae) which come together in dorsal and ventral commissures. The medial wing is concave ventrally and convex dorsally. The dorsal convexity, caused by the lamina of the alar cartilage, is connected caudally with the **alar fold** (Fig. 7-12/1,4). These two structures partially divide the nostril into a large lower part that leads into the nasal cavity and small upper part, the **nasal diverticulum** or "false nostril". Explore the diverticulum with your finger; you may have opened it inadvertently when removing the skin caudal to the nostril. Note that the diverticulum ends at the nasoincisive notch where your finger is stopped. Find the orifice of the **nasolacrimal duct** in the floor of the nostril near the mucocutaneous junction. The orifice occasionally fails to open (congenital atresia) or may be blocked by foreign material, requiring surgical correction.

Examine the **nasal septum,** noting the very vascular mucous membrane covering the cartilage. Remove the septum and study the dorsal and ventral nasal, and the ethmoid conchae. The **conchae** are thin osseous scrolls covered on each side with mucous membrane. They project medially from the lateral wall of the nasal cavity and roll up on themselves, enclosing recesses that freely communicate with the nasal cavity (Fig. 7-12/14). The caudal third of the two large nasal conchae is divided off by an internal septum and houses a conchal sinus. The ventral nasal concha is prolonged rostrally by the basal and alar folds of which the basal is the more ventral. Between the folds is the passage from the nostril to the nasal cavity.

Identify the dorsal, middle, and ventral **nasal meatuses** and note that the ventral is the largest.

Pass a stomach, or nasogastric, tube (demonstration table) through the ventral commissure of the nostril into the ventral nasal meatus. This is harder to do in the embalmed head than in the live horse where the tissues are slippery and more flexible. Note that the tube must be directed ventrally at first to prevent it from entering the middle meatus where it would be blocked, injuring the mucosa and causing hemorrhage. Remove a small piece of conchal mucosa and note its very vascular nature. Examine also the mucosa of the hard palate and the thick venous plexus in its submucosa which is particularly prominent just behind the incisor teeth. (What is the reason for all this blood flow in palate, conchae, and nasal septum?)

Withdraw the apex of the tongue and locate the **sublingual caruncle,** a small papilla opposite the canine teeth (if these are present). The duct of the mandibular salivary gland opens through the papilla.

The **sublingual fold** lies alongside the tongue on the floor of the mouth and presents numerous small papillae through which the ducts of the (polystomatic) **sublingual salivary gland** open. Slit the mucosa alongside the sublingual fold and expose the gland.

The apical portion of the **tongue** is covered on the dorsum and sides with fine filiform **papillae.** Find the round fungiform papillae on the sides of the tongue, and the prominent vallate papillae on the dorsum near the root. The foliate papillae can be located just in front of the palatoglossal arch of the soft palate; they form a rounded prominence marked by transverse fissures.

On the root of the tongue and lateral to the median glossoepiglottic fold the mucosa is thrown into irregular

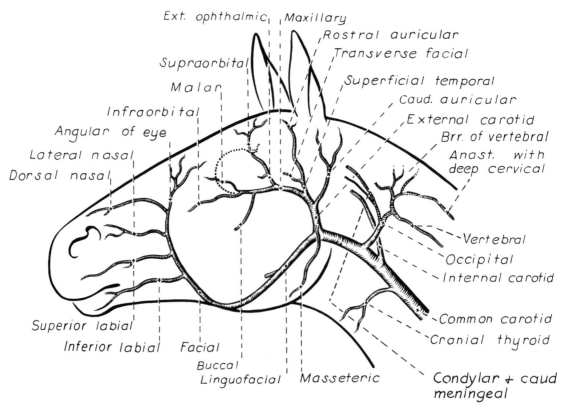

FIGURE 7-9. Arteries of the left half of the head.

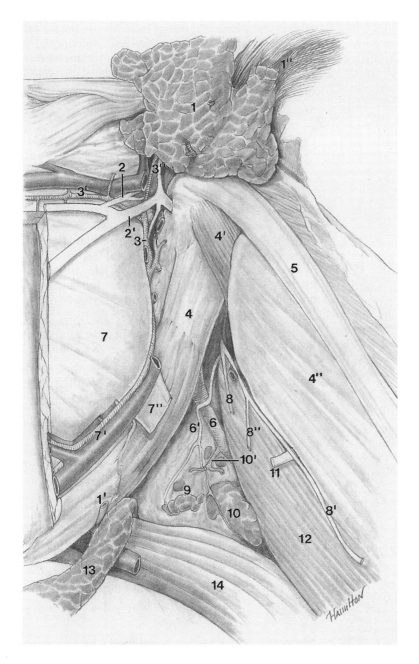

1. Parotid gland reflected dorsally, its duct at 1', base of ear at 1"
2. Transverse facial branch of auriculotemporal nerve (from N.V.)
2' Facial nerve
3. Supf. temporal artery, transverse facial vessels at 3', rostral auricular artery and auriculopalpebral nerve at 3"
4. Occipitomandibular part of digastricus, obliquus capitis cranialis and caudalis at 4' and 4"
5. Tendon of longissimus capitis
6. Common carotid artery, ventral branch of C1 at 6'
7. Masseter, masseteric vessels at 7', insertion of sternocephalicus at 7"
8,8' Ventral and dorsal branches of accessory nerve, communication to C2 at 8"
9. Cranial deep cervical lymph nodes
10. Thyroid gland, cranial thyroid artery at 10'
11. C2
12. Longus capitis
13. Mandibular gland reflected ventrally
14. Fused sterno- and omohyoidei

FIGURE 7-10. Left retromandibular space; the parotid and mandibular salivary glands have been reflected and the veins and sternocephalicus have been removed; lateral view.

elevations that have small orifices at their apices. The deep furrows between the elevations are the crypts of the **lingual tonsils.** The small orifices are the openings of the ducts of mucous glands.

Note how loosely the ample mucous membrane is attached to the rostral surface of the epiglottis. During swallowing, the bolus and the mucous membrane slide up and over the rostral edge of the epiglottis at the same time as the latter is bent caudally. The mucous membrane slides back down again as the epiglottis resumes its normal position after the bolus has passed. (A fresh specimen shows the sliding of the mucous membrane over the edge of the epiglottis much better than your embalmed specimen.)

The **soft palate** is very long in the horse and separates the nasopharynx from the oropharynx. Find the two mucosal folds (palatine arches) by which it is attached to tongue and pharynx. The **palatoglossal arch** passes to the root of the tongue and marks the beginning of the oropharynx. The **palatopharyngeal arch** runs caudally on the lateral wall of the pharynx and meets its mate dorsal to the esophageal orifice. The free border of the soft palate and the palatopharyngeal arches form the intrapharyngeal opening between the nasopharynx and the laryngopharynx. The cranial parts of the larynx project through the opening into the nasopharynx during normal breathing. This puts the free edge of the soft palate ventral to the epiglottis (Fig. 7-13/5,10).

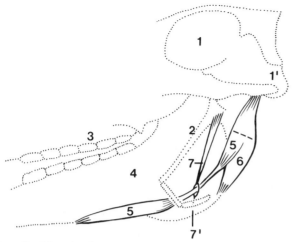

1. Cranial cavity, foramen magnum at 1'
2. Stylohoid bone
3. Cheek teeth
4. Medial surface of right mandible
5. Rostral and caudal bellies of digastricus connected by an intermediate tendon
6. Occipitomandibular part of digastricus
7. Stylohyoideus, its insertion on the thyrohyoid bone at 7'

FIGURE 7-11. The right half of the caudal part of the skull, MEDIAL VIEW. The broken line shows where the occipitomandibular part of the digastricus should be transected.

Delineate the long **palatine tonsil** that lies lateral to the root of the tongue and caudal to the palatoglossal arch. The tonsil is not as obtrusive as in the dog. It consists of mucosal elevations with many invaginations that increase the surface area it presents to the lumen of the oropharynx.

Examine the **pharynx.** On the dorsal wall locate the knobby elevations of the pharyngeal tonsil which may have atrophied in older horses.

Locate the slitlike **pharyngeal opening of the auditory tube** and probe the tube with the finger

499R

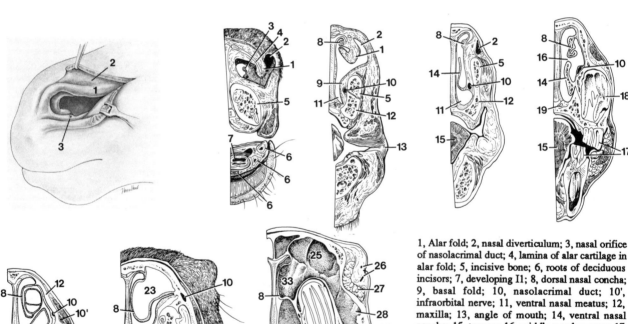

1, Alar fold; 2, nasal diverticulum; 3, nasal orifice of nasolacrimal duct; 4, lamina of alar cartilage in alar fold; 5, incisive bone; 6, roots of deciduous incisors; 7, developing I1; 8, dorsal nasal concha; 9, basal fold; 10, nasolacrimal duct; 10', infraorbital nerve; 11, ventral nasal meatus; 12, maxilla; 13, angle of mouth; 14, ventral nasal concha; 15, tongue; 16, middle nasal meatus; 17, cheek teeth; 18, developing cheek tooth; 19, vomeronasal organ; 20, parotid duct; 21, facial crest; 22, ventral conchal sinus; 23, conchofrontal sinus; 24, levator labii superioris; 25, frontal sinus; 26, lacrimal canaliculi; 27, orbital fat; 28, caudal maxillary sinus; 29, masseter; 30, facial artery and vein; 31 soft palate; 32, mandibular lymph nodes; 33, dorsal conchal sinus

FIGURE 7-12. Topography of the nasolacrimal duct, in transverse sections of the left half of the head. Its nasal orifice is shown in lateral view on the floor of an opened nostril (upper left).

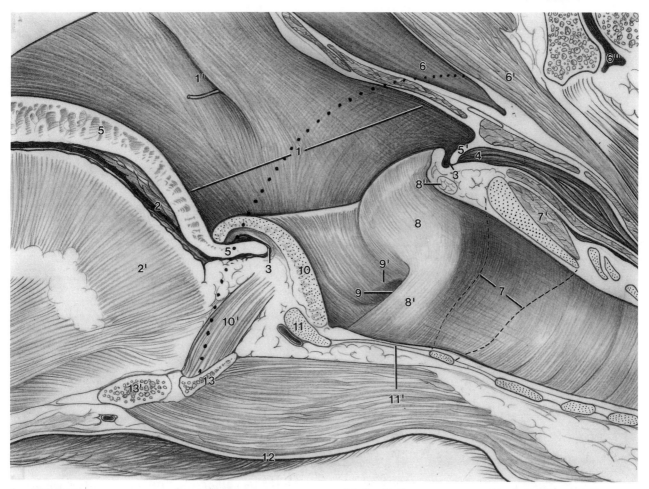

1.	Nasopharynx	5.	Soft palate	
1'	Opening of auditory tube, the wire indicates the ventral extent of the opening	5'	Palatopharyngeal arch	
		6.	Median septum (mucous membrane) separating the two guttural pouches	
2.	Oropharynx, tongue at 2'	6'	Longus capitis	
3.	Laryngopharynx, (collapsed in the present *respiratory* position of 5 and 5')	6"	Atlantoaxial joint cavity	
		7.	Cricoid cartilage	
		7'	Cricoarytenoideus dorsalis	
4.	Beginning of esophagus	8.	Arytenoid cartilage	

8 '	Vocal fold
8"	Arytenoideus transversus
9.	Laryngeal ventricle
9'	Vestibular fold
10.	Epiglottic cartilage
10'	Hyoepiglotticus

11.	Body of thyroid cartilage
11'	Cricothyroid ligament
12.	Skin
13.	Basihyoid
13'	Lingual process of basihyoid

FIGURE 7-13. Median section of pharynx and larynx *in situ*. Rostral is to the left. The dotted line indicates the cut that separates the larynx from the head (p. 170).

(Fig 7-13/1'). About 3 cm caudal to the pharyngeal opening, the tube opens into a large ventral diverticulum, the **guttural pouch.** If the septum separating right and left guttural pouches is on your half of the specimen, remove it so you can probe the full extent of the guttural pouch also from the medial surface. It is related dorsally to the base of the cranium, the ventral straight muscles of the head, and the atlas, and ventrally to the pharynx and to the beginning of the esophagus. The pouch is folded around the rostral border of the stylohoid bone which divides it into medial and lateral compartments. The guttural pouch may be entered in the live horse by passing an endoscope through the nose and the pharyngeal opening. Try to visualize the position of the guttural pouches and the major structures to which it is related on the skull.

The structures of the **POLL** are easily seen on the medial surface of your specimen.

Explore the space between the funicular part of the nuchal ligament and the dorsal arch of the atlas. This is the site of the **cranial nuchal bursa** (Fig. 1-21/A). The bursa is difficult to find: it may be collapsed, or the saw that split the head may have chewed it up.

Now find the **atlanto-occipital space** dorsal to the spinal cord, and the (dorsal) atlanto-occipital membrane that closes the space in the intact animal. Measure, or estimate, the distance from the skin to the atlanto-occipital membrane; to the dura; and to the spinal cord. Note that the needle to collect cerebrospinal fluid from the **cerebellomedullary cistern** is passed in the median plane and therefore penetrates the funicular part of the nuchal ligament.

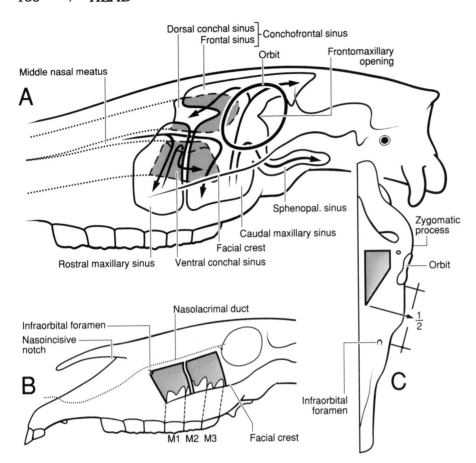

Middle nasal meatus

Dorsal conchal sinus ⎤
Frontal sinus ⎦ Conchofrontal sinus

Orbit

Frontomaxillary opening

A

Sphenopal. sinus

Zygomatic process

Caudal maxillary sinus

Orbit

Facial crest

Rostral maxillary sinus   Ventral conchal sinus

Nasolacrimal duct

Infraorbital foramen
Nasoincisive notch

B

Infraorbital foramen

C

½

M1 M2 M3   Facial crest

FIGURE 7-14. *A:* Left paranasal sinuses, schematic. The entrance to all sinuses is from the middle nasal meatus (arrows). *B:* Surgical boundaries of the maxillary sinuses; also showing the course of the nasolacrimal duct—from a radiograph. *C:* Surgical boundaries of the frontal sinus. (*A* after Nickel, Schummer, Seiferle, 1973.)

Poll evil though rare is still encountered. Its spread from the cranial nuchal bursa may affect the nearby meninges and spinal cord giving rise to nervous symptoms. Surgical correction sometimes involves the resection of the funiculus (if necrotic); the strong attachment of the laminar part of the nuchal ligament to the spinous process of the axis provides sufficient support for the head.

Paranasal Sinuses

Identify the frontal bone on the medial surface of the head and note that it covers the brain and the caudal part of the nasal cavity. The bone is divided into internal and external plates which enclose the **FRONTAL SINUS.** Right and left frontal sinuses are separated by a bony median septum. The median septum is usually not split by the saw and will be found intact on one half of the head or the other (Fig. 7-12/25).

Time saver: The sinuses could be studied on prosected specimens. Ask your instructor whether prosections are available. If so, and if it is decided not to open the sinuses on your half-head, resume using your specimen at the next row of zeroes.

To open the frontal sinus: Remove all the soft tissues from the external surface of the frontal bone. With mallet and chisel (course locker) remove the external plate of the frontal bone. Hold the bevelled side of the chisel down and remove the bone in small pieces. Work from the caudal end of the sinus rostrally and laterally. Try to remove the external plate with as little damage as possible to the bony septa and mucosa of the sinus.*

The **frontal sinus** extends rostrally from the level of the temporomandibular joint to beyond the rostral margin of the orbit. It extends laterally into the root of the zygomatic process of the frontal bone. Note that the frontal sinus is continuous rostrally with the dorsal conchal sinus; the single cavity so formed is called the **conchofrontal sinus** (Figs. 7-12/25,33 and 7-14/A). The dorsal conchal sinus is continuous with the frontal sinus over the ethmoid labyrinth which should be identified. The dorsal conchal sinus extends forward to a plane midway between the rostral margin of the orbit and the infraorbital foramen. It is separated from the nasal cavity medially by the thin plate of the dorsal nasal concha.

The frontal sinus communicates freely with the caudal maxillary sinus through the **fronto-maxillary opening** which is located between the medial angle of the eye and the median plane. Find this large opening and appreciate (by probing) the size of the caudal max-illary sinus into which it leads; this chamber is especially large in older horses.

Except for the caudal limit, the **surgical boundaries of the conchofrontal sinus** are about the same as the actual boundaries (Fig. 7-14/C):

1. *Caudal limit*—transverse plane through zygomatic process of the frontal bone.
2. *Rostral limit*—transverse plane midway between rostral margin of orbit and infraorbital foramen.
3. *Medial limit*—line 2 cm lateral and parallel to dorsal midline.
4. *Lateral limit*—line connecting supraorbital foramen with rostral end of medial limit.

To open the maxillary sinuses: Remove parts of the lacrimal, zygomatic, and maxillary bones rostral to the medial angle of the eye and dorsal to the facial crest. Preserve and expose the nasolacrimal duct which lies just lateral to the frontomaxillary opening; compare this to the position of the lacrimal foramen in the orbit of your half-skull.

Probe the extent of the rostral and caudal **MAXILLARY SINUSES** but do not try to expose them completely. They are separated by an oblique septum which is variable but usually about 5 cm caudal to the rostral end of the facial crest (Fig. 7-14/B).

The **rostral maxillary sinus** communicates medially over the infraorbital canal with the **ventral conchal sinus** (/A). At its highest part, the rostral maxillary sinus communicates with the middle nasal meatus by a narrow slit (nasomaxillary opening). Drainage of the ventral conchal sinus is possible by puncturing the ventral concha through the nasal cavity.

The **caudal maxillary sinus** is divided by the infraorbital canal into medial and lateral chambers. The medial chamber communicates freely with the sphenopalatine sinus (caudoventral to the ethmoid conchae to be seen on the medial cut surface of your specimen). It also communicates with the middle nasal meatus by the narrow nasomaxillary opening. Depending upon the age of the horse, the **roots of the last three or four upper cheek teeth** project variably into the maxillary sinuses. They are covered by mucosa and a thin layer of bone. In old horses, only the last three teeth project for a short distance into the sinuses. The maxillary sinuses can be drained to the outside by trephine.

The **surgical boundaries of the maxillary sinuses** are small compared to their actual size (Fig. 7-14/B):

1. *Caudal limit*—rostral border of orbit.
2. *Rostral limit*—a line from the rostral end of the

facial crest to the infraorbital foramen.
3. *Ventral boundary*—the facial crest.
4. *Dorsal boundary*—a line from the infraorbital foramen parallel to the facial crest. The **nasolacrimal duct** lies just dorsal to this line and must be avoided when the sinus is opened.

0000000000

Surgical access to the nasal cavity for the removal of polyps and foreign bodies, and for resection of the nasal septum involves the following steps and structures. Remove on your specimen a small plate of nasal bone 2-3 cm rostral to the rostral limit of the conchofrontal sinus, as close to the midline as possible. A plate of cartilage extends laterally from the dorsal edge of the nasal septum, closely applied to the deep surface of the nasal bone (Fig. 7-12). Remove some of the cartilage and expose the venous plexus on its deep surface. The plexus appears brown or black and lies between the cartilage and the thick nasal mucosa. Cut through the mucosa, opening the dorsal and common nasal meatuses. The dorsal nasal concha occupies most of the field.

Though enclosed by bone, the paranasal sinuses are subject to trauma, often by a kick from another horse. The overlying bone is fractured and this is commonly followed by infection. Other sources of infection (in the maxillary sinuses primarily) are from diseased upper cheek teeth that project into them, and from diseased airways. Treatment depends heavily on draining accumulated exudate or actual flushing after trephination. Feeding affected horses from the ground puts the head into a more vertical position that promotes natural drainage. Tumors involving the maxillary sinuses are also seen occasionally.

Larynx

Since the larynx of your horse was split with the head, the LARYNGEAL CARTILAGES and the hyoid bones are best studied on demonstration material. You also need the movable "glycerin" horse larynx from your course locker.

The **cricoid cartilage** is shaped like a signet ring with a broad dorsal lamina and a curved lateroventral arch. Note that the dorsal surface of the lamina is divided into two shallow depressions by a median ridge. On the rostral border of the lamina is the articulation with the arytenoid cartilage; and on the lateral border of the lamina is the articulation with the caudal cornu of the thyroid cartilage.

The **thyroid cartilage** consists of two lateral laminae that are united rostroventrally. Each lamina presents a rostral cornu, which articulates with the thyrohyoid bone, and a caudal cornu, which articulates with the cricoid. The thyroid foramen for the cranial laryngeal nerve lies ventral

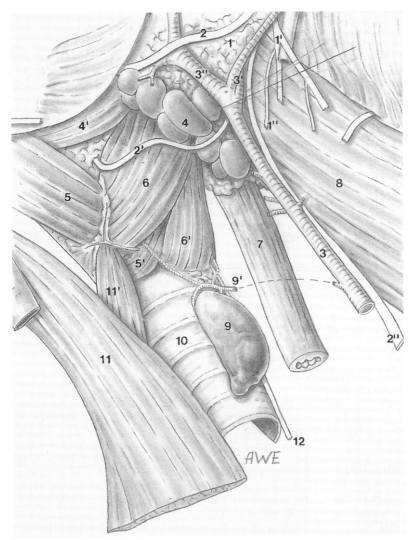

1. Lat. wall of guttural pouch
1'. Accessory nerve and occipital vein
1". Ventral branch of C1
2. Hypoglossal nerve
2'. Cranial laryngeal nerve
2". Vagosympathetic trunk
3. Common carotid artery
3'. Occipital and int. carotid arteries
3". External carotid artery, pulled dorsally
4. Medial retropharyngeal lymph nodes
4'. Hyopharyngeus
5. Thyrohyoideus
5'. Cricothyroideus
6. Thyropharyngeus
6'. Cricopharyngeus
7. Esophagus
8. Longus capitis
9. Thyroid gland
9'. Cranial thyroid artery
10. Trachea
11. Fused omo- and sternohyoidei
11'. Sternothyroideus
12. Recurrent laryngeal nerve

FIGURE 7-15. Larynx and guttural pouch *in situ*, lateral view. The structures occupying the visceral space of the neck have been spread apart; compare with Fig. 7-10.

to the rostral cornu. The clinically important **thyroid notch** is deep and open caudally. It is on the ventral surface of the larynx caudal to the union of the thyroid laminae.

The **epiglottis** is attached by its base to the rostral end of the thyroid cartilage.

The paired **arytenoid cartilage** presents three significant projections. The corniculate process is elastic and curves upward and backward from the rostral border. The rostral and caudal borders of the cartilage converge ventrally to form the vocal process. The muscular process projects from the dorsal part of the lateral surface and with its medial aspect articulates with the lamina of the cricoid.

On radiographs, the thyroid, arytenoid, and cricoid cartilages may show areas of mineralization; these are most pronounced in older horses and best seen in the rostroventral part of the thyroid and may be mistaken for the basihyoid.

The **HYOID APPARATUS** consists of a series of thin bones that articulate with each other to suspend tongue and larynx. The **basihyoid** presents a rostral projection (lingual process) that is embedded in the root of the tongue (Fig. 7-18). The **thyrohyoids** extend caudodorsally from the basihyoid and articulate with the rostral cornua of the thyroid laminae. The **keratohyoids** extend rostrodorsally from the basihyoid. They connect by means of pea-like epihyoids with the long **stylohyoids**. These are directed dorsocaudally to a cartilaginous union with the petrous temporal bones.

Examine the medial cut surface of the larynx. Feel the elasticity of the epiglottis that allows it partly to cover the laryngeal entrance during swallowing. Note the body of the thyroid cartilage (seen in section). The side edges of the epiglottis are attached to the arytenoid cartilages by the **aryepiglottic folds** (palpate). Palpate also the arytenoids and their corniculate processes. Epiglottis, aryepiglottic folds, and arytenoids form the entrance (aditus) of the larynx. Probe the **laryngeal ventricle**. Its entrance is bounded rostrally by the **vestibular fold** and caudally by the **vocal fold**. The vocal fold is attached dorsally to the palpable vocal process of the arytenoid.

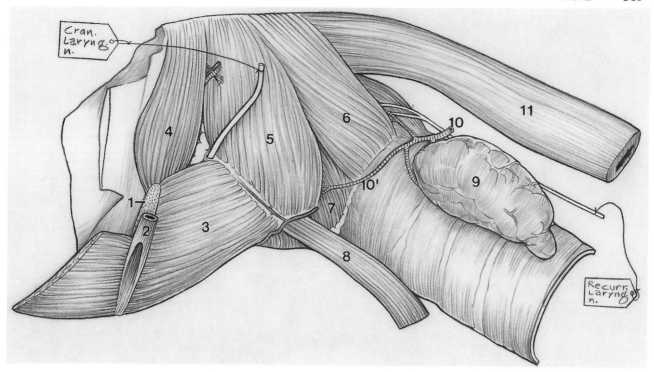

1. Thyrohyoid
2. Stylohyoideus attaching on 1 and forming sleeve for intermediate tendon of digastricus
3. Thyrohyoideus
4. Hyopharyngeus
5. Thyropharyngeus
6. Cricopharyngeus
7. Cricothyroideus
8. Sternothyroideus
9. Thyroid gland
10. Cran. thyroid artery
10' Cran. laryngeal artery
11. Esophagus

FIGURE 7-16. Isolated left half of the larynx showing the entrance of the cranial and caudal (recurrent) laryngeal nerves. Lateral view.

Locate the cut surfaces of the cricoid lamina and arch, and of the first tracheal ring.

Identify the three parts of the **laryngeal cavity:** 1) The **vestibule** extends from the entrance to the vocal folds. 2) The **glottic cleft** is a variable space between the vocal folds and the arytenoid cartilages. These are the structures that form the glottis and regulate the passage of air, or close the larynx completely. 3) The **infraglottic cavity** begins at the caudal edge of the vocal folds and widens to the diameter of the trachea.

On the lateral side: Pick up the **recurrent laryngeal nerve** (N.X, vagus; Fig. 7-15/12). It was tagged close to the thyroid gland—the string of the tag will help you find it. Follow the nerve into the larynx as the dissection proceeds; it passes between the cricopharyngeus laterally and cricoarytenoideus dorsalis medially and enters the larynx medial to the thyroid lamina. **The recurrent laryngeal nerve innervates all the intrinsic muscles of the larynx except the cricothyroideus.** It is not necessary to trace its branches to these muscles.

Locate the **cranial laryngeal nerve** (/2') by pushing the larynx away from the medial aspect of the mandible. It is twice the diameter of the recurrent nerve so you will have no problem finding it. The cranial laryngeal nerve arises also

from the vagus and, lying on the guttural pouch, passes rostroventrally medial to the origin of the internal carotid and occipital arteries from the common carotid. Recall the foramen and its location through which the nerve enters the larynx. **The cranial laryngeal nerve supplies a muscular branch to the cricothyroideus (/5') and is sensory to the mucous membrane of the larynx.** (The muscular branch leaves the cranial laryngeal nerve at its origin; you may see it as a thin strand crossing the pharyngeal constrictors a few cm caudal to the parent nerve.)

Pick up the fused sternothyroideus, sternohyoideus, and omohyoideus muscles (/11',11) and trace them to their insertions. The sternothyroideus is inserted on the thyroid lamina (remove fascia only, do not cut muscles). The fused sternohyoideus and omohyoideus continue rostrally to the basihyoid and its lingual process. This can best be seen on the medial cut surface. Palpate the lingual process; it is unlikely that it was split by the saw.

Hold the head in the extended position and clean the fascia from the surface of the pharyngeal constrictors which are dorsal to the larynx. Identify the muscles without dissection, and outline their borders. The **cricopharyngeus,** the most caudal of the pharyngeal constrictors (/6'), arises from the lateral part of the cricoid arch and

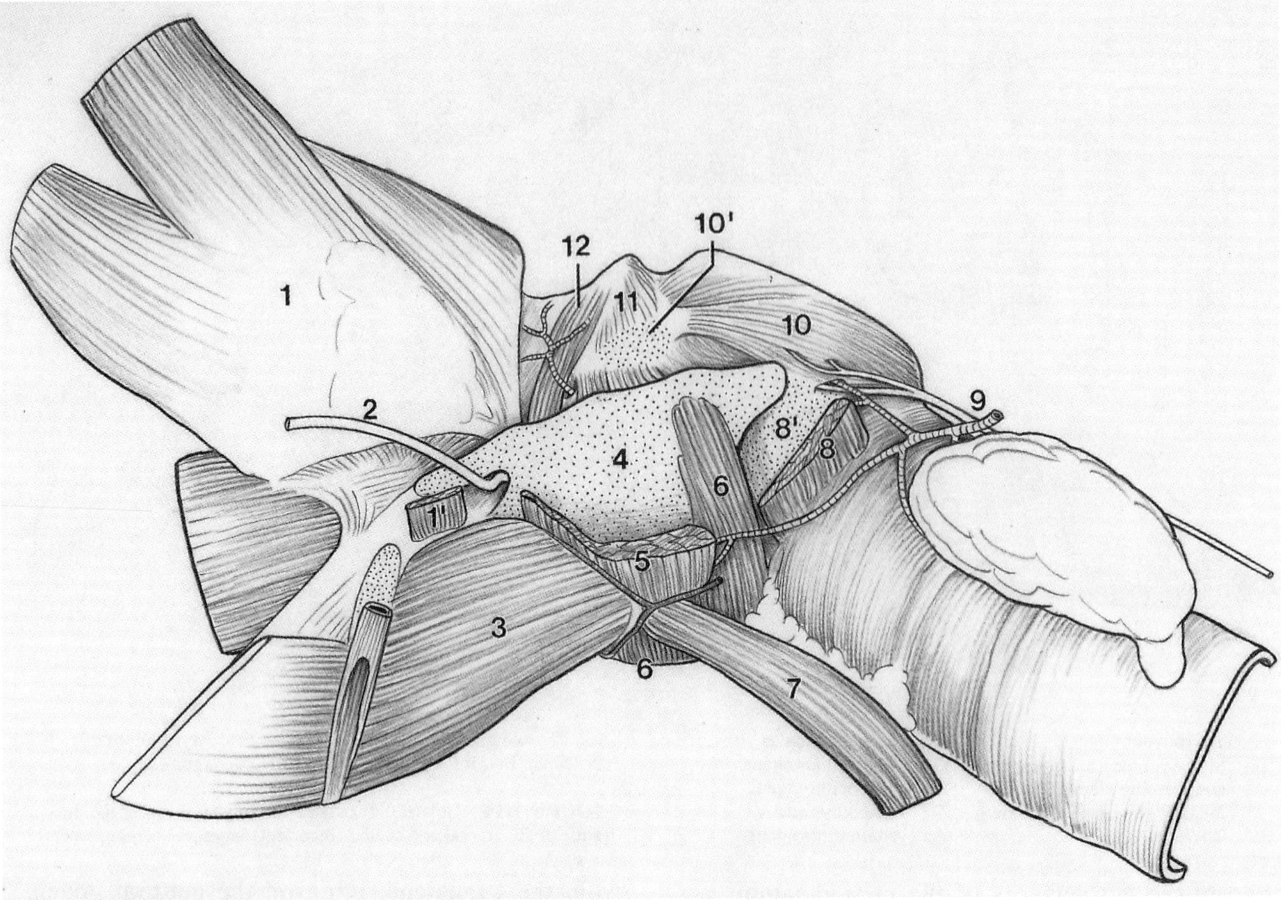

1. Reflected pharyngeal
   constrictors
1' Stump of hyopharyngeus
2. Cran. laryngeal nerve
3. Thyrohyoideus
4. Thyroid cartilage
5. Stump of thyropharyngeus

6. Cricothyroideus
7. Sternothyroideus
8. Stump of cricopharyngeus
8' Arch of cricoid cartilage
9. Cran. thyroid artery and
   recurrent laryngeal nerve

10. Cricoarytenoideus dorsalis
10' Muscular process of
    arytenoid cartilage

11. Arytenoideus transversus
12. Dorsal end of ventricularis

FIGURE 7-17. Isolated left half of the larynx after the reflection of the pharyngeal constrictors. Lateral view.

passes rostrodorsally to the median pharyngeal raphe. The **thyropharyngeus** (/6) arises from the lateral surface of the thyroid lamina and passes dorsomedially to the same raphe. The **hyopharyngeus** (/4') is small and lies rostral to the thyropharyngeus. It arises from the thyrohyoid bone and the thyroid lamina and inserts also on the pharyngeal raphe.

The thyrohyoideus runs rostrally from the thyroid lamina to the basihyoid and thyrohyoid bones (Fig. 7-16/3). It is one of the three **extrinsic muscles of the larynx.** Another, the hyoepiglotticus, may be seen on the medial cut surface running from the basihyoid to the rostral surface of the epiglottis. The third is the sternothyroideus, which should be transected at the third tracheal ring (/8).

To remove the larynx: *Free the esophagus and larynx from the guttural pouches and loose fascia. On the medial side make a curved incision (Fig. 7-13/dotted line) through the pharyngeal mucosa from a point 5 cm rostrodorsal to the esophageal*

opening passing rostroventrally through the caudal end of the soft palate, the palatine tonsil, and the glossoepiglottic fold until the knife strikes bone. Palpate the basihyoid and the thyrohyoid and separate them with bone cutters where they join. Draw the larynx medially, cutting it free from the medial surface of the mandible and remove it.

Time saver: *Half of your group could begin with the dissection of the eye (next section) while the others study the isolated larynx. Demonstrate to each other what you studied separately.*

Orient the larynx on the table with the lateral surface up. Carefully isolate the cricopharyngeus and thyropharyngeus and transect them *close to their origins on the larynx.* Isolate the hyopharyngeus (the less distinct muscle *rostral to the* entry of the cranial laryngeal nerve into the larynx) and cut it from its origin on the thyrohyoid bone; cut also its small slip that attaches to the thyroid lamina. Reflect the three muscles dorsally. Now with the help of Fig. 7-17,

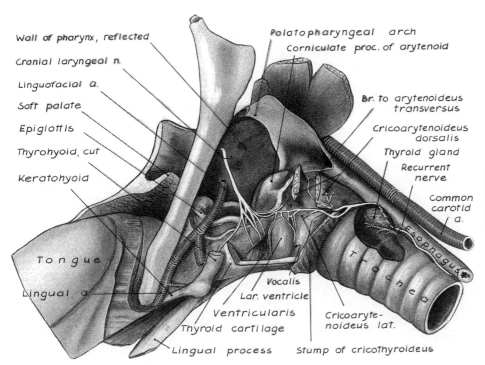

Wall of pharynx, reflected
Cranial laryngeal n.
Linguofacial a.
Soft palate
Epiglottis
Thyrohyoid, cut
Keratohyoid
Tongue
Lingual a.
Palatopharyngeal arch
Corniculate proc. of arytenoid
Br. to arytenoideus transversus
Cricoarytenoideus dorsalis
Thyroid gland
Recurrent nerve
Common carotid a.
Esophagus
Trachea
Vocalis
Lar. ventricle
Ventricularis
Thyroid cartilage
Lingual process
Cricoarytenoideus lat.
Stump of cricothyroideus

FIGURE 7-18. The distribution of the cranial and caudal (recurrent) laryngeal nerves within the larynx, lateral view. (Modified from Hopkins, 1937.)

find (and clean) the cranial laryngeal nerve and see it disappear in the thyroid foramen ventral to the cranial cornu of the thyroid cartilage; and find the stump of the small stylohyoideus tendon inserting on the lateral surface of the thyrohoid bone (examine the stump, it may be long enough to show that it is split (Fig. 7-11/7,7') for the passage of the intermediate tendon of the digastricus).

Next we isolate the **INTRINSIC MUSCLES OF THE LARYNX** that are responsible for the movements of the laryngeal cartilages relative to each other—principally narrowing, closing, or widening the glottic cleft. Find the short **crico-thyroideus** (Figs. 7-17/6). It arises from the lateral surface and caudal edge of the cricoid cartilage and passes dorsorostrally to the caudal edge and lateral surface of the thyroid lamina. It is the only intrinsic muscle that is not innervated by the recurrent nerve. The **cricoarytenoideus dorsalis** (/10) is a fan-shaped muscle that arises on the lamina and median ridge of the cricoid and converges on the muscular process of the arytenoid. Free the esophagus, cricopharyngeus, and thyropharyngeus from the dorsal surface of the larynx and reflect them rostrally, exposing the unpaired **arytenoideus transversus** (/11). This muscle extends transversely across the dorsal surface of the larynx and connects the muscular processes of the two arytenoids.

To see the intrinsic muscles that lie medial to the thyroid lamina, you have two options: the first retains better relationships to the thyroid cartilage, but takes longer; the second is fast. Ask your instructor which you should use. For both methods do first the following: transect the thyrohyoideus muscle (/3) close to its insertion on the thyroid lamina and reflect the stump to the hyoid attachment; scrape what remains of its insertion and the origin of the thyropharyngeus (/5) off the surface of the thyroid lamina.

1. Now, either: palpate the lamina and fenestrate it, leaving a 1 cm strip of cartilage around the borders (Fig. 7-19).
2. Or: cut the thyrohyoid bone from the cranial cornu of the thyroid cartilage; with scissors or cartilage knife cut through the thyroid cartilage near its body that connects it with the lamina on the other side; then reflect the thyroid lamina ventrally, disarticulating its caudal cornu from the cricoid lamina and cutting the cricothyroideus.

Insert a finger into the ventricle and note its position relative to the thyroid lamina. The **ventricularis** lies rostrolateral to the ventricle (Fig. 7-19/2); it arises ventrally on the cricothyroid ligament (to be described shortly) and the ventral border of the thyroid lamina, and passes dorsally to blend with the arytenoideus transversus and to be inserted on the muscular process.

The **vocalis** (/4) lies caudomedial and closely applied to the ventricle. It is partly overlapped by the cricoarytenoideus lateralis caudal to it. The vocalis arises from the cricothyroid ligament and

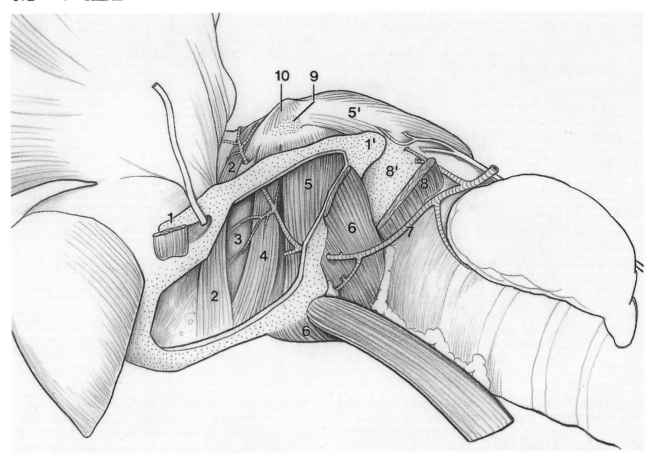

1,1'	Rostral and caudal cornua of thyroid cartilage	5,5'	Cricoarytenoideus lateralis and dorsalis
2.	Ventricularis	6.	Cricothyroideus
3.	Laryngeal ventricle	7.	Cranial laryngeal artery
4.	Vocalis	8.	Stump of cricopharyngeus

8'	Arch of cricoid cartilage		arytenoid cartilage
9.	Muscular process of	10.	Arytenoideus transversus

FIGURE 7-19. Isolated left half of the larynx after fenestrating the thyroid cartilage. Lateral view.

runs dorsally to its insertion on the lateral surface of the arytenoid cartilage, below the muscular process. The **cricoarytenoideus lateralis** (/5) arises from the rostral border of the cricoid arch and passes dorsally to the muscular process.

On your "glycerin" larynx (course locker) or a prepared specimen, see the important **cricothyroid ligament** occupying the **thyroid notch** and attaching caudally to the cricoid arch. The notch and the ligament that closes it have been destroyed by the median saw cut that split the head.

Also find the **cricotracheal ligament** that connects the cricoid cartilage with the first tracheal ring. The **thyrohyoid membrane** connects the rostral borders of the thyroid laminae to the basihyoid and thyrohyoid bones.

Brief consideration of the **ACTION OF THE LARYNGEAL MUSCLES** will aid in understanding the condition (laryngeal hemiplegia, or roaring—see further on) that gives the horse's larynx clinical importance. The ventricularis,

vocalis, and cricoarytenoideus lateralis pull the muscular process ventrally, thereby rotating the arytenoid so that the vocal process carries the vocal fold medially (adduction) closing the glottis. (Which natural body functions require a tightly closed glottis?) The arytenoideus transversus, in addition, draws the two arytenoid cartilages together, aiding in the closure. The cricoarytenoideus dorsalis is the only dilator of the glottis. It pulls the muscular process dorsocaudally, rotating the arytenoid cartilage so that the vocal process and fold are pulled laterally (abduction).

Laryngeal hemiplegia (roaring) is produced by a partial paralysis of the intrinsic laryngeal muscles, notably the cricoarytenoideus dorsalis, which atrophies. The paralysis allows the vocal fold to swing into the air current that passes through the glottis on inspiration. The ventricle fills with air, and a partial occlusion (stenosis) of the laryngeal lumen occurs. The characteristic inspiratory "roar" is due to the stenosis and the vibration of the free edge of the vocal fold. Although the exact cause is still unknown, the consistent involvement of the left vocal fold draws attention to the left recurrent laryngeal nerve. It is thought that the remarkable length of the left recurrent laryngeal nerve makes it vulnerable to the development of this disease.

In one of the surgical treatments of roaring, the larynx is entered by a longitudinal incision through the cricothyroid ligament. The ventricle is everted and cut off. This causes a lateral adhesion of the vocal fold, preventing it from swinging into the lumen of the glottis. In another, the lost function of the cricoarytenoideus dorsalis is simulated: a permanent suture draws muscular process and cricoid lamina toward each other and keeps the vocal process of the arytenoid and the vocal fold abducted.

Eye

The eyeball and its accessory structures (adnexa), though larger than the dog's, must be carefully dissected if all structures are to be exposed for study. Note the stiff **cilia** (eyelashes) on the upper lid; they are shorter and finer on the lower lid.

Reflect the skin to the margin of the eyelids, trim it off, and discard it. The **orbicularis oculi** is now exposed; it is innervated by the auriculopalpebral nerve (Fig. 7-6/54), a branch of the facial, and closes the eye. Preserving the underlying structures, transect the orbicularis in the middle of the upper and lower lids and reflect the stumps to the angles of the eye.

The reflection of the orbicularis exposes the **orbital septum,** the central connective tissue layer of the lid. The septum extends from the margin of the orbit (where it is continuous with the periorbita and the periosteum of the facial bones) to the **tarsi.** These are thickened fibrous plates which may be palpated in the free edge of the eyelid. At the angles of the eye, the orbital septum blends with the medial and lateral **palpebral ligaments** that attach the ends of the tarsi to the bony orbit. The wide tendon of the levator palpebrae superioris (to be seen later) blends with the deep surface of the orbital septum in the upper lid.

The **blood supply of the eyelids** is from the malar, supraorbital, and lacrimal arteries (to be seen later). Branches of these arteries anastomose to form arterial arches that lie in the orbital septum and in front of the tarsi. The arches send branches to the underlying palpebral and bulbar conjunctiva. The arches are difficult to demonstrate on preserved specimens.

The pigmented skin is continuous with the non-pigmented palpebral conjunctiva along the free edge of the eyelid. The orifices of the **tarsal glands** open along the edge. The glands themselves lie immediately deep to the conjunctiva. They are arranged with their long axes perpendicular to the free edge of the eyelid and may shine through the conjunctiva. Place the edge of the lid between the middle portion of the jaws of your thumb forceps and squeeze hard. The white threads of fatty secretion that appear mark the gland orifices. (Why do the lids need to have a fatty edge?)

Evert the lower eyelid near the medial angle and note that the **palpebral conjunctiva** lines the inner surface of the lids and is reflected at the fornix (probe) onto the anterior surface of the eyeball as the **bulbar conjunctiva.** The latter is loosely attached to the sclera, and its epithelium is continuous with the anterior epithelium of the cornea at the **corneoscleral junction** (limbus). When the eye is closed, the conjunctiva and the anterior epithelium of the cornea line a chamber known as the **conjunctival sac.**

At the medial angle a semilunar fold of conjunctiva supported by an enclosed cartilage forms the variably pigmented **third eyelid.** Anterior to the latter the medial angle forms a U-shaped recess, the lacrimal lake, in which is the rounded lacrimal caruncle.

The **lacrimal gland** (to be exposed shortly) lies in the dorsolateral part of the orbit and sheds its secretion into the dorsolateral part of the conjunctival sac through several minute orifices. The secretion washes over the surface of the conjunctiva and cornea and enters the **puncta lacrimalia,** one of which is situated in each lid close to the medial angle. The puncta are the slitlike openings of the lacrimal canaliculi. The canaliculi lead to the lacrimal sac, which lies in the enlarged origin of the bony lacrimal canal (see skull). The sac is drained into the nostril by the nasolacrimal duct.

The ocular adnexa, particularly the eyelids and conjunctiva, are frequently involved in congenital, inflammatory, or traumatic conditions. The conjunctival vessels are of considerable clinical importance, as will be brought out later. The arterial arches in the eyelids, though consisting of narrow vessels, bleed profusely during surgical procedures.

Referring to Fig. 7-20, study the following description of the **ORBITAL FASCIAE** before proceeding with the dissection. The **periorbita** is a conical fibrous membrane that extends from the rim of the orbit to the vicinity of the optic canal. It surrounds the eyeball with its base and the origin of the straight ocular muscles and optic nerve with its apex. The periorbita is thin medially where it lies on bone, and thick caudolaterally (Fig. 7-21/7) where the bony orbit is deficient (see skull). At the orbital rim it is continuous with the orbital septum in the lids and the periosteum of the face.

The periorbita is covered caudolaterally by extraperiorbital fat. Inside the periorbita there is a layer of loose, fatty **supf. fascia** which envelops the lacrimal gland and the levator palpebrae superioris (Fig. 7-20/3,4,5). The heavy, fibrous **deep fascia** (/6) envelops the remaining structures of the orbit. It is attached to the lids and corneal limbus, passes back over the eyeball, and ensheathes the retractor bulbi. The deep fascia reflects around the other muscles of the eyeball as they insert on the sclera

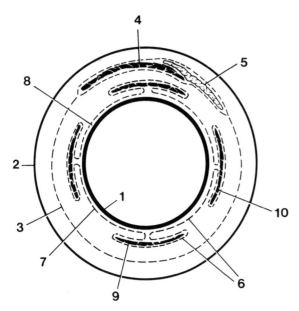

1. Eyeball
2. Periorbita
3. Supf. muscular fascia
4. Levator palpebrae
5. Lacrimal gland
6. Deep muscular fascia
7. Vagina bulbi
8. Episcleral space
9. Ventral rectus
10. Lateral rectus

FIGURE 7-20. Transection of the orbital structures at the level of the eyeball to show the orbital fasciae. Schematic. Part of the deep fascia forms the vagina bulbi.

The purpose of the following dissection is to expose the lateral surface of the orbit and periorbita. The masseter has already been separated from its origin on the facial crest and zygomatic arch (see skull). Reflect the muscle now fully ventrally and keep it out of the way. Remove the remaining muscular and tendinous tissue from the zygomatic arch and facial crest.

Some of the extraperiorbital fat is now exposed. It lies medial to the zygomatic arch and extends dorsocaudally behind the zygomatic process of the frontal bone. On the live horse the fat is palpable as a soft fluctuating mass in a depression (supraorbital fossa) caudal to the process. During mastication the palpable coronoid process of the mandible causes readily observable movements of the fat in the fossa.

Locate the **deep facial vein** (Fig. 7-21/12) ventral to the facial crest and trace it into the orbit, bluntly separating and removing *all* the extraperiorbital fat. The vein perforates the ventral portion of the periorbital cone and joins the ophthalmic vein.

Referring to the skull, saw through the zygomatic arch just rostral to the temporomandibular joint and a second time ventral to the medial angle of the eye. The first is a transverse cut, the second is a caudomedial cut with reference to the longitudinal axis of the head. The second cut should open the maxillary sinus (/10). Saw through the zygomatic process of the frontal bone 1-2 cm lateral to the supraorbital foramen (Fig. 7-22/1). Keeping the scalpel close to the bone carefully separate the lids from all around

and envelops each of them. Inside the retractor bulbi the deep fascia ensheathes the optic nerve from the lamina cribrosa on the back of the eyeball to the optic canal where it is continuous with the dura. The subarachnoid and subdural spaces, therefore, are opened when the optic nerve is cut in enucleation of the eye.

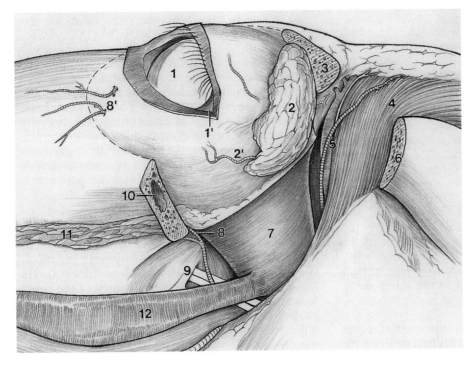

1. Cornea of left eye
1' Lateral angle of the eye
2. Lacrimal gland
2' Branches of lacrimal artery
3. Zygomatic process of frontal bone
4. Temporalis muscle
5. Rostral deep temporal artery and vein
6. Zygomatic arch
7. Periorbita
8. Malar artery, its branches at 8'
9. Maxillary and pterygopalatine nerves
10. Caudal maxillary sinus, opened by removal of zygomatic arch
11. Origin of masseter from the ventral surface of the facial crest
12. Deep facial vein

FIGURE 7-21. Left periorbital cone and lacrimal gland exposed after the removal of the zygomatic arch and extraperiorbital fat.

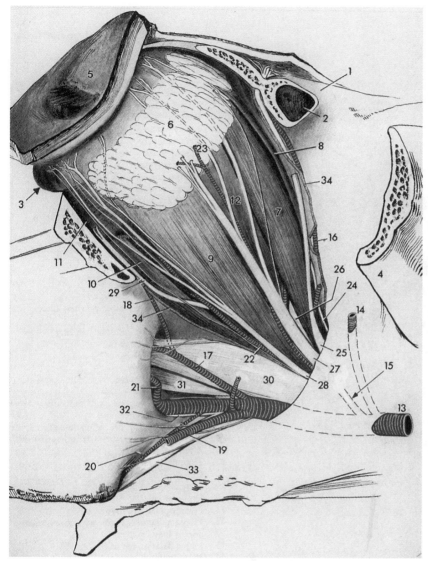

1. Zygomatic process of frontal bone
2. Frontal sinus
3. Margin of orbit
4. Zygomatic arch, partly removed
5. Upper eyelid
6. Lacrimal gland
7. Dorsal rectus
8. Levator palpebrae superioris
9. Lateral rectus
10. Ventral rectus
11. Ventral oblique
12. Retractor bulbi
13. Maxillary artery
14. Rostral deep temporal artery
15. External ophthalmic artery
16. Supraorbital artery
17. Infraorbital artery
18. Malar artery
19. Buccal artery
20. Minor palatine artery
21. Sphenopalatine artery
22. Muscular branch of ext. ophthalmic artery
23. Lacrimal artery
24. Trochlear nerve
25. Supraorbital nerve
26. Nasociliary nerve
27. Lacrimal nerve
28. Zygomatic nerve
29. Branch of oculomotor to ventral oblique
30. Maxillary nerve
31. Pterygopalatine nerve
32. Major palatine nerve, covered by major palatine artery
33. Minor palatine nerve
34. Edge of reflected periorbita

FIGURE 7-22. Superficial dissection of the left orbit, lateral view. (Modified from Hopkins, 1937.)

the orbital margin so they are connected to the eyeball by the conjunctiva only. Carefully remove the isolated segment of bone, stripping it away from the underlying periorbita. Avoid damaging the periorbita as much as possible. Your specimen should look like Fig. 7-21 now.

Dissect bluntly rostromedially from the point where the deep facial vein perforates the periorbita and locate the **malar artery.** It is a branch of the infraorbital artery (dorsal branch of the maxillary; Fig. 7-22/18,17,13). Displace the periorbita and eyeball dorsomedially and trace the artery rostrodorsally between the periorbita and the bony orbit to the medial angle. Its branches are distributed to the eyelids, conjunctiva, and to the area around the medial angle of the eye.

Displace the eyeball and periorbita ventrolaterally and bluntly expose the **supraorbital artery.** It passes to the supraorbital foramen between the periorbita and the medial wall of the bony orbit. It is derived from the external ophthalmic artery, a branch of the second part of the maxillary. The **supraorbital nerve** (N.V, ophthalmic) perforates the periorbita and accompanies the artery to the

foramen (Fig. 7-22/16,25). Artery and nerve ramify in the skin of the forehead and upper eyelid.

Remove the remaining extraperiorbital fat and examine the exposed caudolateral portion of the periorbita. It is reinforced by a wide yellow band of elastic tissue. Incise the periorbita along this band and reflect the flaps. Bluntly outline the **lacrimal gland** in the dorsolateral part of the orbit (Fig. 7-22/6). Note that the lacrimal gland extends ventrally below the lateral angle of the eye.

The **lacrimal artery** and **lacrimal nerves** (N. V, ophthalmic) are exposed passing from the depths of the orbit to the lacrimal gland. The artery is derived from the external ophthalmic artery (maxillary) and supplies the lacrimal gland and twigs to the eyelids. The nerve receives secretory fibers (derived from the facial nerve) by communication with the zygomatic nerve and ramifies in the lacrimal gland, upper eyelid, and conjunctiva. Ventral to the lacrimal vessels and nerves, the **zygomatic nerve** (N. V, maxillary), accompanied by branches of the external ophthalmic artery, passes rostrolaterally to the lateral angle. It ramifies in the conjunctiva, lower eyelid, and adjacent skin (Fig. 7-22/28).

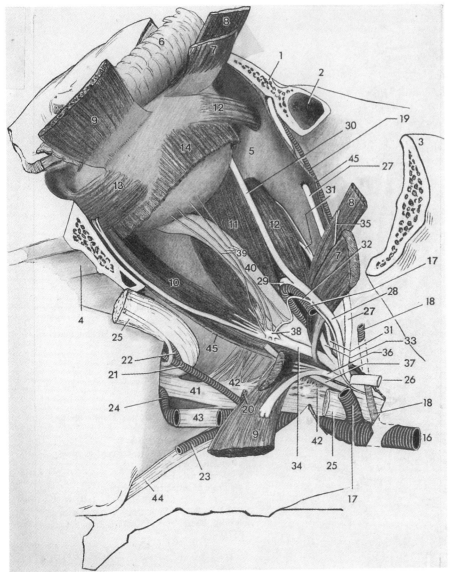

1. Cut surface of zygomatic process of frontal bone
2. Frontal sinus
3,4 Zygomatic arch, partly removed
5. Trochlea
6. Lacrimal gland, reflected
7. Dorsal rectus
8. Levator palpebrae superioris
9. Lateral rectus
10. Ventral rectus
11. Medial rectus
12. Dorsal oblique
13. Ventral oblique
14. Retractor bulbi
16. Maxillary artery
17. External ophthalmic artery
18. Rostral deep temporal artery
19. Supraorbital artery
20. Small branch to temporal fossa
21. Infraorbital artery
22. Malar artery
23. Buccal artery
24. Sphenopalatine artery
25. Maxillary nerve, cut and rostral stump reflected rostrally
26. Lacrimal nerve, reflected caudally
27. Supraorbital nerve
28. Nasociliary nerve
29. Ethmoidal nerve
30. Infratrochlear nerve
31. Trochlear nerve
32. Communicating branch of nasociliary nerve to ciliary ganglion
33,34 Dors. and ventr. brr. of oculomotor nerve
35. Branch of oculomotor of levator palpebrae
36. Abducent nerve
37. Zygomatic nerve
38. Ciliary ganglion, a little too large
39. Long and short ciliary nerves
40. Optic nerve
41. Pterygopalatine nerve
42. Pterygopalatine ganglia with many small nerves leaving them
43. Major palatine nerve
44. Minor palatine nerve
45. Edge of reflected periorbita

FIGURE 7-23. Deep dissection of the left orbit, lateral view. (Modified from Hopkins, 1937.)

The **infratrochlear nerve** (do not look for it now) arises from the nasociliary, the third branch of the ophthalmic (N. V). It passes rostrodorsally through the medial part of the orbit to the medial angle (Fig. 7-23/30). It is distributed to the skin, third eyelid, conjunctiva, and the lacrimal structures at the medial angle.

Summary of blood supply and innervation of eyelids and conjunctiva: The major *blood supply* is by branches of the malar, supraorbital, and lacrimal arteries.

The *sensory innervation* consists of a network of fibers derived from the following nerves:

    N. V, ophthalmic
       a. lacrimal
       b. supraorbital
       c. infratrochlear
    N. V, maxillary
       d. zygomatic

The *motor innervation* is by the auriculopalpebral nerve (N. VII) for the orbicularis oculi (Fig. 7-6/54). The oculomotor nerve (N. III) innervates the levator palpebrae.

Reflect the lacrimal gland rostrally and remove the supf. fascia from the dorsal surface of the eyeball. This will expose the flat **levator palpebrae superioris** (Fig. 7-22/8). It arises on the pterygoid crest (see skull; the crest forming the lateral edge of the orbital fissure), runs upward and forward, and widens as it passes under the lacrimal gland. The levator terminates by a wide tendon on the orbital septum of the upper eyelid.

Before beginning the dissection of the **BULBAR MUSCLES** that move the eyeball, it should be remembered that the deep orbital fascia attaches to the lids and corneal limbus, envelops the eyeball, and ensheathes the bulbar muscles.

Identify the belly of the **lateral rectus** posterior to the eyeball, and by reflecting the branches of the lacrimal and zygomatic nerves (Fig. 7-22/27,28) determine its borders. The rostral half of the muscle is covered by thick, deep fascia which should be incised in the direction of the muscle fibers and reflected. The lateral rectus is now fully exposed. Note that it inserts by a wide tendon close to the corneal limbus (incise and reflect the deep fascia to see the insertion). The tendon may be differentiated by its silky glistening appearance from the dull white of the sclera. Free the ventral border of the tendon and note the **ventral oblique muscle** passing deep to it. By reflecting the deep fascia, expose the ventral oblique as far as possible toward its origin from the medial wall of the orbit in a small depression caudal to the lacrimal fossa (see skull). Transect the lateral rectus and reflect the rostral stump to see the fleshy insertion of the ventral oblique on the lateral surface of the eyeball (Fig. 7-23/13).

Transect the ventral oblique at the middle of its belly and reflect the stumps. This exposes the tendon of the **ventral rectus** (/10) which inserts on the sclera deep (dorsal) to the oblique muscle.

Do not disturb the fat in the spaces around the muscles any more than necessary.

Transect the levator palpebrae and reflect the stumps. Identify the **dorsal rectus** and slit the deep fascia that covers it in the direction of the muscle fibers. Reflect the fascial flaps and cut them off close to the eyeball. The dorsal rectus (/7) is now fully exposed. It lies immediately ventral to the levator and with its wide glistening tendon inserts close to the corneal limbus.

Transect the dorsal rectus at the musculotendinous junction, exposing the tendon and belly of the **dorsal oblique** (/12). Trace the dorsal oblique medially to its right-angle turn over the cartilaginous **trochlea** (part of the periorbita). Transect the muscle between eyeball and trochlea, close to the latter. Draw the eyeball laterally and note the course of the muscle. It arises near the ethmoid foramen, passes rostrodorsally, and curves over the trochlea to reach the eyeball.

With the eyeball still retracted note the course of the **infratrochlear nerve** (/30). Displace the nerve and the supf. fascia and slit the deep fascia to expose the medial rectus (/11).

With the reflection of some of the bulbar muscles you will have noticed the **retractor bulbi** on the deep surface of the recti. The bundles of the retractor form a cone, the apex of which arises from the bone around the optic canal and the base of which inserts posterior to the equator of the eyeball (/14). The retractor bulbi, not present in ourselves, is well developed in the large herbivores.

The motor **nerves to the bulbar muscles** that move the eyeball are difficult to expose without removing the mandible. Their distribution may be summarized as follows:

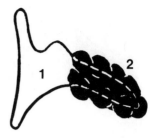

1. Free part of the cartilage forming the edge of the third eyelid

2. Gland of the third eyelid, surrounding the deep part of the cartilage

FIGURE 7-24. Isolated cartilage of the third eyelid and its gland. Most of the free part of the cartilage is covered by conjunctiva.

N. III   ventral oblique
         dorsal rectus
         medial rectus
         ventral rectus
         (retractor bulbi)
N. IV   dorsal oblique   (The innervation of the
N. VI   lateral rectus   retractor bulbi is still
         (retractor bulbi)   controversial.)

Displace the eyeball laterally and examine the bulbar surface of the **third eyelid,** noting the raised lymph nodules that give it a granular appearance (similar to what you have seen in the dog). Now, in the mass of fat and fascia in the depth of the medial angle between the eyeball and the periorbita locate the **cartilage** of the third eyelid (Fig. 7-24/1). The part of the cartilage closest to the angle of the eye is wide and thin. The deep part is thicker and narrower and is surrounded by the (lacrimal) **gland of the third eyelid.** The gland opens by small ducts on the bulbar surface of the third eyelid. Cut the cartilage away from the orbital fat and remove it (the cartilage). The third eyelid may be protruded in the live horse by gently pressing on the upper lid between the eyeball and the bony orbital margin. A similar increased tension caused by tonic spasm of the ocular muscles protrudes the third eyelid in cases of tetanus.

The dorsal and ventral **anterior ciliary arteries** are small and difficult to demonstrate unless special injection techniques are employed. They are of considerable clinical importance, however, and warrant description and study. The dorsal anterior ciliary artery arises from the external ophthalmic and runs rostrally in the fat on the deep surface of the dorsal rectus. It winds around the medial border of the muscle and breaks up into many branches at the corneoscleral junction. These branches connect with similar branches of the ventral anterior ciliary artery to form an annular pericorneal network. Branches from this network join the conjunctival network derived from the arterial arches in the lids. Other branches perforate the sclera to contribute to the **greater arterial circle of the iris,** an annular network of vessels at the junction of the iris and the ciliary body; it

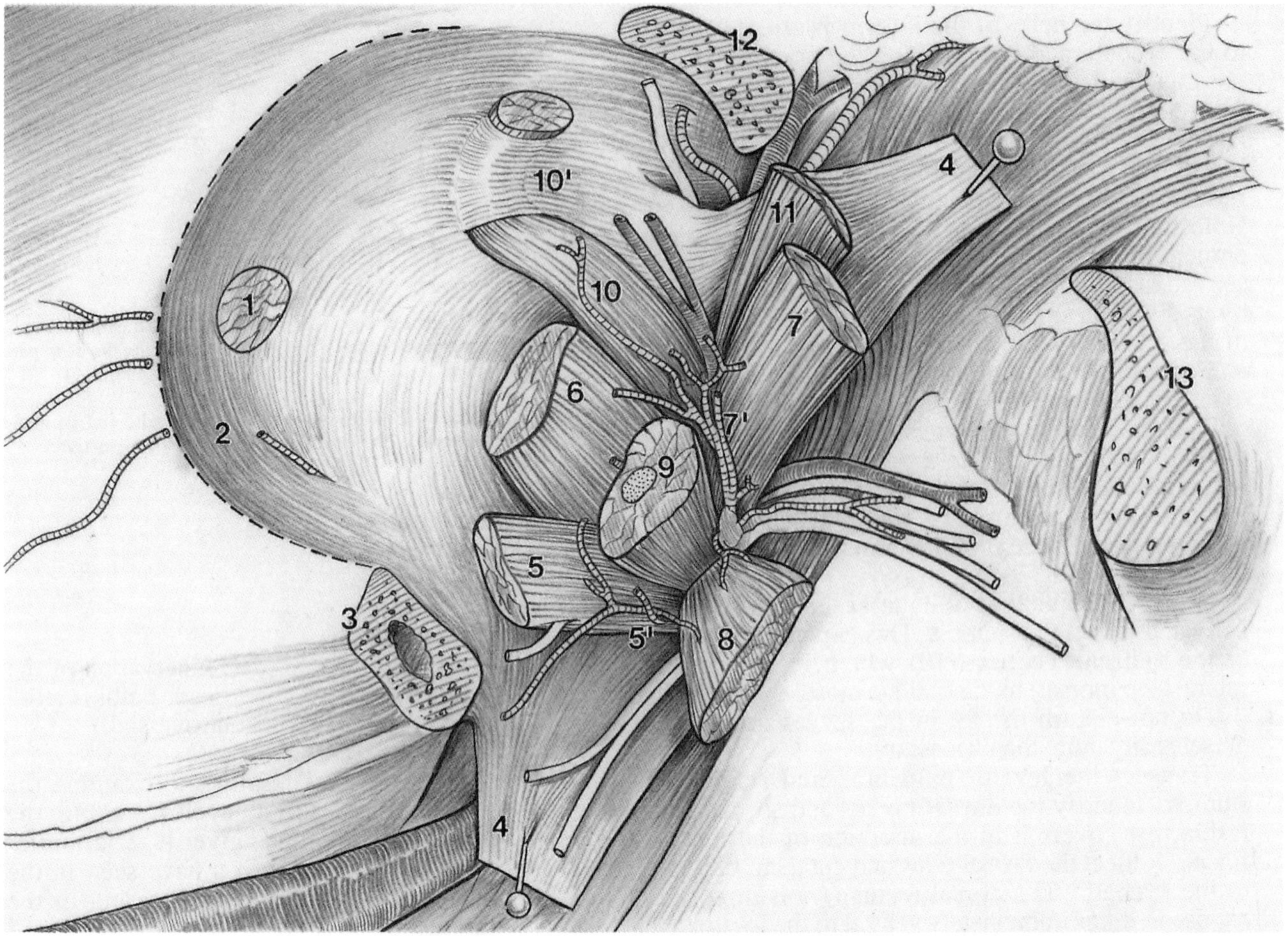

1. Stump of ventral oblique
2. Malar artery and its branches
3. Caudal maxillary sinus opened by removal of zygomatic arch
4. Periorbita, reflected
5. Ventral rectus
5' Ant. and post. ciliary arteries
6. Medial rectus
7. Dorsal rectus
7' Ant. and post. ciliary arteries
8. Lateral rectus
9. Optic nerve within retractor bulbi
10. Dorsal oblique, its trochlea at 10'
11. Levator palpebrae
12. Zygomatic process of frontal bone
13. Zygomatic arch

FIGURE 7-25. Left orbit after the removal of the eyeball. Lateral view.

will be mentioned again later. The ventral anterior ciliary artery passes along the lateral border of the ventral rectus, then between the ventral oblique and the eyeball, and breaks up to form the ventral portion of the annular pericorneal network.

Inflammation of the conjunctiva can be differentiated from inflammation of deeper structures by reference to the arterial supply. Although the two systems anastomose, the conjunctiva is supplied *mainly* by the arterial arches in the lids, while the pericorneal network and, in part, the ciliary body and iris are supplied by the anterior ciliary arteries. In conjunctivitis, vascular congestion colors the bulbar conjunctiva brick-red, and the redness increases toward the fornix and decreases toward the cornea. The vessels move with the conjunctiva. In inflammation of the iris and ciliary body, or of the cornea, a characteristic rose-pink band of congestion of the pericorneal network appears around the corneoscleral junction. These vessels do not move with the conjunctiva.

The other vessels examined in the live subject are the **retinal arteries** visible through an ophthalmoscope. These are derived from (short) posterior ciliary arteries,

branches (like the anterior ciliary aa.) of the external ophthalmic artery. The latter is the main ocular supply; it enters the periorbital cone and supplies the eyeball and all structures within the cone caudal to the eyeball (Fig. 7-23/17).

Reflect the dorsal and lateral recti caudally and remove fat and deep fascia to see the retractor bulbi more fully. Two of the four or five **vorticose veins** are now also exposed as they perforate the sclera near the equator of the eyeball. They drain the vascular coat of the eye (choroid, ciliary body, and iris) and pass caudally. They need not be traced. Consult your textbook for a complete description of the blood supply of the eye.

Cut the medial and ventral recti, the rest of the retractor, and the optic nerve and remove the eyeball.

With the aid of Fig. 7-25 examine the orbit and identify

the stumps of the four recti and the two oblique muscles, the optic nerve, and the malar and supraorbital arteries.

Clean the exterior of the **EYEBALL** by removing adherent fat and muscles, but leave the optic nerve. Note that the optic nerve is ventral to the posterior pole of the "globe", as the eyeball is often called.

The **wall of the eyeball** consists of three concentric coats:
1. External or fibrous coat, composed of sclera and cornea
2. Middle or vascular coat, composed of choroid, ciliary body, and iris
3. Internal coat or retina, divided into nervous and pigmented layers.

The four **refractive media** are:
1. Cornea
2. Aqueous humor
3. Lens
4. Vitreous body

Examine the dense white **sclera** and the bulging transparent **cornea**. The latter is opaque in embalmed subjects and is oval in the horse and ox (our own and the dog's are round). Its layers are shown in Fig. 7-26. The cornea is avascular and receives nutrition by diffusion from capillaries at the limbus and from the aqueous humor and lacrimal fluid. Sensory nerve filaments in the cornea reach it by way of the ophthalmic nerve through the nasociliary and ciliary nerves.

Incise the cornea close to the limbus and remove it. This opens the **anterior chamber** of the eye, releasing the **aqueous humor.** The **iris** is a dark brown or black diaphragm with a variable aperture, the **pupil.** The pupil in the embalmed eye is dilated and almost round; in the live animal it is a mediolaterally oriented oval. The black **iridic granules** on the dorsal and ventral margins of the iris are normal and are thought to contribute to the production of the aqueous humor, or act as "shades".

Through the pupil, the **lens** may be seen. It is transparent in the normal state but is rendered opaque by embalming. Opaque areas in the lens of live animals are known as cataracts. The **posterior chamber** of the eye lies between the iris and the lens. The anterior and posterior chambers contain the aqueous humor and communicate freely through the pupil (Fig. 7-26). With a sharp scalpel (new blade) divide the eyeball at the

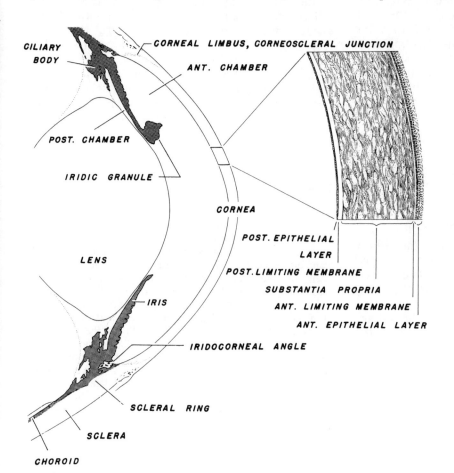

CILIARY BODY
CORNEAL LIMBUS, CORNEOSCLERAL JUNCTION
ANT. CHAMBER
POST. CHAMBER
IRIDIC GRANULE
CORNEA
LENS
IRIS
IRIDOCORNEAL ANGLE
SCLERAL RING
SCLERA
CHOROID
POST. EPITHELIAL LAYER
POST. LIMITING MEMBRANE
SUBSTANTIA PROPRIA
ANT. LIMITING MEMBRANE
ANT. EPITHELIAL LAYER

FIGURE 7-26. Meridian (superior-inferior) section through the anterior pole of the eye, schematic.

equator into anterior and posterior halves. Do not exert pressure or distort the eyeball while making the cut.

Look into the posterior half first. The opaque **optic part of the retina** is the innermost layer. It is closely attached at the **optic disc** but is usually detached from the rest of the wall in the embalmed specimen. In the live animal the optic part is transparent and closely held to the wall by the **vitreous body**, a transparent, semigelatinous mass composed of water, salts, and protein. The vitreous is in contact also with the posterior surface of the lens. Supf. to the optic part is a thin black pigmented layer that belongs to the retina developmentally but remains on the choroid when the optic part detaches after death. It is non-pigmented (translucent) in albinos.

The **vascular coat (uvea) of the eyeball** lies between the retina and the sclera and consists of choroid, ciliary body, and iris.

The **choroid** is a thin membrane loosely attached to the sclera and tightly adherent to the pigmented layer of the retina. The blood in the capillary layer of the choroid causes the reddish color of the **fundus** (posterior part of the interior of the eyeball) that may be seen with the ophthalmoscope. The choroid is often heavily pigmented, obscuring the presence of the rich vascular network. Dorsal to the optic disc the choroid contains a blue-green light-reflecting area, the **tapetum lucidum.** The pigment layer of the retina is nonpigmented over the tapetum so the tapetum can shine through. It is the iridescence of the tapetum that causes the eyes of some animals to "shine" when struck by light.

Examine the anterior half of the eyeball and begin by gently scooping out the vitreous with the scalpel handle. The opaque optic part of the retina extends anterior to the equator and ends at a slightly scalloped margin (ora serrata). Anterior to this the retina is "blind" and simply lines the posterior surface of the ciliary body and iris.

The second part of the vascular coat, the **ciliary body**, is a raised ring of radially arranged processes converging on the lens. (The medial quadrant of the ring is narrower than the rest.) Gently press the lens sideways and note the fine fibers (zonula ciliaris) that connect the ciliary processes with the capsule of the lens and hold the lens in place.

Remove the **lens** and strip the capsule off the onion-like lamellae that form its substance.

Examine the black posterior surface of the **iris.** It is continuous with the ciliary body where the latter is attached to a slight thickening (scleral ring) of the sclera (Fig. 7-26). The iris contains sphincter and dilator muscles controlled respectively by parasympathetic and sympathetic nerve fibers.

Incise the iris, ciliary body, and sclera parallel to the ciliary processes. On the cut surface identify the corneoscleral junction. The anterior surface of the iris is attached to the sclera by a delicate meshwork of fibers, the pectinate ligament. The interstices of the meshwork form spaces which receive aqueous humor from the anterior chamber and drain into a microscopic circular venous plexus. The plexus is connected with the pericorneal blood vessels. The **iridocorneal angle** between the anterior surface of the iris and the corneoscleral junction is, therefore, of considerable physiological and pathological importance.

Blockage of the drainage of the aqueous humor through the iridocorneal angle may produce increased intraocular tension known as *glaucoma*.
In the horse *recurrent iridocyclitis* (simultaneous inflammation of iris and ciliary body; also known as periodic ophthalmia or moon blindness) is the most common disease of the eyeball.

Grasp the iris and gently pull it backward so that the ciliary muscle tears loose from its attachment to the sclera. The muscle may be identified as a grayish band on the scleral surface of the ciliary body. The muscle is attached to the ciliary body such that when it contracts, it pulls the ciliary body and processes toward the lens, releasing the tension on the zonula ciliaris. This allows the elastic lens to become more convex (near vision). For far vision the muscle relaxes and the natural tension of the zonula decreases the convexity of the lens. The ciliary muscle is more highly developed in animals with good accommodation.

Teeth

Before we start studying the teeth we should find the **orifice of the parotid duct** in the mouth. Detach the masseter from the mandible. Saw through the ramus of the mandible parallel and 8 cm ventral to the zygomatic arch. Then with the scalpel placed into the saw cut, incise soft tissue (pterygoid muscle) until the lower part of the mandible can be folded dorsally against the lateral surface of the face. Turn the head over and probe the buccal mucosa that lies against the upper 2nd and 3rd cheek teeth. In the embalmed state the orifice does not open on a papilla—as does that of the mandibular duct (sublingual caruncle)—but has to be found among the crevices of the wrinkled mucosa. If you cannot locate the orifice, re-identify the duct on the lateral side and introduce a flexible probe in a rostromedial direction, pushing it through the cheek. The orifice is occasionally blocked by food particles or stones (sialoliths).

Study the teeth on demonstration material, utilize also your specimen and estimate your horse's age. But read the next three paragraphs before you begin.

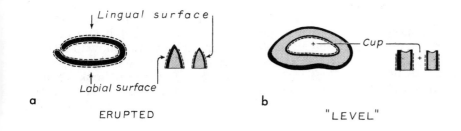

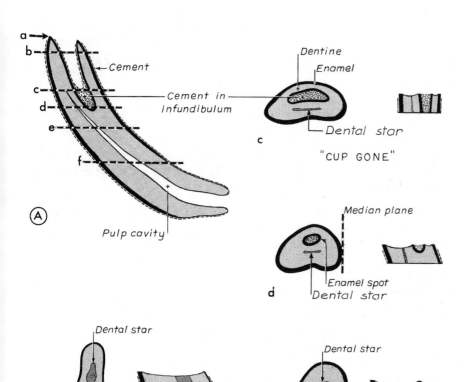

FIGURE 7-27. Wear of the horse's incisor teeth, based on the lower right I1. A, Lower incisor in sagittal section showing different levels of wear (a-f). For each level the occlusal surface and a sagittal section are shown.

The horse has long teeth (hypsodont) with much of the long body of the tooth embedded in the jaws. In contrast, the dog has short-crowned teeth (brachydont). These cease to grow when they reach the level of the adjacent teeth; and since a carnivorous diet is not very abrasive they usually last for the life of the animal.

The horse's rough plant diet is very abrasive and wears the teeth at the occlusal surface. In order to keep up with this wear the teeth continue to grow for several years and continuously push out into the mouth. At about five years of age small roots form and the body of the tooth ceases to grow, but is still pushed out into the mouth to be worn away. Such a tooth has to last the horse for the rest of its life.

For this reason the teeth of the horse are never available for study in their entirety: when the distal portion is present, the proximal end of the tooth has not yet developed; and when the proximal end is present and the tooth has finished growing, the distal portion—indeed most of the tooth—has been worn away.

The formula for the **deciduous teeth** of the horse is:

$$2 \left(Di\,\frac{3}{3} - Dc\,\frac{0}{0} - Dp\,\frac{3}{3} \right) = 24$$

The deciduous teeth are erupted at birth or within a few weeks thereafter. Di3 does not erupt until the sixth to the ninth month. **The deciduous incisors are smaller than the permanent incisors and have a distinct neck at the junction of the root and crown.** For the purpose of aging horses, it is important to be able to distinguish deciduous from permanent incisors.

The formula for the **permanent teeth** is:

$$2 \left(I \frac{3}{3} - C \frac{1}{1} - P \frac{3 \text{ or } 4}{3} \quad M \frac{3}{3} \right) = 40 \text{ or } 42$$

The canine teeth are usually absent or rudimentary in the mare. The first upper premolar ("wolf tooth" ; also present occasionally in the lower jaw) is a much-reduced, inconstant vestige (1-2 cm in length). Wolf teeth are usually pulled because of perceived interference with the bit that may result in inflammation of the gums.

Both the deciduous and permanent incisors present a deep invagination of enamel, the **infundibulum**, which extends from the occlusal surface a considerable distance into the body of the tooth (Fig. 7-28/A). The infundibulum is partially filled with cement, leaving a lumen darkened by food deposits. This is the **cup** (Fig. 7-27/b).

AGING OF HORSES BY THE TEETH utilizes eruption and wear of the lower incisors. The **eruption** of the permanent incisors is a quite constant phenomenon and an accurate indication of age. A tooth is erupting when it breaks through the gums. It must be remembered however that it takes about 6 months for the tooth to grow out far enough to be in wear. After five years, when all permanent incisors are present, age determination is based upon **wear**. But this, unfortunately, is influenced by genetic, environmental, and management factors; hence it is less reliable than eruption. At best, age determination after five years is skilled estimation.

A tooth is **"in wear"** when it has risen to the masticatory level, and the enamel begins to wear on the occlusal surface. When the entire outer enamel ring is in wear and separated from the inner enamel ring by dentine, the tooth is said to be **"level"** (Fig. 7-27). The disappearance of the cup, **"cup gone"**, means that the black cavity of the cup is gone. The thick bottom of the infundibulum remains for some time as the raised **"enamel spot"**.

1 year—Di1 and Di2 are in wear. Di3 is erupted.

2 years—Di1 and Di2 are level.

2.5 years—I1 erupts.

3.5 years—I2 erupts.

4.5 years—I3 erupts.

5 years—All permanent incisors are in wear. The canines erupt between 3.5 and 5 years.

6 years—Lower I1 cup is gone. (The disappearance of the *upper incisor* cups is of no value in the estimation of age.)

7 years—Lower I2 cup is gone. All lower incisors are level. The cement has worn off, changing the color from yellow to bluish-white. There is a **"hook"** on upper I3 (Fig. 7-28/B). The 7-year hook, though included in this outline, is of doubtful value. Moreover, it may reappear at age 11.

8 years—Lower I3 cup is gone. The **"dental star"** appears in lower I1. The star is the remnant of the obliterated dental (pulp) cavity and appears first as a dark yellow transverse line in the dentine on the labial side of the infundibulum.

9 years—Lower I1 is **"round"**; that is, the occlusal surface is no longer elliptical with the long diameter transverse but is more strongly curved on the lingual side. The transverse diameter is about the same as the labiolingual diameter.

10 years—Lower I2 is round. **Galvayne's groove** emerges from the gum on upper I3 (Fig. 7-28/C). Although the appearance and

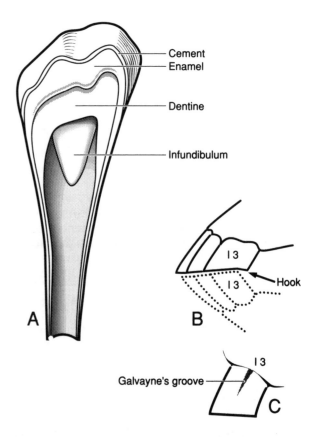

FIGURE 7-28. *A*, Sculptured right lower I2 of a 3.5 year old horse; labial (front) view. *B*, The position and appearance of the hook on upper I3. *C*, The positon of Galvayne's groove on the labial surface of the upper I3.

progression of Galvayne's groove are not accurate criteria for aging horses, Galvayne's name has survived. Sydney Frederick Galvayne (1851?-1913) was an Australian horse trainer who worked also in England and South Africa.

13 years—The enamel spot is small and round in the lower incisors. The dental stars are in the middle of the occlusal surfaces.

15 years—Galvayne's groove is halfway down upper I3. The dental stars are round, dark, and distinct in the lower incisors.

16 years—I1 is **"triangular"**. The transverse diameter of the occlusal surface is now shorter than the labiolingual diameter.

17 years—I2 is triangular. The enamel spots are gone from the lower incisors.

A general idea of age may be obtained by looking at the animal as a whole and by parting the lips to note the **angle of the incisors in profile.** In young horses the incisors are vertical. With increasing age the incisors progressively approach the horizontal.

It is helpful in dentistry to know the eruption dates of the permanent premolar and molar teeth:

P1 (wolf tooth) at 5-6 months	M1 at 1 year
P2 at 2.5 years	M2 at 2 years
P3 at 3 years	M3 at 3.5- 4 years
P4 at 4 years	

Exercises on the Live Animal

Students at Cornell should view the videotape on the HEAD to appreciate how many structures can actually be palpated. (The tape is "Part 8: Head," in the series Equine Anatomy Reviewed on the Live Animal.

1---Palpate the groove on the rostral border of the masseter; from here find the facial artery where it crosses the ventral border of the mandible and attempt to feel the pulse. At this level palpate the soft mandibular lymph nodes on the medial aspect of the mandible, and, deep to where the two chains of nodes join, find the lingual process of the basihyoid, and the basihyoid itself. Move rostrally on the lateral surface of the mandible and locate the mental foramen and nerve—you have to push the depressor labii inferioris dorsally a little. If you are working on a thin-skinned horse, palpate

(or see) the buccal branches of the facial nerve as they cross the masseter. With the aid of Fig. 7-7 attempt to take the pulse on the subcutaneous segment of the masseteric artery (/13).Follow the facial crest to its rostral end. From here move rostrodorsally, push the levator labii superioris dorsally and find the infraorbital foramen; remember that it lies a little caudal to the midpoint on a line connecting the rostral end of the facial crest with the nasoincisive notch.

2---Palpate the caudal border of the mandible and the wing of the atlas and, between the two, outline the parotid gland. Visualize the position of the long, curved mandibular gland and, deep to its dorsal end, the guttural pouch. Locate Viborg's triangle by extending the animal's head and distending the jugular vein.

3---Wash your hands before examining the nostril. Feel the lamina of the alar cartilage in the dorsal convexity of the medial wing and palpate the alar fold. Carefully insert a finger into the nasal diverticulum dorsal to the alar fold. Insert the finger into the ventral nasal meatus. See the opening of the nasolacrimal duct in the floor of the nostril.

4---With the aid of Fig. 7-14/B,C trace the surgical boundaries of the frontal and maxillary sinuses on the surface of the head, palpating and identifying the respective landmarks.

5---Palpate cranially on the trachea until the much larger diameter of the cricoid arch is felt. Locate the (median) thyroid notch rostral to the cricoid arch. Rostral to the notch is the laryngeal prominence (our Adam's apple) where the two thyroid laminae are joined; and rostral to that is the transverse bar of the basihyoid. Identifying more dorsal features of the larynx is difficult for the novice: follow the caudal border of the thyroid lamina to the caudal cornu; find the hard, rounded muscular process of the arytenoid cartilage dorsal to the cornu; caudal to the muscular process is the cricoarytenoideus dorsalis. This muscle atrophies in the roarer, leaving a distinct hollow.

6---Note that the horse's pupil is oval. *Very gently* press on the upper eyelid between eyeball and upper margin of the orbit to protrude the third eyelid. The blinking that occurs is from the orbicularis oculi, innervated by the palpebral branch of the auriculopalpebral branch of the facial nerve. Try to palpate the thin palpebral branch as it crosses the highest point of the zygomatic arch.

7---Part the lips on the left side and see the angle of the incisors in profile. Have you been palpating a young, middle-age, or old horse? If you think it was a young horse, were you looking at deciduous or permanent incisors?

APPENDIX A

Converting a Fresh Hindlimb into a Specimen that Demonstrates the Passive Stay-Apparatus

This does not need to be a careful dissection; do most of the cutting with a sharp post mortem knife. Disregard and remove all vessels and nerves as they are encountered. The object is to retain only the bones and the collateral ligaments that connect them, and certain other ligaments, tendons, and "ligamentous muscles" (supf. digital flexor, peroneus tertius, and interosseus).

1. The limb (preferably from the light horse) should have been disarticulated at the hip joint. Skin the limb down to the fetlock joint.
2. With reference to Exercises on the Live Animal (following the Chapter on the Hindlimb) and to Figure 5-30/B, palpate the three patellar ligaments and carefully remove the deep fascia that covers them. The fascia attaches to the medial and lateral ligaments, but not to the intermediate one. Do not cut the ligaments when you remove the fascia.
3. Detach all muscles where they insert on the medial and lateral patellar ligaments, so that the two ligaments are fully exposed from patella to tibial tuberosity.
4. Detach the quadriceps from the patella and remove that muscle. Sparing the gastrocnemius, totally remove also the sartorius, gracilis, semimembranosus, adductor, semitendinosus, biceps, and the small muscles near the hip joint.
5. Remove the fat and femoropatellar joint capsule from in between, and deep to, the patellar ligaments.
6. Isolate the medial head of the gastrocnemius and, sparing the supf. digital flexor, cut it off the back of the femur and at its musculotendinous junction.
7. Recognizing that the supf. digital flexor is enclosed by the belly of the lateral gastrocnemius, carefully detach only the gastrocnemius from the femur, leaving the slender supf. digital flexor in place. Remove now the entire gastrocnemius by cutting its tendon at the calcanean tuber.
8. Remove the deep fascia over the long digital extensor. Isolate the belly of the muscle and transect it very carefully so as not to injure the tendinous peroneus tertius deep to it. Remove the long extensor by separating it proximally from its common tendon with the underlying peroneus tertius. Cutting retinacula at the hock, free its long tendon from tarsus and metatarsus, and transect the tendon at the fetlock to remove the rest of the muscle. The tendinous peroneus tertius is now exposed and must remain intact.
9. The entire tibialis cranialis should be removed because it is not part of the stay-apparatus, but it can be left in place if time is limited.
10. Identify and remove the lateral digital extensor as you did the long extensor.
11. Preserving the supf. digital flexor that connects the femur with the calcanean tuber, remove the muscle mass, including the popliteus, that lies on the caudal surface of the tibia.
12. Stand the limb on the floor. With the patella ready to assume the gliding position, it should be possible to force the limb to collapse when heavy pressure is applied to the head of the femur. Conversely, holding the patella in the locked position, the limb should support any weight you care to place on the femoral head. Put a little sand or chalk dust on the resting surface of the femoral trochlea, if the resting surfaces are too slippery to hold the patella in place with one hand.
13. Again preserving the supf. flexor (and the interosseus) cut the deep flexor tendon in midmetatarsus. Do number 12 again.
14. Cut also the superficial flexor tendon in midmetatarsus and do number 12 once more. When the limb collapses, the hoof stays now planted on the ground. With the stifle locked, the limb still supports weight. Note how the system gives a little when maximum weight is placed on the limb.

APPENDIX B

The Nerve Supply of the Hindlimb Muscles grouped according to their Primary* Actions

Action on Joint	Muscles	Nerve Supply
HIP JOINT		
Extensors	Gluteus medius Biceps femoris Semitendinosus Semimembranosus Quadratus femoris	Gluteals Caudal gluteal, sciatic Caudal gluteal, sciatic Sciatic Sciatic
Flexors	Iliopsoas 　Iliacus 　Psoas major Sartorius Tensor fasciae latae Gluteus superficialis	 Lumbar, femoral Lumbar, femoral Saphenous Cranial gluteal Gluteals
Adductors	Adductor Gracilis Pectineus Obturator externus	Obturator
Abductors	Gluteus profundus Gluteus superficialis Gluteus medius	Gluteals
Outward rotators (supinators)	Obturator internus Gemellus	Sciatic
Inward rotators (pronators)	Gluteus profundus Semitendinosus Adductor	Cranial gluteal Caudal gluteal, sciatic Obturator
STIFLE JOINT		
Extensors	Quadriceps femoris Caudal thigh muscles	Femoral Caudal gluteal, sciatic
Flexors	Popliteus Biceps Semitendinosus	Tibial Caudal gluteal, sciatic
TARSUS		
Extensors	Gastrocnemius Supf. digital flexor	Tibial
Flexors	Peroneus tertius (transmits action of stifle flexors) Long digital extensor Lateral digital extensor Tibialis cranialis	 Peroneal

Action on Joint	Muscles	Nerve Supply
DIGIT		
Extensors	Long digital extensor Lateral digital extensor	Peroneal
Flexors	Supf. digital flexor Deep digital flexor	Tibial

* Note that only the *primary* action on the one joint is indicated. Most muscles have several actions, and many act on more than one joint.

APPENDIX C

Summary of the Innervation of the Fetlock and Digit (Forelimb)

Nerve degeneration and electrophysiologic studies, and histologic studies on fetal limbs indicate that the structures of the fetlock and digit are innervated in the following manner (both medial and lateral):

1. **Palmar Nerves**—before branching—supply the palmar part of the fetlock joint capsule.

2. **Palmar Metacarpal Nerves**—innervate the entire fetlock joint capsule. These nerves are not desensitized by the usual block for the palmar nerve; the deposit has to be enlarged dorsally, across the palpable interosseus, to infiltrate the area distal to the ends of the splint bones (Figs. 6-17 and 6-31).

3. **Dorsal Branches of the Digital Nerves**
   Totally innervate:
   1) most of the skin of the fetlock
   2) dorsal part of the pastern joint
   3) coronary dermis

   Partially innervate:
   5) small part of the fetlock joint
   6) collateral part of the laminar dermis
   7) cartilage of the hoof

4. **Digital Nerves**
   Totally innervate:
   1) navicular bursa
   2) deep digital flexor distal to the level of the pastern joint
   3) palmar and dorsal parts of the coffin joint capsule
   4) palmar part of the cartilage of the hoof
   5) palmar part of the pastern joint
   6) laminar dermis
   7) dermis of the bars
   8) dermis of the frog
   9) dermis of the sole
   10) digital cushion
   11) skin on the palmar surface of the pastern and digital cushion

In addition, the branches of the palmar nerves overlap in the cutaneous innervation of the fetlock, pastern, and coronary region. The palmar nerves and the digital nerves also supply fine branches (vaso-motor nerves) to the adventitia of the digital arteries.

APPENDIX D

The Nerve Supply of the Forelimb Muscles grouped according to their Primary* Actions

Action on Joint	Muscles	Nerve Supply
SHOULDER JOINT		
Extensor	Supraspinatus	Suprascapular
Flexors	Teres major Deltoideus Teres minor	Axillary
Adductors	Subscapularis Coracobrachialis The four pectorals	Subscapular, Axillary Musculocutaneous Pectoral nerves
Abductor	Infraspinatus	Suprascapular
ELBOW JOINT		
Extensors	Triceps Anconeus Tensor fasciae antebrachii	Radial
Flexors	Biceps Brachialis	Musculocutaneous Musculocutaneous, Radial
CARPUS		
Extensors	Extensor carpi radialis Extensor carpi obliquus	Radial
Flexors	Flexor carpi radialis Flexor carpi ulnaris Ulnaris lateralis	Median Ulnar Radial
DIGIT		
Extensors	Comm. digital extensor Lat. digital extensor	Radial
Flexors	Deep digital flexor Supf. digital flexor	Median, Ulnar Ulnar

* Note that only the *primary* action on one joint is indicated. Most muscles have several actions, and many act on more than one joint.

APPENDIX E

The Prominences of the Digital Skeleton and the Tendons and Ligaments attaching on them—a Review best done on an Articulated Specimen

Distal end of Mc3—medial and lateral fossae surmounted by tubercles. They provide proximal attachment for the collateral ligaments of the fetlock. The articular surface presents a sagittal ridge.

PROXIMAL SESAMOID BONES:

1. **Flexor surfaces**—provide attachment for the palmar ligament
2. **interosseus (abaxial) surfaces**—concave and provide the main attachment for the interosseus
3. **basal (distal) surfaces**—provide the proximal attachment for:
   a. straight sesamoid ligament
   b. oblique sesamoid ligaments
   c. cruciate sesamoid ligaments
   d. short sesamoid ligaments
4. **palmar borders** (rough borders separating interosseus and flexor surfaces)—provide attachment for the palmar annular ligament and the collateral sesamoid ligaments
5. **articular surfaces**—conform to the distal articular surface of Mc3. The sesamoids articulate with Mc3 only and not with PI.

PROXIMAL PHALANX (PI):

1. **Triangular area on the proximal middorsal surface**—insertion of the lateral extensor tendon and partial insertion of the common extensor tendon
2. **palmar margin of the proximal articular surface**—distal attachment of the short sesamoid ligaments
3. **triangular rough area on the palmar surface**—proximally, the distal attachment of the cruciate ligaments; distally, the distal attachment of the oblique sesamoid ligaments; proximal attachments of the axial palmar ligaments of the pastern joint are medial and lateral to the triangular area
4. **proximal collateral tubercles**—distal attachments of the collateral ligaments of the fetlock joint and collateral sesamoid ligaments; proximal attachments of the proximal digital annular ligament
5. **distal collateral tubercles**—distal attachments of the proximal digital annular ligament; proximal attachments of the collateral ligaments of the pastern joint

6. **rough oval areas on palmar surface palmar to distal tubercles**—insertion of part of the superficial digital flexor
7. **depression and roughness on the distal end dorsal to the distal tubercles**—proximal attachment of the collateral ligament of the navicular bone
8. **intermediate tuberosities**, rough oval areas in the middle of each border—proximal attachments of the abaxial palmar ligaments of the pastern joint
9. **oblique crest on the distal half of each border**, connecting the intermediate tuberosities with the distal collateral tubercles—attachments of the distal digital annular ligament and of a ligament (lig. chondrocompedale) going to the hoof cartilage.

MIDDLE PHALANX (PII):

1. **Transverse flattened area on the proximal palmar border**—attachment of the complementary fibrocartilage which provides the distal attachment for the straight sesamoid ligament and for the palmar ligaments of the pastern joint
2. **rough area on the proximal dorsal surface**—partial insertion of the common digital extensor tendon
3. **proximal collateral tubercles**—distal attachments of the collateral ligaments of the pastern joint; partial insertion of the superficial flexor tendon
4. **depressions on each side of the distal end**—proximal attachments of the collateral ligaments of the coffin joint
5. **rough eminences dorsal to the depressions**—attachments of a ligament (lig. chondrocoronale) going to the hoof cartilage
6. **oblique groove** between the proximal collateral tubercles and the depressions on each side of the distal end—provides passage for the collateral (suspensory) ligament of the navicular bone.

DISTAL PHALANX (PIII):

1. **Extensor process** on coronary border—insertion of the common extensor tendon
2. **depressions on the sides of the bone**—distal attachments of the collateral ligaments of the coffin joint
3. **palmar processes**—the hoof cartilages attach to the palmar processes
4. **foramina of the palmar processes**—(may be only notches) perforate the palmar processes and lead to the
5. **parietal grooves**—carry the dorsal arterial branch to PIII and a nerve branch (Fig. 6-31)

6. **semilunar line and the flexor surface proximal to it**—insertion of the deep flexor tendon

7. **sole foramina**—transmit the terminations of the digital arteries into the **sole canal**.

NAVICULAR BONE—a shuttle-shaped (distal) sesamoid bone which articulates with PII and PIII. The **flexor surface** is covered with cartilage in the fresh state and acts as a bearing surface for the deep flexor tendon. The collateral (suspensory) ligament of the navicular bone attaches to the two extremities and the **proximal border**. The distal navicular ligament extends from the **distal border** to the flexor surface of PIII.

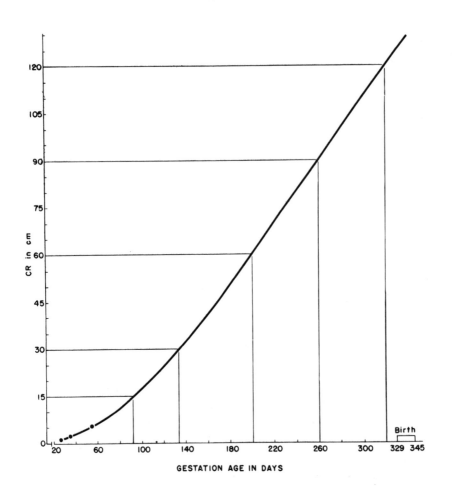

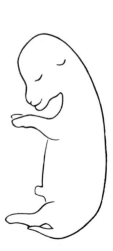

Early Fetus
55 days

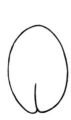

Primitive Streak
15 days

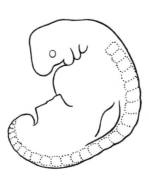

Tailbud Embryo
26 days

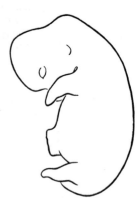

Late Embryo
35 days

APPENDIX F

Growth Curve and Developmental Stages of the Horse
(Evans and Sack, 1973)

◄ EXTERNAL CHARACTERISTICS OF HORSE EMBRYOS AND FETUSES

Days of
Gestation

20	Allantois forming; optic vesicle and heart present
21	Amnion complete
24	Embryo crescent-shaped
26	Pontine fissure present; *forelimb bud* present; three branchial arches present; eye appears 0.5 mm in diameter
30	Genital tubercle present; lens visible
36	Pontine fissure closed;feet tapered with rudiments of three digits; eyes pigmented; facial clefts closing; acoustic meatus forming
40	Pinna forming; nostrils visible; elbow and stifle regions evident; eyelids developing
42	Pinna triangular and pointing rostrally, mammary ridge present
45	External genitals differentiated
47	*Palate fused*
49	Teats present
55	Eyelids almost closed; pinna covers acoustic meatus
63	*Eyelids fused;* wall, sole, and frog of hoof recognizable
75	Clitoris prominent
80	Scrotum present
95	Pinna curls rostrally and ventrally; hoof is yellow; coronary dermis present as ridge
112	Tactile hairs on lips; teats well formed
120	Fine hair on muzzle, chin, and around eyes; orbital area prominent; ergot prominent
150	Eyelashes emerging; udder forming
180	Mane and tail hair present
210	Mane hair 2.5 mm long
240	Hair appears on poll, pinnae, throat, chin, and muzzle; mane hair 5 mm long; hair covers distal half of tail
270	Body covered with fine hair; mane hair 1.5 cm long; short switch on tail
335	Birth

(Data from Bergin et al., 1967, 93 specimens; Ewart, 1897; and the review by Zietzschmann and Krölling, 1955.)

SELECTED BIBLIOGRAPHY

(Compiled by M. Susan Hackett, DVM, PhD.)

General References:

Ashdown, R.R. and S.H. Done: Color atlas of veterinary anatomy: the horse. Philadelphia: J.B. Lippincott Co., 1987.

Auer, J.A.: Equine surgery. Philadelphia: W.B. Saunders Co., 1992.

Budras, K.D., W.O. Sack and S. Röck: Anatomy of the horse: an illustrated text, 3rd ed. Hannover: Schlütersche, 2001.

Butler, J.A., et al.: Clinical radiology of the horse. Oxford: Blackwell Scientific Publications, 1993.

DeLahunta, A. and R.E. Habel: Applied veterinary anatomy. Philadelphia: W.B. Saunders Co., 1986.

Denoix, J.M.: The eqine distal limb: Atlas of clinical anatomy and comparative imaging. London: Mason Publishing/Veterinary Press, 2000.

Dyce, K.M., W.O. Sack and C.J.G. Wensing: Textbook of veterinary anatomy, 3rd ed. Philadelphia: W.B. Saunders Co., 2002.

Ellenberger, W. and H. Baum: Handbuch der vergleichenden Anatomie der Haustiere, 18th ed. Berlin: Springer, 1943.

Ellenberger, W., H. Dittrich and H. Baum: An atlas of animal anatomy for artists. New York: Dover Publications, 1956.

Evans, H.E. and W.O. Sack: Prenatal development of domestic and laboratory mammals. Growth curves, external features and selected references. Anat. Histol. Embryol. 2: 11-45, 1973.

Evans, J.W. et al.: The horse, 2nd ed. New York: W.H. Freeman and Company, 1990.

Habel, R.E., J. Frewein, and W.O. Sack: Nomina anatomica veterinaria, 4th ed. Ithaca, NY: Internat. Comm. Vet. Gross Anat. Nomencl., 1994.

Hopkins, G.S.: Guide to the dissection and study of the blood vessels and nerves of the horse, 3rd ed. Ithaca, NY: Author, 1937.

Hutchison, C.P. and P.D. Garrett: Equine anatomy: an illustrated guide for dissection. Auburn, Alabama: by authors, 1994.

McIlwraith, C.W. and A.S. Turner: Equine surgery advanced techniques. Philadelphia: Lea & Febiger, 1987.

Nickel, R. et al.: The anatomy of the domestic animals, V. 1: The locomotor system of the domestic mammals. Berlin: Paul Parey, 1986.

Nyland, T.G. and J.S. Mattoon: Veterinary diagnostic ultrasound. Philadelphia: W.B. Saunders Co., 1995.

Rantanen, N.W. and A.O. McKinnon: Equine diagnostic ultrasonography. Baltimore: Williams & Wilkins, 1998.

Reef, V.B.: Equine diagnostic ultrasound. Philadelphia: W.B. Saunders Co., 1998.

Schebitz, H. and H. Wilkens: Atlas of radiographic anatomy of the horse, 4th ed. Berlin: Paul Parey Scientific Publishers, 1986.

Schmaltz, R.: Atlas der Anatomie des Pferdes. Vol I-V, Berlin: Richard Schoetz, 1905-1929.

Schummer, A., R. Nickel and W.O. Sack: The viscera of the domestic mammals, 2nd ed. Berlin: Paul Parey, 1979.

Schummer, A. et al.: The anatomy of the domestic animals, V. 3: The circulatory system, the skin, and the cutaneous organs of the domestic mammals. New York: Springer, 1981.

Sisson, S. and J.D. Grossman: Anatomy of the domestic animals, V. 1, 5th ed. Philadelphia: W.B. Saunders Co., 1975.

Smith, B.P.: Large animal internal medicine, 2nd ed. Baltimore: Mosby, 1996.

Speirs, V.C. and R. H. Wrigley: Clinical examination of horses. Philadelphia: W.B. Saunders Co., 1997.

Taylor, F.G.R. and M.H. Hillyer: Diagnostic techniques in equine medicine. Philadelphia: W.B. Saunders Co., 1997.

Thrall, D.E.: Textbook of veterinary diagnostic radiology, 3rd ed. Philadelphia: W.B. Saunders Co., 1998.

Turner, A.S. and C.W. McIlwraith: Techniques in large animal surgery, 2nd ed. Philadelphia: Lea & Febiger, 1989.

Wissdorf, H., H. Gerhards and B. Huskamp: Praxisorientierte Anatomie des Pferdes, 2nd ed. Hannover: M & H Schaper, 2002.

Chapter 1 Neck:

Garrett, P.D.: Anatomy of the dorsoscapular ligament. JAVMA, 196: 446-448, 1990.

Gaughan, E.M., S.L. Fubini and A. Dietze: Fistulous withers in horses: 14 cases (1978-1987). JAVMA 193: 964-966, 1988.

Harrison, I.W. and C.W. Raker: Sternothyrohyoideus myectomy in horses: 17 cases (1984-1985). JAVMA 193: 1299-1302, 1988.

Jamdar, M.S. and A.N. Ema: A note on the vertebral formula of the donkey. Br. Vet. J. 138: 209-211, 1982.

Martin B.B. and A.M. Klide: Physical examination of horses with back pain. Vet. Clin. North Am. Equine Pract. 15: 61-70, 1999.

Mayhew, I.G.: Collection of cerebrospinal fluid from the horse. Cornell Vet, 65: 500-511, 1975.

Premiani, B.B.: El Caballo. Buenos Aires: Ediciones Centauro, 1957.

Sisson, S. and J.D. Grossman: Anatomy of the domestic animals, 4th ed. Philadelphia: W.B. Saunders Co., 1953.

Tomizawa, N. et al.: Relationships between radiography of cervical vertebrae and histopathology of the cervical cord in 19 wobbling foals. J. Vet. Med. Sci. 56: 227-233, 1994.

Tomizawa, N. et al.: Morphological analysis of cervical vertebrae in ataxic foals. J. Vet. Med. Sci. 56: 1081-1085, 1994.

Chapter 2 Thorax:

McKibben, J.S. and R. Getty: Innervation of the heart of domesticated animals: horse. Am. J. Vet. Res. 30: 193-202, 1969.

Miller, P.J. and J.R. Holmes: Observations on structure and function of the equine mitral valve. Eq. Vet. J. 16: 457-460, 1984.

Nakakuki, S.: The bronchial tree and lobular division of the horse lung. J. Vet. Med. Sci. 55: 435-438, 1993.

Pipers, R.S., R.L. Hamlin and V. Reef: Echocardiographic detection of cardiovascular lesions in the horse. J. Eq. Med. Surg. 3: 68-77, 1979.

Vachon, A.M. and A.T. Fischer: Thoracoscopy in the horse: diagnostic and therapeutic indications in 28 cases. Equine Vet. J. 30: 467-475, 1998.

Voros, K., J.R. Homres and C. Gibbs: Anatomical validation of two-dimensional echocardiography in the horse. Equine Vet. J. 22: 392-397, 1992.

Chapter 3 Abdomen:

Andrews, R.M. and J.T. Robertson: Diagnosis and surgical treatment of functional obstruction of the right dorsal colon in a horse. JAVMA 193: 956-958, 1988.

Beard, W.L., C.L. Lohse and J.T. Robertson: Vascular anatomy of the descending colon of the horse. Vet. Surg. 18: 130-134, 1989.

Bernard, W.V. et al.: Ultrasonographic diagnosis of small intestinal intussusception in three foals. JAVMA, 194: 395-397, 1989.

Blue, M.G.: Enteroliths in horses – a retrospective study of 30 cases. Equine Vet. J., 11: 76-84, 1979.

Dart, A.J., J.R. Snyder and J.R. Pascoe: Resection and anastomosis of the small colon in four horses. Aust. Vet. J. 69: 5-7, 1992.

Dart, A.J. et al.: Abnormal conditions of the equine descending (small) colon: 102 cases (1979-1989). JAVMA 200: 971-978, 1992.

Ducharme, N.G. et al.: Surgical treatment of colic – results in 181 horses. Vet. Surg. 12: 206-209, 1983.

Fontaine, G.L. et. al.: Ultrasound evaluation of equine gastrointestinal disorders. Comp. Cont. Ed. Pract. Vet. 21: 253-262, 1999.

Ford, T.S. et al.: Ileocecal intussusception in horses: 26 cases (1981-1988). JAVMA 196: 121-126, 1990.

Galuppo, L.D., J.R. Snyder and J.R. Pascoe: Laparoscopic anatomy of the equine abdomen. Am. J. Vet. Res. 56: 518-531, 1995.

Hackett, R.P.: Nonstrangulated colonic displacement in horses. JAVMA 182: 235-240, 1983.

Hackett, M.S. and R.P. Hackett: Chronic ileocecal intussusception in horses. Cornell Vet. 79: 353-361, 1989.

Hance, S.R. and R.M. Embertson: Colopexy in broodmares: 44 cases (1986-1990). JAVMA 201: 782-787, 1992.

Harrison, I.W.: Equine large intestinal volvulus. A review of 124 cases. Vet. Surg. 17: 77-81, 1988.

Horowitz, A.: Guide for the laboratory examination of the anatomy of the horse. Columbus, Ohio: Author, 1965.

Kiper, M.L., J. Traub-Dargatz and C.R. Curtis: Gastric rupture in horses: 50 cases (1979-1987). JAVMA 196: 333-336, 1990.

McCarthy, P.H.: Eyes at the Tips of our Fingers. The Anatomy of the Abdominal and Pelvic Viscera of the Narcotized Horse as perceived by Palpation during Exploratory Laparotomy. Melbourne: Australian Equine Research Foundation. 1986.

Milne, D.W. et al.: Left dorsal displacement of the colon in the horse. J. Equine Med. Surg. 1: 47-52, 1977.

Milne, E.M. et al.: Cecal intussusception in two ponies. Vet. Rec. 125: 148-150, 1989.

Ross, M.W.: Surgical diseases of the equine cecum. Vet. Clin. North Amer. Equine Pract. 5: 363-375, 1989.

Ross, M.W., J.A. Orsini and S.J. Ehnen: Jejunocolic anastomosis for the surgical management of recurrent cecal impaction in a horse. Vet Surg. 16: 265-268, 1987.

Santschi, E.M., D.E. Slone Jr. and W.M. Frank 2d.: Use of ultrasound in horses for diagnosis of left dorsal displacement of the large colon and monitoring its nonsurgical correction. Vet. Surg. 22: 281-284, 1993.

Snyder, J.R. et al.: Strangulating volvulus of the ascending colon in horses. JAVMA 195: 757-764, 1989.

Turner, T.A., S.B. Adams and N.A. White: Small intestine incarceration through the epiploic foramen of the horse. JAVMA 184: 731-734, 1984.

Wallace, K.D. et al.: Transrectal ultrasonography of the cranial mesenteric artery of the horse. Am. J. Vet. Res. 50: 1699-1703, 1989.

White, N.A.: Intestinal infarction associated with mesenteric vascular thrombotic disease in the horse. JAVMA 178: 259-262, 1981.

Chapter 4 Pelvis:

Aanes, W.A.: Surgical management of foaling injuries. Vet. Clin. North Amer. Equine Pract. 4: 417-438, 1988.

Blanchard, T.L. et al.: Management of dystocia in mares: examination, obstetrical equipment, and vaginal delivery. Comp. Cont. Ed. Pract. Vet. 11: 745-753, 1989.

Clem, M.F. and R.M. DeBowes: Paraphimosis in horses – Part I. Comp. Cont. Ed. Pract. Vet. 11: 72-75, 1989.

Colbern, G.T. and W.J. Reagan: Ovariectomy by colpotomy in mares. Comp. Cont. Ed. Pract. Vet. 9: 1035-1040, 1987.

Dalin, G. and L.B. Jeffcott: Sacroiliac joint of the horse. 1. Gross morphology. Anat. Histol. Embryol. 15: 80-94, 1986.

Dalin, G. and L.B. Jeffcott: Sacroiliac joint of the horse. 2. Morphometric features. Anat. Histol. Embryol. 15: 97-107, 1986.

Desjardins, M.R. et al.: Surgical repair of rectovaginal fistulae in mares: twelve cases (1983-1991). Can. Vet. J. 34: 226-231, 1993.

Fischer, A.T. and A.M. Vachon: Laparoscopic intra-abdominal ligation and removal of cryptorchid testes in horses. Equine Vet J. 30: 105-108, 1998.

Gatewood, D.M., J.H. Cox and R.M. DeBowes: Diagnosis and treatment of acquired pathologic conditions of the equine penis and prepuce. Comp. Cont. Ed. Pract. Vet. 11: 1498-1504, 1989.

Ginther, O.J. et al.: Anatomy of the vasculature of uterus and ovaries in the mare. Am. J. Vet. Res. 33: 1561-1568, 1972.

Hopkins, G.S.: The correlation of anatomy and epidural anesthesia in the domestic animals. Cornell Vet. 25: 263-270, 1935.

Love, C.C.: Ultrasonographic evaluation of the testis, epididymis, and spermatic cord of the stallion. Vet. Clin. North Am. Equine Pract. 8: 167-182, 1992.

McAllister, R.A. and W.O. Sack: Identification of anatomic features of the equine clitoris as potential growth sites for *Taylorella equigenitalis*. JAVMA 196: 1965-1966, 1990.

McKinnon, A.O. and J.L. Voss: Equine reproduction. Philadelphia: Lea & Febiger, 1993.

McKinnon, A.O., E.L. Squires and J.L. Voss: Ultrasonic evaluation of the mare's reproductive tract – part I. Comp. Cont. Ed. Pract. Vet. 9: 336-344, 1987.

Moll, H.D. et. al.: A survey of equine castration complications. J. Equine Vet. Sci. 15: 522-526, 1995.

Schneider, R.K., D.W. Milne and C.W. Kohn: Acquired inguinal hernia in the horse: a review of 27 cases. JAVMA 180: 317-320, 1982.

Taylor, T.S. et al.: Management of dystocia in mares: uterine torsion and Caesarean section. Comp. Cont. Ed. Pract. Vet. 11: 1265-1272, 1989.

Valdez, H. et al.: Abdominal cryptorchidectomy in the horse, using inguinal extension of the gubernaculum testis. JAVMA 174: 1110-1112, 1979.

Van der Velden, M.A. and L.J.E. Rutgers: Visceral prolapse after castration in the horse: a review of 18 cases. Equine Vet. J. 22: 9-12, 1990.

Wissdorf, H. and C. Poulsen Nautrup: Beitrag zur Nomenklatur von Klitoris und Präputium bei der Stute im Hinblick auf die Klitorissinusektomie gemäss CEM-Bestimmungen. Tierärztl. Praxis 14: 371-375, 1986.

Chapter 5 Hindlimb:

Adoux, D.M.: Some biomechanical aspects of the structure of the equine tarsus. Anat. Anz. 164: 53-61, 1987.

Back W. et al.: How the horse moves: 2. Significance of graphical representations of equine hind limb kinematics. Equine Vet. J. 27: 39-45, 1995.

Brama, P.A.J. et al.: Thrombosis of the aorta and the caudal arteries in the horse: additional diagnostics and a new surgical treatment. Vet. Quart. 18: S85-S89, 1996.

Cahill, J.I. and B.E. Goulden: Stringhalt – current thoughts on etiology and pathogenesis. Equine Vet. J. 24: 161-162, 1992.

Dyson, S.J. and J.M. Romero: An investigation of injection techniques for local analgesia of the equine distal tarsus and proximal metatarsus. Equine Vet. J. 25: 30-35, 1993.

Engelbert, T.A. et al.: Lateral patellar luxation in miniature horses. Vet. Surg. 22: 293-297, 1993.

Foland, J.W., C.W. McIlwraith and G.W. Trotter: Arthroscopic surgery for osteochondritis dissecans of the femoropatellar joint of the horse. Equine Vet. J. 24: 419-423, 1992.

Habel, R.E. and K.D. Budras: Anatomy of the prepubic tendon in the horse, cow, sheep, goat, and dog. Am. J. Vet. Res. 53: 2183-2195, 1992.

Hendrickson, D.A. and A.J. Nixon: Comparison of the cranial and a new lateral approach to the femoropatellar joint for aspiration and injection in horses. JAVMA 205: 1177-1179, 1994.

Honnas, C.M. et al.: Arthroscopy of the coxofemoral joint of foals. Vet. Surg. 22: 115-121, 1993.

Jansson, N.: Treatment for upward fixation of the patella in the horse by medial patellar desmotomy: indications and complications. Equine Pract. 18: 24-29, 1996.

Kraus-Hansen, A.E. et al.: Arthrographic analysis of communication between the tarsometatarsal and distal intertarsal joints of the horse. Vet. Surg. 21: 139-144, 1992.

Martin, G.S. and C.W. McIlwraith: Arthroscopic anatomy of the equine femoropatellar joint and approaches for treatment of osteochondritis dissecans. Vet. Surg. 14: 99-104, 1985.

Prades, M. et al.: Injuries to the cranial cruciate ligament and associated structures: summary of clinical, radiographic, arthroscopic and pathological findings from 10 horses. Equine Vet. J. 21: 354-357, 1989.

Preuss, R., K.D. Budras, and W. Traeder: Arcus inguinalis und Tendo praepubicus des Pferdes und deren vergleichend anatomische Bedeutung. Acta Anat. 82: 47-74, 1972.

Reeves, M.J., G.W. Trotter and R.A. Kainer: Anatomical and functional communications between the synovial sacs of the equine stifle joint. Equine Vet. J. 23: 215-218, 1991.

Ross, M.W. et. al.: First-pass radionuclid angiography in the diagnosis of aortoiliac thromboembolism in a horse. Vet. Radiol. & Ultrasound 38: 226-230, 1997.

Sack, W.O. and S. Ferraglio: Clinically important structures of the equine hock. JAVMA 172: 277-280, 1978.

Sack, W.O. and P.G. Orsini: Distal intertarsal and tarsometatarsal joints in the horse: communication and injection sites. JAVMA 179: 355-359, 1981.

Schneider, R.K., P. Jenson and R.M. Moore: Evaluation of cartilage lesions on the medial femoral condyle as a cause of lameness in horses: 11 cases (1988-1994). JAVMA 210: 1649-1652, 1997.

Shoemaker, R.S. et al.: Disruption of the caudal component of the reciprocal apparatus in two horses. JAVMA 198: 120-122, 1991.

Tietje, S: Computed tomography of the stifle region in the horse: a comparison with radiographic, ultrasonographic and arthroscopic evaluation. Pferdeheilkunde 13: 647-658, 1997.

Trumble, T.N. et al.: Consideration of anatomic and radiographic features of the caudal pouches of the femorotibial joints of horses for the purpose of arthroscopy. Am. J. Vet. Res. 55: 1682-1689, 1994.

Updike, S.J.: Functional anatomy of the equine tarsocrural collateral ligaments. Am. J. Vet. Res. 45: 867-874, 1984.

Updike, S.J.: Anatomy of the tarsal tendons of the equine tibialis cranialis and peroneus tertius muscles. Am. J. Vet. Res. 45: 1379-1382, 1984.

Updike, S.J.: Fascial compartments of the equine crus. Am. J. Vet. Res. 46: 692-696, 1985.

Vacek, J.R., T.S. Ford and C.M. Honnas: Communication between the femoropatellar and medial and lateral femorotibial joints in horses. Am. J. Vet. Res. 53: 1431-1434, 1992.

Valentino, L.W. et al.: Radiographic prevalence of osteochondrosis in yearling feral horses. Vet. Comp. Orthop. Traumatol. 12: 151-155, 1999.

Chapter 6 Forelimb:

Adams, M.N. and T.A. Turner: Endoscopy of the intertubercular bursa in horses. JAVMA 214: 221-225, 1999.

Adams, O.R. et al.: A surgical approach to treatment of suprascapular nerve injury in the horse. JAVMA 187: 1016-1018, 1985.

Back, W. et al.: How the horse moves: 1. Significance of graphical representations of equine forelimb kinematics. Equine Vet. J. 7: 31-38, 1995.

Back W., H.C. Schamhardt and A. Barneveld: Are kinematics of the walk related to the locomotion of a warmblood horse at the trot? Vet. Quart. 18 Suppl 2: S79-S84, 1996.

Bertone, A.L. and C.W. McIlwraith: Arthroscopic surgical approaches and intraarticular anatomy of the equine shoulder joint. Vet. Surg. 16: 312-317, 1987.

Blythe, L.L. and R.L. Kitchell: Electrophysiologic studies of the thoracic limb of the horse. Am. J. Vet. Res. 43: 1511-1524, 1982.

Bowker, R.M. et al.: Immunocytochemical and dye distribution studies of nerves potentially desensitized by injections into the distal interphalangeal joint or the navicular bursa of horses. JAVMA 203: 1708-1714, 1993.

Bowker, R.M. et al.: Sensory innervation of the navicular bone and bursa in the foal. Equine Vet. J. 27: 60-65, 1995.

Bowker, R.M. et al.: Anatomy of the distal interphalangeal joint of the mature horse: relationships with navicular suspensory ligaments, sensory nerves and neurovascular bundle. Equine Vet. J. 29: 129-135, 1997.

Bowker, R.M. et al.: Functional anatomy of the cartilage of the distal phalanx and digital cushion in the equine foot and a hemodynamic flow hypothesis of energy dissipation. Am.

J. Vet. Res. 59: 961-968, 1998.

Budras, K.D., R.L. Hullinger and W.O. Sack: Light and electron microscopy of keratinization in the laminar epidermis of the equine hoof with reference to laminitis. Am. J. Vet. Res. 50: 1150-1160, 1989.

Colles, C.M. and J. Hickman: The arterial supply of the navicular bone and its variations in navicular disease. Equine Vet. J. 9: 150-154, 1977.

Cornelissen, B.P.M., A.B.M. Rijkenhuizen and A. Barneveld: The diagnostic nerve block of the sesamoidean nerve: desensitized structures and possible clinical applications. Vet. Quart.18: S97-S102, 1996.

Crabill, M.R., M.K. Chaffin and D.G. Schmitz: Ultrasonographic morphology of the bicipital tendon and bursa in clinically normal Quarter Horses. Am. J. Vet. Res. 56: 5-10, 1995.

Crevier-Denoix, N. et al.: Mechanical correlations derived from segmental histologic study of the equine superficial digital flexor tendon, from foal to adult. Am. J. Vet. Res. 59: 969-977, 1998.

DeBowes, R.M. and J.V. Yovich: Penetrating wounds, abscesses, gravel, and bruising of the equine foot. Vet. Clin. North Am. Equine Pract. 5: 179-194, 1989.

Denoix, J.M.: Functional anatomy of tendons and ligaments in the distal limbs (manus and pes). Vet. Clin. North Am. Equine Pract. 10: 273-322, 1994.

Dyson, S.J.: Shoulder lameness in horses: an analysis of 58 suspected cases. Equine Vet. J. 18: 29-36, 1986.

Ehrlich, P.J. et al.: Results of bone scintigraphy in horses used for show jumping, hunting, or eventing: 141 cases (1988-1994). JAVMA 213: 1460-1467, 1998.

Genovese, R.L. et. al.: Diagnostic ultrasonography of equine limbs. Vet. Clin. North Am. Equine Pract. 2: 145-226, 1986.

Gray, B.W. et al.: Clinical approach to determine the contribution of the palmar and palmar metacarpal nerves to the innervation of the equine fetlock joint. Am. J. Vet. Res. 41: 940-943, 1980.

Kainer, R.A.: Clinical anatomy of the equine foot. Vet. Clin. North Am. Equine Pract. 5: 1-27, 1989.

Kannegieter, N.J.: Chronic proliferative synovitis of the equine metacarpophalangeal joint. Vet. Rec. 127: 8-10, 1990.

Keg, P.R. et al.: The effect of diagnostic regional nerve blocks in the forelimb on the locomotion of clinically sound horses. Vet. Quart. 18: S106-S109, 1996.

Kneller, S.K. and J.M. Losonsky: Misdiagnosis in normal radiographic anatomy: nine structural configurations simulating disease entities in horses. JAVMA, 195: 1272-1282, 1989.

Lamb, C.R.: Contrast radiography of equine joints, tendon sheaths, and draining tracts. Vet. Clin. North Am. Equine Pract. 7: 241-257, 1991.

McIlwraith, C.W. and J.F. Fessler: Evaluation of inferior check ligament desmotomy for treatment of acquired flexor tendon contracture in the horse. JAVMA 172: 293-298, 1978.

Molyneuz, G.S. et al.: The structure, innervation and location of arteriovenous anastomoses in the equine foot. Equine Vet. J. 26: 305-312, 1994.

Moyer, W. and J.P. Anderson: Lamenesses caused by improper shoeing. JAVMA 166: 47-52, 1975.

Navarro, M. et al.: Vascularization of the equine hoof: a macroscopic and scanning electron microscopy study of vascular casts. Revue Med. Vet. 145: 953-959, 1994.

Nickels, R.A., B.D. Grant and S.D. Lincoln: Villonodular synovitis of the equine metacarpophalangeal joint. JAVMA 168: 1043-1046, 1976.

O'Callaghan, M.W.: The integration of radiography and alternative imaging methods in the diagnosis of equine orthopedic disease. Vet. Clin. North Am. Equine Pract. 7: 339-364, 1991.

Pleasant, R.S. et al.: Intra-articular anesthesia of the distal interphalangeal joint alleviates lameness associated with the navicular bursa in horses. Vet. Surg. 26: 137-140, 1997.

Pohlmeyer, K. and R. Redecker: Die für die Klinik bedeutsamen Nerven an den Gliedmassen des Pferdes einschliesslich möglicher Varianten. Deutsche Tierärztl. Wschr. 81: 501-505, 1974.

Pollitt, C.C.: The basement membrane at the equine hoof dermal epidermal junction. Equine Vet. J. 26: 399-407, 1994.

Pollitt, C.C.: Basement membrane pathology: a feature of acute equine laminitis. Equine Vet. J. 28: 38-46, 1996.

Pollitt, C.C. and C.T. Davies: Equine laminitis: its development coincides with increased sublamellar blood flow. Equine Vet. J. Suppl.: 125-132, 1998.

Premiani, B.B.: El Caballo. Buenos Aires: Ediciones Centauro, 1957.

Rijkenhuizen, A.B. et al.: The arterial supply of the navicular bone in the normal horse. Equine Vet. J. 21: 399-404, 1989.

Rose, R.J.: Navicular disease in the horse. J. Equine Vet. Sci. 16: 18-24, 1996.

Sack, W.O.: Nerve distribution in the metacarpus and front digit of the horse. JAVMA 167: 298-305, 1975.

Sack, W.O.: Subtendinous bursa on the medial aspect of the equine carpus. JAVMA 168: 315-316, 1976.

Soana, S. et al.: Anatomic-radiographic study on the osteogenesis of carpal and tarsal bones in horse fetus. Anat. Histol. Embryol. 27: 301-305, 1998.

Stashak, T.S.: Adams' Lameness in horses, 4th ed. Philadelphia: Lea & Febiger, 1987.

Trout, E.R., W.J. Hornof and T.R. O'Brien: Soft tissue- and bone-phase scintigraphy for diagnosis of navicular disease in horses. JAVMA 198: 73-77, 1991.

Wilson, D.A. et al.: Composition and morphologic features of the interosseous muscle in Standardbreds and Thoroughbreds. Am J. Vet. Res. 52: 133-139, 1991.

Chapter 7 Head:

Bohanon, T.C., W.L. Beard and J.T. Robertson: Laryngeal hemiplegia in draft horses – a review of 27 cases. Vet. Surg. 19: 456-459, 1990.

Boles, C.L., C.W. Raker and J.D. Wheat: Epiglottic entrapment by arytenoepiglottic folds in the horse. JAVMA 172: 338-342, 1978.

Cook, W.R.: The clinical features of guttural pouch mycosis in the horse. Vet. Rec. 83: 336-345, 1968.

Cook, W.R.: Some observations on diseases of the ear, nose and throat in the horse, and endoscopy using a flexible fibreoptic endoscope. Vet. Rec. 94: 533-541, 1974.

Cook, W.R., R.S.F. Campbell and C. Dawson: The pathology and aetiology of guttural pouch mycosis in the horse. Vet. Rec. 83: 422-428, 1968.

Ducharme, N.G. and R.P. Hackett: The value of surgical treatment of laryngeal hemiplegia in horses. Comp. Cont. Ed. Pract. Vet. 13: 472-275, 1992.

Duncan, I.D. et al.: The pathology of equine laryngeal hemiplegia. Acta Neuropathol. (Berl.) 27: 337-348, 1974.

Engelke, E. et al.: Opening of the auditory tube in horses – anatomical basics and endoscopical findings.

Pferdheilkunde 13: 639-646, 1997.

Freeman, D.E. and W.J.Donawick: Occlusion of internal carotid artery in the horse by means of a balloon-tipped catheter: evaluation of a method designed to prevent epistaxis caused by guttural pouch mycosis. JAVMA 176: 232-235, 1980.

Freeman, D.E. et. al.: Occlusion of the external carotid and maxillary arteries in the horse to prevent hemorrhage from guttural pouch mycosis. Vet. Surg. 18: 39-47, 1989.

Galvayne, S.F.: Horse dentition: showing how to tell exactly the age of a horse up to thirty years. Glasgow: Thomas Murray & Son (no year given, but published ca. 1886).

Griffiths, I.R.: The pathogenesis of equine laryngeal hemiplegia. Equine Vet. J. 23: 75-76, 1991.

Hackett, R.P. et al.: The reliability of endoscopic examination in assessment of arytenoid cartilage movement in horses. Part 1: subjective and objective laryngeal evaluation. Vet. Surg. 20: 174-179, 1991.

Hilbert, B.J. et al.: Tumors of the paranasal sinuses in 16 horses. Aust. Vet. J. 65: 86-88, 1988.

Kainer, R.A.: Clinical anatomy of the equine head. Vet. Clin. North Am. Equine Pract. 9: 1-23, 1993.

Lindsay, F.L. and H.M. Clayton: An anatomical and endoscopic study of the nasopharynx and larynx of the donkey (*Equus asinus*). J. Anat. 144: 123-132, 1986.

Marks, D. et al.: Observations on laryngeal hemiplegia in the horse and treatment by abductor muscle prosthesis. Equine Vet. J. 23: 86-90, 1970.

McCarthy, P.H.: Anatomy of the laryngeal and adjacent regions as perceived by palpation of clinically normal standing horses. Am. J. Vet. Res. 51: 611-618, 1990.

McCarthy, P.H.: Subcutaneous part of the masseteric ramus of the external carotid artery as a proposed site of pulse-taking in Thoroughbreds. JAVMA 197: 751, 1990.

McCarthy, P.H.: The triangle of Viborg (*Trigonum viborgi*) and its anatomical relationships in the normal standing horse. Anat. Histol. Embryol. 19: 303-313, 1990.

Mueller, P.O.E.: Equine dental disorders: cause, diagnosis, and treatment. Comp. Cont. Ed. Pract. Vet. 13: 1451-1461, 1991.

Richardson, J.D., J.G. Lane and K.R. Waldron: Is dentition an accurate indication of the age of a horse? Vet. Rec. 135: 31-34, 1994.

Robinson, N.E. and R. Wilson: Airway obstruction in the horse. Equine Vet. Sci. 9: 155-160, 1989.

Russell, A.P. and D.E. Slone: Performance analysis after prosthetic laryngoplasty and bilateral ventriculectomy for laryngeal hemiplegia in horses: 70 cases (1986-1991). JAVMA 204: 1235-1241, 1994.

Tietje, S. M. Becker and G. Bockenhoff: Computed tomographic evaluation of head diseases in the horse: 15 cases. Equine Vet. J. 28: 98-105, 1996.

INDEX

Page numbers set in *italics* refer to illustrations.